Handbook of Endocrinology and Metabolism

Handbook of Endocrinology and Metabolism

Edited by Roose Ware

hayle
medical

New York

Hayle Medical,
750 Third Avenue, 9th Floor,
New York, NY 10017, USA

Visit us on the World Wide Web at:
www.haylemedical.com

ISBN: 978-1-63241-818-0

Cataloging-in-Publication Data

Handbook of endocrinology and metabolism / edited by Roose Ware.
    p. cm.
Includes bibliographical references and index.
ISBN 978-1-63241-818-0
1. Endocrinology. 2. Metabolism. 3. Hormones. 4. Internal medicine. I. Ware, Roose.
RC648 .H36 2019
616.4--dc23

Table of Contents

Preface

Metabolism is essential for the conversion of food into energy and building blocks of lipids, proteins and nucleic acids. It is also responsible for the elimination of nitrogenous wastes. The field of medicine concerned with the study of hormones along with the functioning and disorders of the endocrine system is called endocrinology. It also studies the psychological or behavioral activities, growth and development, mood, stress, lactation, reproduction and sensory perception caused by hormones. The endocrine system constitutes of several glands that secrete hormones, which affect the actions of several organ systems in the body. Some of the common hormones include insulin, thyroid hormone and growth hormone. The various advancements in endocrinology and metabolism are glanced at in this book, and their applications as well as ramifications are looked at in detail. It strives to provide a fair idea about these disciplines and to help develop a better understanding of the latest researches in these domains. Students, researchers, experts and all associated with these fields will benefit alike from this book.

The information contained in this book is the result of intensive hard work done by researchers in this field. All due efforts have been made to make this book serve as a complete guiding source for students and researchers. The topics in this book have been comprehensively explained to help readers understand the growing trends in the field.

I would like to thank the entire group of writers who made sincere efforts in this book and my family who supported me in my efforts of working on this book. I take this opportunity to thank all those who have been a guiding force throughout my life.

Editor

Expression of miR-155, miR-146a, and miR-326 in T1D patients from Chile: relationship with autoimmunity and inflammatory markers

Diego F. García-Díaz[1], Carolina Pizarro[1], Patricia Camacho-Guillén[1],
Ethel Codner[2], Néstor Soto[2], Francisco Pérez-Bravo[1]

ABSTRACT

Objective: The aim of this research was to analyze the expression profile of miR-155, miR-146a, and miR-326 in peripheral blood mononuclear cells (PBMC) of 47 patients with type 1 diabetes mellitus (T1D) and 39 control subjects, as well as the possible association with autoimmune or inflammatory markers. Subjects and methods: Expression profile of miRs by means of qPCR using TaqMan probes. Autoantibodies and inflammatory markers by ELISA. Statistical analysis using bivariate correlation. Results: The analysis of the results shows an increase in the expression of miR-155 in T1D patients in basal conditions compared to the controls ($p < 0.001$) and a decreased expression level of miR-326 ($p < 0.01$) and miR-146a ($p < 0.05$) compared T1D patients to the controls. miR-155 was the only miRs associated with autoinmmunity (ZnT8) and inflammatory status (vCAM). Conclusion: Our data show a possible role of miR-155 related to autoimmunity and inflammation in Chilean patients with T1D.
Arch Endocrinol Metab. 2018;62(1):27-33

Keywords
miRNAs; inflammation; type 1 diabetes; autoimmunity

[1] Laboratorio de Nutrigenómica, Departamento de Nutrición, Facultad de Medicina, Universidad de Chile
[2] Instituto de Investigaciones Materno Infantil (IDIMI), Hospital San Borja Arriarán, Facultad de Medicina, Universidad de Chile

Correspondence to:
Francisco Pérez Bravo
Laboratorio de Nutrigenómica
Departamento de Nutrición
Facultad de Medicina
Universidad de Chile
Santiago, Chile.
fperez@med.uchile.cl

INTRODUCTION

Type 1 diabetes (T1D) is an autoimmune disease triggered by T cells that destroy pancreatic beta cells. This destruction takes place by means of a complex interaction between active lymphocytes, cytokines, and macrophages (1). During the initial step of the disease, β cells are exposed to high levels of cytokines that cause the activation of the immune system and trigger the insulitis process. This inflammatory environment results in β cell damage, decreased insulin production, and the consequent destruction of β cells through apoptosis (2).

The first indication that miRNAs may be involved in regulating the β cell function was the identification of miRNAs specifically expressed in human pancreatic islets – miR-375 and miR-376 (3). In the last decade, a number of miRNAs have been described that are capable of regulating pancreatic function (4).

The expression of miRNAs may be induced by a variety of stimuli-including cell stress and inflammation, which either induce or suppress its expression in response to different stimuli, which may influence some biological processes and have pro- or anti-inflammatory effects (5) – such as hyperglycemia in patients with T1D – which increases the inflammatory response by increasing cytokines. This effect is associated with increased expression of Toll receptors (6,7), and has been correlated with studies on PBMC cultures stimulated with high glucose concentrations, which showed an increase in the expression levels of TNF-α, IL-1β, and IL-6 (8). It has been shown that stimulation by TNF-α induces the expression of certain miRNAs, including miR-146a and miR-155, which affect the pathogenesis of some diseases such as rheumatoid arthritis (6,9). Studies show the involvement of miR-155 in the activation and maturation of T and B lymphocytes. This is why it has been associated with many autoimmune diseases, such as rheumatoid arthritis; thus, an increase in the expression level of this miRNA is observed both in fibroblasts and in the PBMC of patients with this disease (10). miR-146a and miR-155 are described to be altered in T lymphocytes of patients with rheumatoid arthritis (9). miR-326 is observed to be altered in PBMC of multiple sclerosis patients (10) and shows higher expression levels in T1D patients from Italy (11,12). The aim of this study was to analyze the expression levels of the miRNAs miR-146a, miR-155, and miR-326 in PBMC from T1D and healthy patients, and to estimate their possible relationships with inflammatory or autoimmunity status in Chilean children with T1D.

SUBJECTS AND METHODS

Subjects

This study involves 47 T1D patients aged 6–11 years from the metropolitan region of Santiago in Chile, recruited from the Institute of Maternal and Child Research (IDIMI) of the San Borja Arriarán Hospital. T1D was diagnosed based on the American Diabetes Association (ADA) criteria. In all cases, a survey was applied to gather the patient's family medical and clinical history. The presence of possible chronic complications in T1D patients was corroborated through a survey and through the hospital clinical history; this included normal renal function (microalbuminuria) and normal eye fundus. In addition, 39 samples from healthy individuals (control group) aged 13–30 years were used. During the blood sample collection, patients and controls who declared the presence of previous febrile state (three days) or some inflammatory process were excluded from the study. The blood samples of T1D patients and controls were collected in the hospital after an informed consent was signed by parents of patients younger than 10 years and/or directly by patients older than 10 years. This study has been approved by the Ethics Committee of IDIMI and Faculty of Medicine, University of Chile.

Extraction and culture of PBMC

The 10 ml of drawn blood was diluted with phosphate buffered saline (PBS) at a ratio of 1:1 to facilitate the handling of the sample. The PBMC was extracted and incubated, as previously described (13).

Extraction of total RNA and miRNAs analysis

Total RNA extraction was performed using the TRIZOL method (Invitrogen) following the manufacturer's instructions. Single-stranded cDNA was synthesized from 300 ng of total RNA taken at dilutions of 2–10 ng of RNA in each sample. To assess the relative expression of miRNAs, stem-loop RT real-time PCR was performed (Applied Biosystems, Foster City, CA, USA) with specific primers for each miRNA. Expression levels were determined using TaqMan MGB probes and TaqMan Universal PCR Master Mix II (2x) in triplicate in an equipment from Agilent Technologies (CA, USA). The expression levels of miRNAs – miR-155, miR-146a, and miR326 – were normalized to a small RNA called RNU48, as an internal control.

Serological analysis

Anti-GAD65, anti-IA2, and anti-ZnT8 antibodies were determined through enzyme immunoassay (ELISA) using the Medizym commercial kits (Berlin, Germany). Antibody detection was carried out semi-quantitatively through reference to the value of 5 IU/mL for GAD65, 10 IU/mL for IA2, and 15 IU/ml for ZnT8. The analysis of inflammatory markers included human ultrasensitive C Reactive Protein (usCRP, BioVendor, Czech Republic) and the measurements of TNFα, IL-6, vCAM, and C-peptide concentrations determined by ELISA (R&D Quantikine Human ELISA Assay, UK). HbA1c levels were measured using a commercially available automatic system (DCA 2000, Bayer Diagnostics, Tarrytown, NY, USA).

Statistical analyses

We used the REST© (Relative Expression Software Tool) program, designed especially for analyzing the results of qPCR using the Pfaffl equation. Afterwards, tests were performed to evaluate the statistical significance or non-significance of the results, regarding the variations in expression observed between patients and controls. All subsequent calculations were performed using the Graph Pad Prism 6 (Graph Pad Software, Inc. San Diego CA, USA). The Shapiro-Wilk normality test was used and the effect of glucose was studied in GraphPad using the Kruskal-Wallis test. To determine the relationship between gene expression and clinical records, the bivariate correlation test was used. A p value of < 0.05 was considered as statistically significant.

RESULTS

Table 1 describes the clinical, immunological, and inflammatory characteristics of all individuals included in this study. T1D patients showed a high pattern of autoimmunity and a pattern of 28% inflammation by mean of usCRP over 3 mg/dL. This was not observed in the control group. All controls subjects tested negative to autoantibodies profile. TNFα, usPCR, IL-6, and vCAM were significantly elevated in T1D patients compared to control subjects.

Overall, miR-155 expression was significantly higher in T1D patients than in controls (Figure 1A). On the contrary, miR-326 and miR-146a expressions were lower in T1D subjects (Figures 1B and 1C). In order to find relationships in miRNAs expression regarding autoantibody and inflammatory profile in T1D patients, 2x2 ANOVA was performed (Figures 2, 3 and 4). Regarding miR-155, only a significant interaction between Znt8 low or high titer and VCAM low or high

expression was observed (p < 0.01), presenting the Znt8 H/VCAM H (the higher) and the Znt8 L/VCAM L (the lower) miR-155 expression (Figure 2A). On the other hand, miR-326 presents a significant interaction when contrasted in the presence of at least two positive autoantibodies in serum with either low/high IL6 or VCAM presence (Figures 3B and C), although these interactions seem to have come from a different pattern of expression between factors (lower expression at IL-6 H and higher at VCAM H in the two positive autoantibody conditions, although no significant differences between groups were found). Finally, miR-146a expression only showed a tendency toward a higher expression induced by higher IL-6 presence (Figures 4B and D). This is especially significant when the sample is dichotomized in presence of three positive autoantibodies (Figure 4D).

Table 1. Clinical, immunological and inflammatory parameters in T1D patients and controls

	T1D patients (n = 47)	Healthy controls (n = 39)	p-value
Age (years)	15.5 ± 3.9	19.5 ± 7.7	NS
BMI (kg/m²)	23.8 ± 3.3	25.6 ± 3.2	NS
Glycemia at debut (mmol/L)	31.3 (17.7 – 58.3)	-	-
HbA1c (%)	8.6 (6.7 – 15.5)	-	-
C-peptide (pmol/L)	94 ± 29	762 ± 314	0.01
Disease duration (years)	3.4 ± 1.9	-	-
Chronic complications*	Negative	-	-
Positive anti-ZnT8 (%)	67	Negative	-
Positive anti-GAD65 (%)	76	Negative	-
Positive anti-IA2 (%)	81	Negative	-
TNF-α (pg/mL)	4.2 ± 1.6	2.4 ± 1,3	0.01
usCRP (ng/mL)	1.71 (0.19 – 14.1)	1.28 (0.4 – 2.7)	0.03
IL-6 (pg/mL)	2.16 (0.93 – 5.61)	0.87 (0.72 – 1.44)	0.05
vCAM (ng/mL)	276.5 (101.6 – 567.9)	139.4 (91.7 – 349.2)	0.01

* Renal function (normal microalbuminuria); diabetic retinophaty: eye fundus examination.

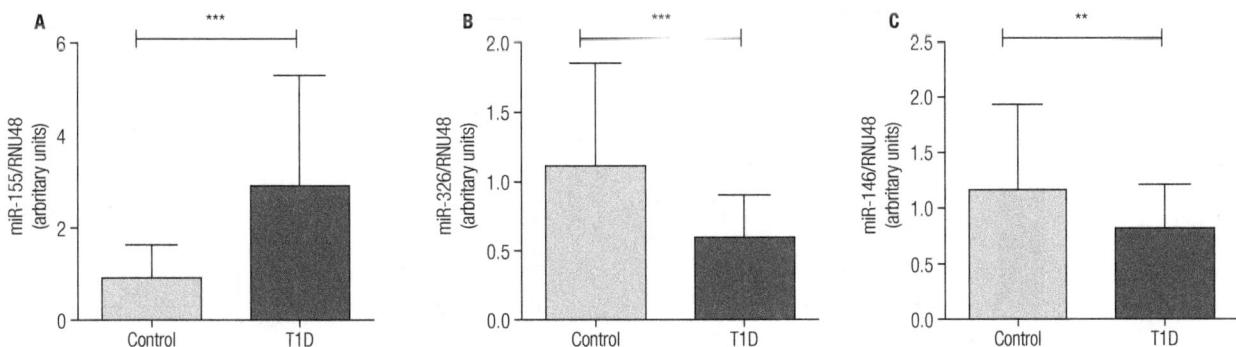

Figure 1. Expression of miR-146a (a); miR-55 (b) and miR-326 in control subjects (n = 37) and T1D patients (n = 47) in baseline conditions. Kruskal Wallis, Dunn post hoc test. ** p < 0.01; *** p < 0.001.

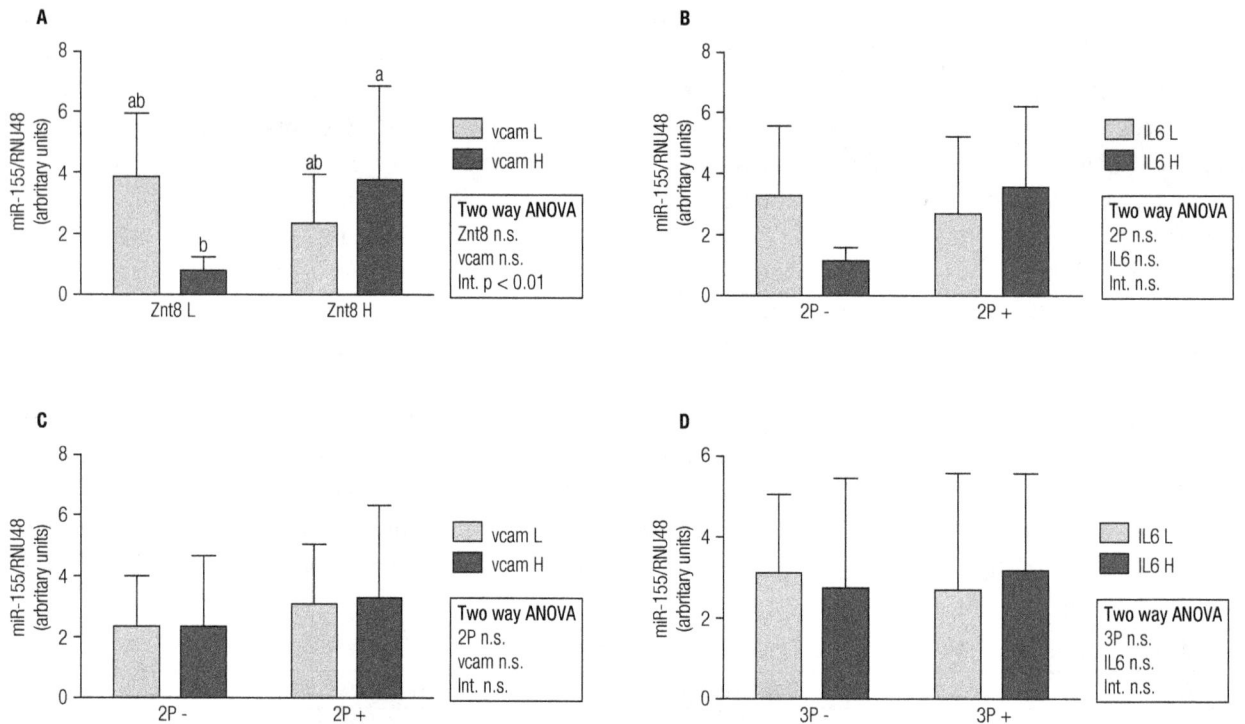

Figure 2. miR-155 gene expression and relationship with autoimmune and inflammatory status in T1D patients (L = low; H = high; 2P- = two negative autoantibodies; 2P+ = two positive autoantibodies; 3P- = three negative autoantibodies; 3P+ = three positive autoantibodies).

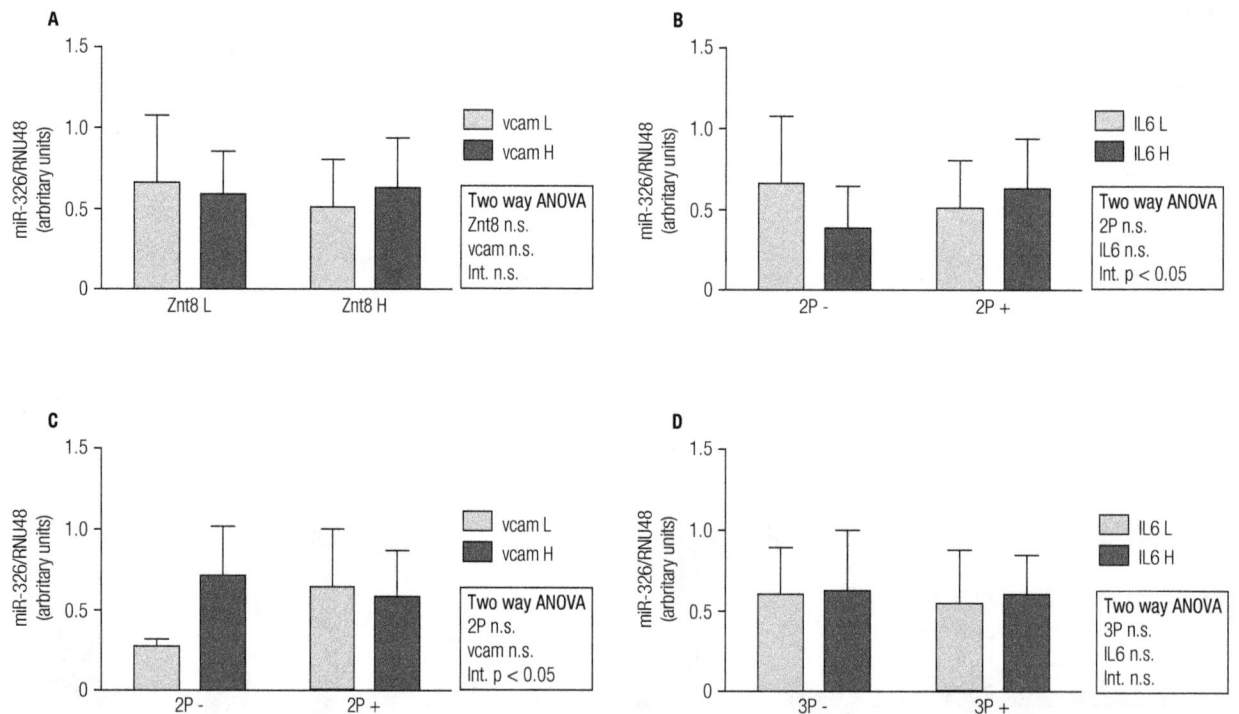

Figure 3. miR-326 gene expression and relationship with autoimmune and inflammatory status in T1D patients (L = low; H = high; 2P- = two negative autoantibodies; 2P+ = two positive autoantibodies; 3P- = three negative autoantibodies; 3P+ = three positive autoantibodies).

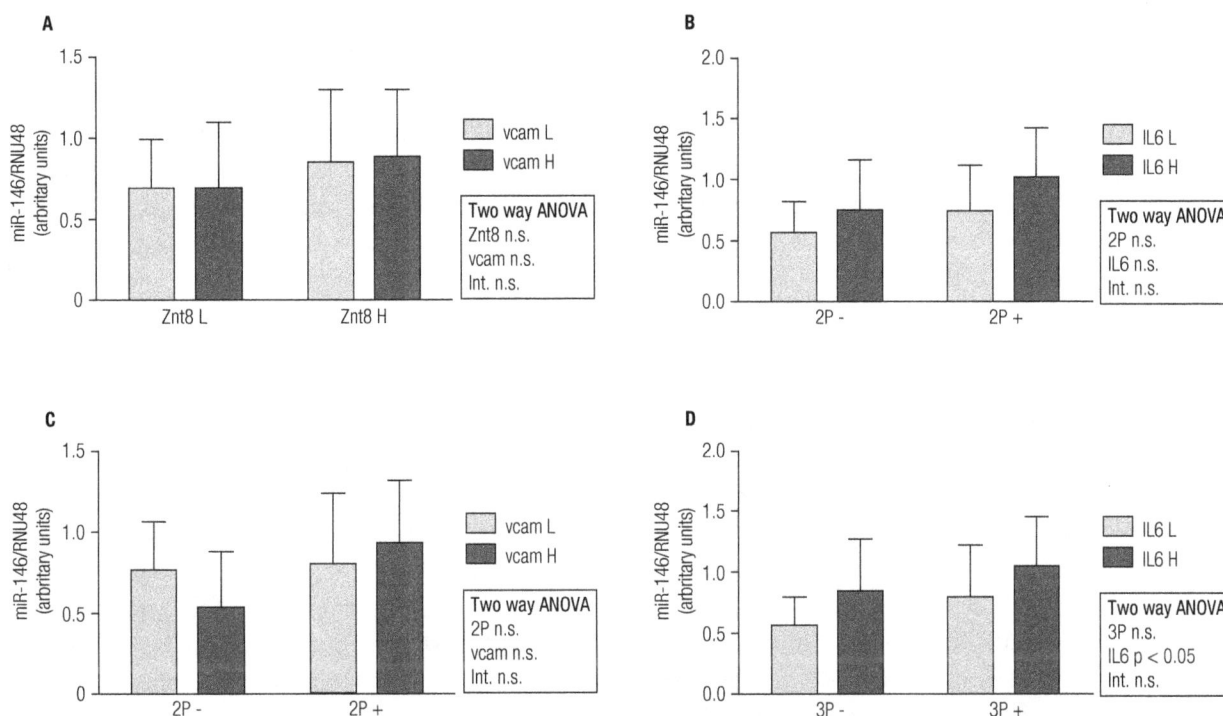

Figure 4. miR-146a gene expression and relationship with autoimmune and inflammatory status in T1D patients (L = low; H = high; 2P- = two negative autoantibodies; 2P+ = two positive autoantibodies; 3P- = three negative autoantibodies; 3P+ = three positive autoantibodies).

DISCUSSION

Despite the massive expansion in miRNAs studies and extensive investigation in several diseases, the role of miRNAs in T1D has only recently been explored. T1D – an eminent autoimmune disease – suggests a possible connection between these miRNAs and the immune system components.

The relationship between miRNAs and the various components of the immune system has been addressed in different autoimmune pathologies previously. miR-155 is related with the immune response of macrophages to different types of inflammatory mediators, such as TNF-α, which can induce the expression of miR-155 in macrophages and monocytes (14,15). miR-146a is associated with innate immunity and inflammation (16). In mice, these miRNAs have shown a deficiency in accordance with cytokine production after LPS stimulation (17,18). miR-146a acts by stimulating TLR4 toll-like receptors that activate TRAF6 and IRAK1 and genes that control cytokine production, thus suggesting that miR-146a participates in regulating cytokines release (19). miR-146a expression has been described as decreased in patients with T1D and is associated with high levels of GADA (20). In our previous studies, we analyzed several miRNAs in

T1D and control subjects. We obtained a different expression profile in PBMC submitted to increase concentrations of glucose (13,21). The above point opens up the possibility of searching miRNAs that are capable of sensing subtle changes in glucose profiles.

It is known that hyperglycemia increases the production of pro-inflammatory cytokines like TNF-α, IL-1β, and IL-6, which act by way of NF-kB (22). The medium in which T cells are found in T1D patients is a hyperglycemic environment leading to a sustained inflammatory state. This altered environment in which T cells are found could change the expression of some miRNAs (12,14). miR-155 is a microRNA that has been previously studied in rheumatoid arthritis, where there has been an increase in the expression levels (14), as well as in the PBMC of patients with systemic lupus erythematosus (SLE) (23). miR-155 is also a miRNA that is linked to inflammation and acts through the signaling of Toll receptors, which activate TAB 2, Ik-B and whose final objective is NF-kB, which is responsible for producing pro-inflammatory cytokines such as TNF-α and IL-1β (13). TNF-α is a potent inflammatory mediator produced by T cells; it has been linked to T1D and it is over-expressed in the inflammatory phenomena (insulitis). This inflammatory phase is characterized by an infiltrate composed mainly of CD4 and CD8 T lymphocytes β cells (24). In our study, the basal expression of miR-155 is elevated in T1D patients compared than control subjects. Our results are similar to what has been reported in viral myocarditis in myocardial cells, where the increased expression of miR-155 has been described (25). The low expression of miR-146a observed in T1D patients could be associated with an overproduction of inflammatory cytokines, as observed in studies with mice, which show that the decrease in the expression levels of miR-146a is associated with an excessive increase in proinflammatory cytokines (TNF-α and |IL-6) in response to LPS or cytokines, as in the case of sepsis and asthma (26). Our observation is consistent with the effect that occurs in vesicular stomatitis, where the low expression of miR-146a induces the production of pro-inflammatory cytokines such as TNF-α, |IL-1β, and IL-8. All these antecedents make us presume that miR-146a could regulate inflammation through a negative feedback through NF-kB to maintain a controlled immune response (15).

Regarding miR-326, in 2011, Sebastiani and cols. (12) reported a high positive correlation between this miRNA and autoimmunity. However, this analysis was carried out only for a group of T1D patients, without comparing their miRNA levels with that of healthy subjects, as was done in the work of Du and cols. (27) on multiple sclerosis. Our study shows differences between miR-326 expression between T1D patients and controls, and no relationship based on the number of positive autoantibodies. Finally, our study shows a tendency for possible relationships between the expression of miR-22 and ZnT8 antibodies among a group of patients who tested positive for this autoantibody, which could indicate an association effect. A recent study reports that 32 miRNAs located in the same genomic region (Chromosome 14q32) could act on the mRNA of several T1D autoantigens; 12 of these miRNAs were sensitive to changes in glucose. This study shows no data on ZnT8 (28). The relationship between miRNAs and the environmental factors (virus, diet) – related with the T1D and the immune system regulation – is a field of research that is currently being explored (29).

Our study describes an increase in the expression of miR-155 and a decrease in the expression of miR-146a and miR-326 in T1D patients, compared to control subjects. A possible interaction was observed between miR-155 and ZnT8 autoantibody, but no interaction was described to inflammatory status in T1D (related with vCAM and IL-6 levels). Regarding our cell model, PBMC represent a diverse population of cells; as such, each distinct cell type may have a unique miRNA expression profile. Finally, an important aspect to be considered in our study is the age of the disease among patients with T1D. This study includes young patients with a short evolution of their disease. In general, during this period, the patients have a metabolically stable picture. Our findings should be interpreted with caution if we consider advanced stages of the disease. Several microRNAs have been linked to complications of T1D. There is evidence of changes in proinflammatory cytokines and oxidative stress in these patients, consistent with changes in glycemic stability and with changes in the miRNAs profile in according with long-standing hyperglycemia (30,31). This would be an interesting point for corroboration in future studies, with cell subpopulations to establish the true benefits and limitations of circulating miRNA as biomarkers of T1D.

Statement of human and animal rights: all procedures followed were in accordance with the ethical standards of the responsible committee on human experimentation (institutional and national) and with the Helsinki Declaration of 1975, as revised in 2008.

Statement of informed consent: informed consent was obtained from all patients for inclusion in the study.

Acknowledgements: we thank all participants for their cooperation.

Funding: this project was supported by FONDECYT Grant 1130240.

REFERENCES

1. Van Belle T, Coppieters K, von Herrath M. Type 1 diabetes: etiology, immunology, and therapeutic strategies. Physiol Rev. 2011;91(1):79-118.
2. Eizirik D, Colli M, Ortis F. T The role of inflammation in insulitis and beta-cell loss in type 1 diabetes. Nat Rev Endocrinol. 2009;5(4):219-26.
3. Poy M, Eliasson L, Krutzfeldt J, Kuwajuma S, Ma X, Macdonald P, et al. A pancreatic islet-specific microRNA regulates insulin secretion. Nature. 2004;432(7014):226-30.
4. Guay C, Regazzi R. Circulating microRNAs as novel biomarkers for diabetes mellitus. Nat Rev Endocrinol. 2013;9(9):513-21.
5. Marques-Rocha JL, Samblas M, Milagro FI, Bressan J, Martínez JA, Marti A. Noncoding RNAs, cytokines, and inflammation-related diseases. FASEB J. 2015;29(9):3595-611.

6. Taganov K, Boldin M, Chang K. NFk-B-dependent induction of microRNA miR-146, an inhibitor targeted to signaling proteins of innate immune responses. Proc Natl Acad Sci U S A. 2006;103(33):12481-6.

7. Wade E. Hyperglycemia may alter cytokine production and phagocytosis by means other than hyperosmotic stress. Crit Care. 2008;12(5):182.

8. Dasu MR, Devaraj S, Zhao L, Hwang DH, Jialal I. High glucose induces toll-like receptor expression in human monocytes: mechanism of activation. Diabetes. 2008;57(11):3090-8.

9. Devaraj S, Venugopal S, Singh U. Hyperglycemia induces monocytic release of interleukin-6 via induction of protein kinase c-{alpha} and -{beta}. Diabetes. 2005;54(1):85-91.

10. Pauley K, Satoh M, Chan A, Bubb MR, Reeves WH, Chan EK. Upregulated miR-146a expression in peripheral blood mononuclear cells from rheumatoid arthritis patients. Arthritis Res Ther. 2008;10(4):R101.

11. Volinia S, Calin GA, Liu CG, Ambs S, Cimmino A, Petrocca F, et al. A microRNA expression signature of human solid tumors defines cancer gene targets. Proc Natl Acad Sci U S A. 2006;103(7):2257-61.

12. Sebastiani G, Grieco FA, Spagnuolo I, Galleri L, Cataldo D, Dotta F. Increased expression of microRNA miR-326 in type 1 diabetic patients with ongoing islet autoimmunity. Diabetes Metab Res Rev. 2011;27(8):862-6.

13. Salas-Pérez F, Codner E, Valencia E, Pizarro C, Carrasco E, Pérez-Bravo F. MicroRNAs miR-21a and miR-93 are down regulated in peripheral blood mononuclear cells (PBMCs) from patients with type 1 diabetes. Immunobiology. 2013;218(5):733-7.

14. O'Connell RM, Taganov KD, Boldin MP, Cheng G, Baltimore D. MicroRNA-155 is induced during the macrophage inflammatory response. Proc Natl Acad Sci U S A. 2007;104(5):1604-9.

15. O'Neill L, Frederick J, Sheedy C. MicroRNAs: the fine-tuners of Toll-like receptor signalling. Nat Rev Immunol. 2011;11(3):163-75.

16. Saba R, Sorensen DL, Booth SA. MicroRNA-146a: A Dominant, Negative Regulator of the Innate Immune Response. Front Immunol. 2014;5:578.

17. Boldin M, Taganov K, Rao D, Yang L, Zhao, J, Kalwani M. miR-146a is a significant brake on autoimmunity, myeloproliferation, and cancer in mice. J Exp Med. 2011;208(6):1189-201.

18. Jiang M, Xiang Y, Wang D, Gao J, Liu D, Liu Y, et al. Dysregulated expression of miR-146a contributes to age related dysfunction of macrophages. Aging Cell. 2012;11(1):29-40.

19. Nahid MA, Pauley KM, Satoh M, Chan EK. mir-146a is critical for endotoxin-induced tolerance: implication in innate immunity. J Biol Chem. 2009;284(50):34590-9.

20. Yang M, Ye L, Wang B, Gao J, Liu R, Hong J, et al. Decreased miR-146 expression in peripheral blood mononuclear cells is correlated with ongoing islet autoimmunity in type 1 diabetes patients 1miR-146. J Diabetes. 2015;7(2):158-65.

21. Estrella S, Garcia-Diaz DF, Codner E, Camacho-Guillén P, Pérez-Bravo F. Expression of miR-22 and miR-150 in type 1 diabetes mellitus: possible relationship with autoimmunity and clinical characteristics. Med Clin (Barc). 2016;147(6):245-7.

22. Li J, Huang M, Shen X. The association of oxidative stress and proinflammatory cytokines in diabetic patients with hyperglycemic crisis. J Diabetes Complications. 2014;28(5):662-6.

23. Lashine Y, Salah S, Aboelenein H, Albdelaziz A. Correcting the expression of miRNA-155 represses PP2Ac and enhances the release of IL-2 in PBMCs of juvenile SLE patients. Lupus. 2015;24(3):240-7.

24. Willcox A, Richardson SJ, Bone AJ, Foulis AK, Morgan NG. Analysis of islet inflammation in human type 1 diabetes. Clin Exp Immunol. 2009;155(2):173-81.

25. Bao J, Lin L. MiR-155 and miR-148a reduce cardiac injury by inhibiting NF-kB pathway during acute viral myocarditis. Eur Rev Med Pharmacol Sci. 2014;18:2349-56.

26. Comer BS, Camoretti-Mercado B, Kogut PC, Halayko AJ, Solway J, Gerthoffer WT. MicroRNA-146a and microRNA-146b expression and anti-inflammatory function in human airway smooth muscle. Am J Physiol Lung Cell Mol Physiol. 2014;307(9):L727-34.

27. Du C, Liu C, Kang J, Zhao G, Ye Z, Huang S. MicroRNA miR-326 regulates TH-17 differentiation and is associated with the pathogenesis of multiple sclerosis. Nat Immunol. 2009;10(12):1252-9.

28. Abuhatzira L, Xu H, Tahhan G, Boulougoura A, Schaffer AA, Notkins AL. Multiple microRNAs within the 14q32 cluster target the mRNAs of major type 1 diabetes autoantigens IA-2, IA-2β, and GAD65. FASEB J. 2015;29(10):4374-83.

29. Isaacs SR, Wang J, Kim KW, Yin C, Zhou L, Mi QS, et al. MicroRNAs in Type 1 Diabetes: Complex Interregulation of the Immune System, β Cell Function and Viral Infections. Curr Diab Rep. 2016;16(12):133.

30. Barutta F, Bruno G, Matullo G, Chaturvedi N, Grimaldi S, Schalkwijk C, et al. MicroRNA-126 and micro-/macrovascular complications of type 1 diabetes in the EURODIAB Prospective Complications Study. Acta Diabetol. 2017;54(2):133-9.

31. Pezzolesi MG, Satake E, McDonnell KP, Major M, Smiles AM, Krolewski AS. Circulating TGF-β1-Regulated miRNAs and the Risk of Rapid Progression to ESRD in Type 1 Diabetes. Diabetes. 2015;64(9):3285-93.

2

Relationship between adiponectin and leptin on osteocalcin in obese adolescents during weight loss therapy

Raquel Munhoz da Silveira Campos[1], Deborah Cristina Landi Masquio[2], Flávia Campos Corgosinho[3], Joana Pereira de Carvalho-Ferreira[4], Bárbara Dal Molin Netto[5], Ana Paula Grotti Clemente[6], Lian Tock[7], Sergio Tufik[8], Marco Túlio de Mello[5,8,9], Ana Raimunda Dâmaso[5]

[1] Departamento de Fisioterapia, Laboratório de Recursos Terapêuticos, Universidade Federal de São Carlos (UFSCar), São Carlos, SP, Brasil
[2] Centro Universitário São Camilo, São Paulo, SP, Brasil
[3] Universidade Federal de Goiás (UFG), Goiânia, GO, Brasil
[4] Programa de Pós-Graduação Interdisciplinar em Ciências da Saúde, Universidade Federal de São Paulo (Unifesp), Santos, SP, Brasil
[5] Programa de Pós-Graduação em Nutrição, Universidade Federal de São Paulo (Unifesp), São Paulo, SP, Brasil
[6] Universidade Federal de Alagoas (Ufal), Maceió, AL, Brasil
[7] Weight Science, São Paulo, SP, Brasil
[8] Departamento de Psicobiologia, Universidade Federal de São Paulo (Unifesp), São Paulo, SP, Brasil
[9] Escola de Educação Física, Fisioterapia e Terapia Ocupacional, Universidade Federal de Minas Gerais (UFMG), Belo Horizonte, MG, Brasil

ABSTRACT

Objectives: Obesity is a multifactorial disease characterized by the presence of the pro-inflammatory state associated with the development of many comorbidities, including bone turnover marker alterations. This study aimed to investigate the role of the inflammatory state on bone turnover markers in obese adolescents undergoing interdisciplinary weight loss treatment for one year. **Subjects and methods:** Thirty four post-pubescent obese adolescents with primary obesity, a body mass index (BMI) greater than > 95th percentile of the CDC reference growth charts, participated in the present investigation. Measurements of body composition, bone turnover markers, inflammatory biomarkers and visceral and subcutaneous fat were taken. Adolescents were submitted to one year of interdisciplinary treatment (clinical approach, physical exercise, physiotherapy intervention, nutritional and psychological counseling). **Results:** Reduction in body mass, body fat mass, visceral and subcutaneous fat, as well as, an increase in the body lean mass and bone mineral content was observed. An improvement in inflammatory markers was seen with an increase in adiponectin, adiponectin/leptin ratio and inteleukin-15. Moreover, a positive correlation between the adiponectin/leptin ratio and osteocalcin was demonstrated. Further, both lean and body fat mass were predictors of osteocalcin. Negative associations between leptin with osteocalcin, adiponectin with Beta CTX-collagen, and visceral fat with adiponectin were observed. **Conclusions:** It is possible to conclude that the inflammatory state can negatively influence the bone turnover markers in obese adolescents. In addition, the interdisciplinary weight loss treatment improved the inflammatory state and body composition in obese adolescents. Therefore, the present findings should be considered in clinical practice. Arch Endocrinol Metab. 2018;62(3):275-84

Keywords
Inflammation; bone turnover markers; obesity; adolescents; weight loss

Correspondence to:
Raquel Munhoz da Silveira Campos
Laboratório de Recursos Terapêuticos,
Departamento de Fisioterapia,
Universidade Federal de São Carlos
Rodovia Washington Luís, km 235
13565-905 – São Carlos, SP, Brasil
raquelmunhoz@hotmail.com

INTRODUCTION

Obesity is a multifactorial disease associated with a pro-inflammatory state including a lower adiponectinemia and hyperleptinemia framework. Many comorbidities are associated with obesity, including bone mineral alterations, metabolic syndrome, cardiovascular complications, non-alchoolic fatty liver disease, sleep disorders and asthma (1,2).

Concomitant with this, body fat distributions, especially visceral adipocytes, are linked to the secretion of pro-inflammatory adipokines that can act negatively on bone metabolism (3). In a previous study, it was shown that visceral fat, as well as the visceral/ subcutaneous ratio, were independent, negative predictors of bone mineral density (BMD) (4).

Beta-CTx collagen and osteocalcin are bone metabolism biomarkers that may represent bone turnover. Beta-CTx collagen is the C-terminal telopeptide of type I collagen, the main component (approximately 90%) of the protein matrix of bone. Beta-CTx collagen is released into the bloodstream during bone resorption and is almost entirely excreted by the kidneys. Its quantification serves as a specific marker for the degradation of mature type I collagen from bone (5). Osteocalcin is the major noncollagenous protein that acts locally in the bone mineralization. It is synthesized by the osteoblasts and has been utilized as a marker of bone formation or bone turnover (6).

Leptin, an adipokine that is primarily expressed by adipose tissue, is considered to be involved in neuroendocrine control of energy balance. However, in human obesity, hyperleptinemia was associated with a reduction of bone formation biomarkers, especially osteocalcin (7). On the other hand, adiponectin seems to improve bone formation (8), promoting the proliferation, differentiation, and mineralization of osteoblastic cells (9). In addition, serum osteocalcin levels were significantly associated with plasma adiponectin levels and inversely related to leptin levels, in the presence of metabolic syndrome (10).

The adiponectin/leptin ratio is associated as a better inflammatory biomarker of inflammation in metabolic syndrome patients than these adipokines analyzed in isolation (11). However, the relationship between the adiponectin/leptin ratio and bone biomarkers, mostly considering its role in osteocalcin in obese adolescents, has yet to be explored. Moreover, considering obesity to be a multifactorial disease, clinical strategies to promote weight loss, associated with physical exercise, nutrition and psychological interventions can be an interesting approach to promote weight loss and health benefits (12). In this way, the aim of the present investigation is to analyze the effects of interdisciplinary weight loss therapy on pro/anti-inflammatory adipokines and their role in bone turnover markers in obese adolescents.

SUBJECTS AND METHODS

Population

For this study, it was involved 34 post-puberty obese adolescents of both genders, with age of 15-19 years. Inclusion criteria were Tanner stage five (13), primary obesity, body mass index BMI > 95th percentile of the CDC reference growth charts (14). Non-inclusion criteria were the use of birth control pills, cortisone, anti-epileptic drugs, history of renal disease, alcohol intake, smoking and secondary obesity due endocrine disorders. There were no obese adolescents with diagnoses of ferritin alteration, autoimmune diseases and virus of Hepatitis A, B and C.

The main reasons for dropping out (n = 4) in our study were financial and family problems, followed by school and job opportunities. No sex differences were observed in adherence rates. The study was conducted

with the principles of the Declaration of Helsinki and was approved by the ethics committee on research at the *Universidade Federal de São Paulo* (Unifesp) (0135/04; 152.281), Clinical Trial: NCT01358773. All procedures were clear to those responsible for the volunteers and it was obtained consent for research. All evaluations were performed at two different times (baseline and after interdisciplinary intervention).

Anthropometric measurements

Weight was measured by plethysmography scale (BODPOD equipment), where patients wore minimum clothing possible and height was measured using a stadiometer (Sanny – model ES 2030). After obtaining the data was calculated using the body mass index (BMI) by dividing the weight by height squared (kg/m^2). Body composition, including body fat mass (percentage and kilograms) and body lean mass (percentage and kilograms), was obtained through air displacement pletismography (BODPOD).

Bone mineral density (BMD) and bone mineral content (BMC)

A whole-body DXA absorptiometry scan was performed per unit of bone densitometry to determine the whole-body of bone mineral density-BMD (g/cm^2) and bone mineral content-BMC (grams) using a Lunar Prodigy Advance System (GE Healthcare). The whole-body scan required the subjects to be placed in a supine position with their arms and legs positioned according to the manufacturers' specifications (15). Quality control was performed daily using a phantom, and measurements were maintained within the manufactures standards of ≤ 1%. In order to obtain statistically precise measurements, 68% of the exams were repeated within a coefficient of variation of 1DP ($\pm 0.010 \ g/cm^3$ for total body size).

Serum analysis

Blood samples were collected at the outpatient clinic at approximately 8:00 A.M. after an overnight fast (12 hours). The adipokines concentrations (adiponectin, leptin and interleukin-15) were measured using a commercially available multiplex assay (EMD Millipore: HMHMAG-34K; HCYTOMAG-60K). Manufacture-supplied controls were included to measure assay variation and all samples were analyzed on the same day to minimize day-to-day variation. A minimum of 100 beads were collected for each analyzed using a Luminex MagPix System (Austin, Texas), which was calibrated and verified prior to sample analysis. Unknown sample values were calculated offline using Milliplex Analyst Software (EMD Millipore) (16). Serum osteocalcin and Beta CTx-collagen levels were obtained using the ECLIA (Electrochemiluminescent immune Assay). For the leptin hormone, the following values were adopted: males, between 1 and 20 ng/mL and females, between 4.9 and 24 ng/mL previously described by Gutin and cols. (17).

Visceral and subcutaneous adiposity measurements

The abdominal ultrasonography procedures and the measurements of visceral and subcutaneous fat tissue and fatty liver were performed by the same physician, who was blinded to the subject assignment groups at the baseline time-point and following 1 year therapy. This physician was a specialist in imaging diagnostics. A 3.5-MHz multifrequency transducer (broad band) was used to reduce the risk of misclassification. The intra-examination coefficient of the variation for ultrasound (US) was 0.8%. US measurements of intra-abdominal (visceral) and subcutaneous fat were obtained. US determined subcutaneous fat was defined as the distance between the skin and external face of the rectus abdominal muscle, and visceral fat was defined as the distance between the internal face of the same muscle and the anterior wall of the aorta. The cut-off points for the definition of visceral obesity by ultrasonography were based on the previous methodological descriptions made by Ribeiro-Filho and cols. (18).

Descriptive methodology of interdisciplinary weight loss therapy

All sessions were conducted by an interdisciplinary group of health professionals. Three times of week during two hours per day not consecutive, the adolescents participated of supervised therapy in physical exercise, nutrition and psychological attendances during one year. Once each month the adolescents were followed by an endocrinologist (Figure 1).

Clinical intervention

All obese adolescents visited the endocrinologist with their parents once each month. In all of these visits, the entire GEO team (Study Group of Obesity) was also present. The doctor monitored and evaluated all clinical exams of adolescents and treated health problems

during therapy. The medical follow-up included the initial medical history and a physical examination of blood pressure, cardiac frequency and body mass, and the adolescents were checked for their adherence to all interdisciplinary therapies. The team discussed with the adolescents and their parents some possible changes in lifestyle to promote their health (Figure 1).

Physical exercise intervention: aerobic plus resistance training (AT + RT)

During the 1-year therapy period, the adolescents followed a combined exercise training therapy. The protocol was performed three times per week for 1 year and included 30 min of aerobic training plus 30 min of resistance training per session. The subjects were instructed to reverse the order of the exercises (aerobic and resistance) at each training session. The aerobic training consisted of running on a motor-driven treadmill (Life Fitness – model TR 9700HR) or bicycle at a cardiac frequency intensity representing the ventilatory threshold I (± 4 bpm), which was determined by the results of an initial oxygen uptake test for aerobic exercises (ergoespirometry). The exercise therapy was based on the guidelines from the American College of Sports Medicine (ACSM). Resistance training was also designed based on ACSM recommendations (19,20) (Figure 1).

Nutrition intervention

Energy intake was set at the levels recommended by the dietary reference intake for subjects with low levels of physical activity and of the same age and gender following a balanced diet (21). No pharmacotherapies or antioxidants were recommended. Once a week, adolescents had dietetics lessons educating participants on the food pyramid, diet record assessment, weight loss diets and fad diets, food labels, dietetics, fat-free and low-calorie foods and other related topics. Monthly, they had individual consultations (Figure 1).

Physiotherapy intervention

The adolescents were accompanied by a physiotherapist during the therapy, in order to prevent musculoskeletal injuries. Once a week, the volunteers had lessons regarding such topics as the postural orientation, prevention of musculoskeletal injuries, diaphragmatic breathing, hydrotherapy, isostretching, and balance.

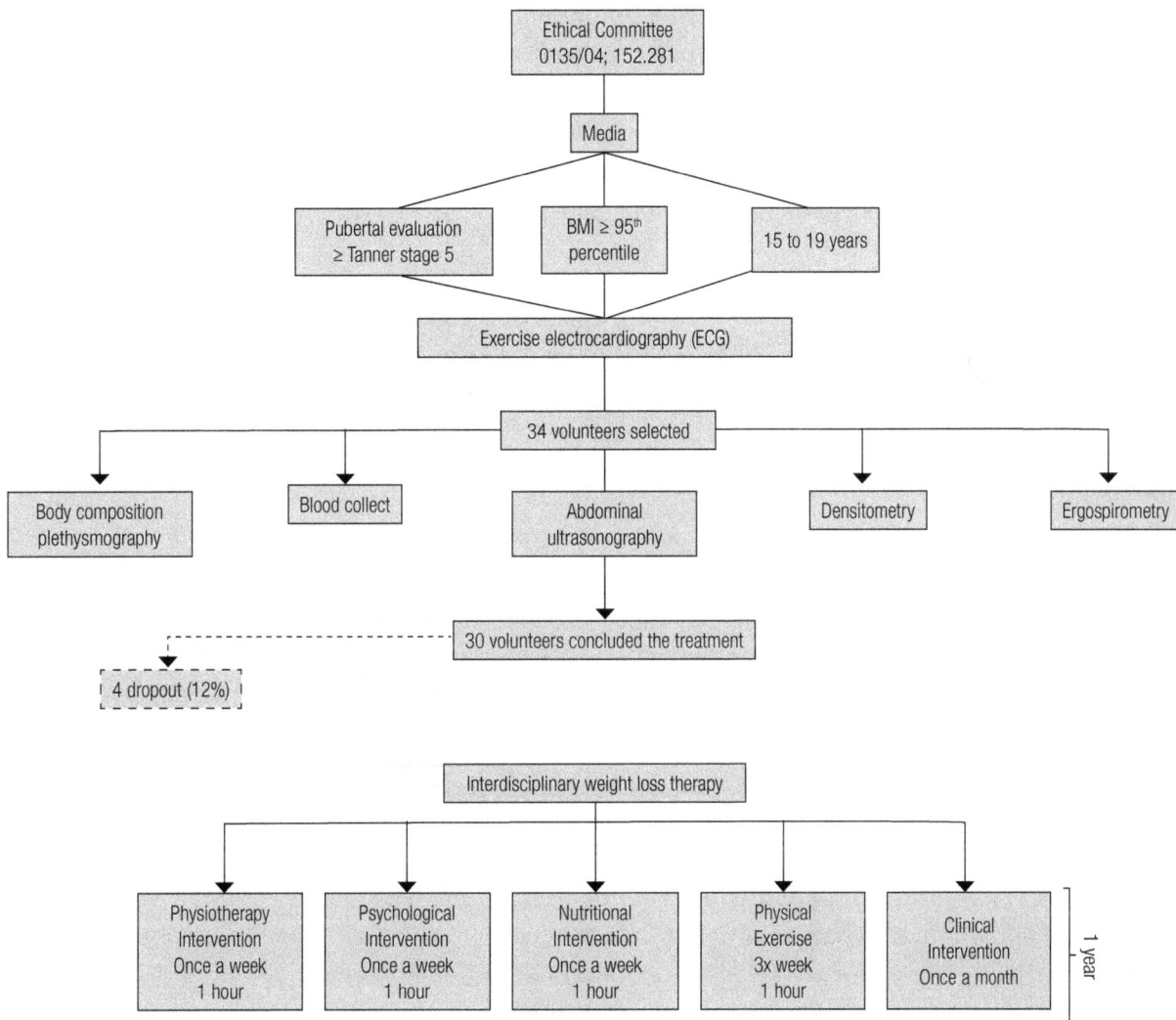

Figure 1. Descriptive methodology of study.

Psychological intervention

Psychological therapy treatment plans were established on the basis of validated questionnaires that considered some of the psychological problems caused by obesity, as described in the literature. These include depression, eating disorders, anxiety, decreased self-esteem and body image disorders. Interdisciplinary therapy consisted of a weekly 1h group session. Individualized psychological therapy was recommended when it was necessary according psychological assessment (Figure 1).

Statistical analysis

Statistical analysis was performed using the program STATISTICA version 7.0 for Windows Vista. The adopted significant value was $\alpha \leq 5\%$. Data normality was verified with the Shapiro Wilk test. Parametric data were expressed as mean ± SD, and non-parametric data were expressed as median, minimum and maximum values. The effects of interdisciplinary therapy during 1 year were analyzed by t test dependent by samples. For the non-parametric data the Wilcoxon test was applied. Correlations were established through the Pearson test for parametric data and Spearman for nonparametric data. Finally, it was verified the dependencies of variables by simple linear regression. The correlations and regression test were analyzed with baseline and final values.

RESULTS

The present study was composed by 34 obese adolescents: 18 girls (11 ± 1age of menarche) and 16 boys with 16 ± 1 years old, primary obesity (diagnosis of obesity around 10 ± 3 years old), body mass 94.5 ± 15.45 (kg) and body mass index 33.21 ± 3 (kg/m²).

Effects of interdisciplinary weight loss therapy

One year of interdisciplinary weight loss therapy demonstrated significantly reduction in body mass (kg), BMI (kg/m²), body fat mass (kg and %), visceral fat (cm), subcutaneous fat (cm) and visceral/subcutaneous ratio. Increases in the values of body lean mass (%), bone mineral content (g), adiponectin (μg/L), adiponectin/leptin ratio, and interleukin-15 (IL-15) (pg/mL) were observed (Tables 1 and 2).

Correlations analysis

Baseline values

Negative correlations were showed between bone mineral content (g) with body fat mass (%), visceral fat (cm) with adiponectin (ng/mL) and Beta CTX-collagen (ng/ml) with adiponectin (ng/mL). Positive correlations were

demonstrated between bone mineral content (g) with body lean mass (% and kg), visceral fat (cm) with body mass index (kg/m²) and body fat mass (kg), leptin (ng/mL) with body mass index (kg/m²) and body fat mass (kg) (Table 3).

Final values

Negative correlations were showed between bone mineral content (g) with body fat mass (%); osteocalcin (ng/mL) with leptin (ng/mL); and adiponectin/leptin ratio with subcutaneous fat (cm). Positive correlations were demonstrated between bone mineral content (g) with body lean mass (% and kg) (Table 3).

Regression analysis

As shown in the Figure 2 leptin (β -0.41; p = 0.04), adiponectin/leptin ratio (β 0.79; p < 0.001), body fat mass (β -0.66; p < 0.001) and body lean mass (β 0.66; p < 0.001) were predictors for changes in osteocalcin concentration.

Table 1. Effects of interdisciplinary weight loss therapy in body composition of obese adolescents

Variables	Baseline	1 year	p value	Δ value
Body mass (kg)	94.50 ± 15.45	88.70 ± 14.62*	< 0.001	-5.27 ± 4.5
Height (m)	1.68 ± 0.10	1.69 ± 0.12	0.60	0 ± 0.002
Body mass index (kg/m²)	33.21 ± 3.09	31.52 ± 3.19*	< 0.001	-1.90 ± 1.61
Body fat mass (%)	40.40 ± 6.50	37.35 ± 7.03*	< 0.001	-3.31 ± 2.98
Body fat mass (kg)	38.19 ± 8.75	33.17 ± 8.32*	< 0.001	-4.98 ± 4.22
Body lean mass (%)	59.60 ± 6.50	62.65 ± 7.03*	< 0.001	3.32 ± 2.98
Body lean mass (kg)	56.38 ± 10.89	57.55 ± 10.84	0.36	1.17 ± 2.00
Bone mineral density (g/cm²)	1.25 ± 0.08	1.26 ± 0.08	0.82	0 ± 0.02
Bone mineral content (g)	3192.21 ± 465.89	3338.12 ± 547.06*	< 0.001	140.34 ± 121.74
Visceral fat (cm)	4.46 ± 1.34	3.69 ± 1.20*	< 0.001	-0.66 ± 0.87
Subcutaneous fat (cm)	3.66 ± 0.79	3.40 ± 0.84*	0.01	-0.44 ± 0.54
Visceral/subcutaneous ratio	1.27 ± 0.45	0.29 ± 1.46*	0.001	-0.91 ± 1.20

* Statistical difference p ≤ 0.05. Effects of therapy: comparison between baseline and 1 year of therapy.

Table 2. Effects of interdisciplinary weight loss therapy in bone turnover markers and inflammation biomarkers of obese adolescents

Variables	Baseline	1 year	p value	Δ value
Beta-CTx collagen (ng/mL)	0.77 ± 0.46	0.64 ± 0.18	0.26	-0.16 ± 0.54
Osteocalcin (ng/ml)	30.3 (19/57.20)	34.60 (23.10/56.20)	0.28	3.60 (-7.2/43.3)
Adiponectin (μg/L)	1.9 ± 1.06	3.2 ± 1.2*	< 0.001	1.3 ± 1.4
Leptin (ng/ml)	24.65 ± 13.12	24.66 ± 14.53	0.50	-1.16 ± 8.53
Adiponectin/leptin ratio	0.09 ± 0.06	0.17 ± 0.16*	< 0.001	0.08 ± 0.13
IL-15 (pg/mL)	0.05 (0/1.23)	0.10 (0/1.28)*	0.04	0.06 (-0.98/0.81)

Beta-CTx collagen: C-terminal telopeptides of type I collagen; IL-15: interleukin-15.
* Statistical difference p ≤ 0.05. Effects of therapy: comparison between baseline and 1 year of therapy.

Table 3. Correlations analysis

Variables	r	p value
Baselines values		
Bone mineral content (g)		
Body fat mass (%)	-0.48	0.012
Body lean mass (%)	0.48	0.012
Body lean mass (kg)	0.56	0.003
Visceral fat (cm)		
Body mass index (kg/m²)	0.64	0.0001
Body fat mass (kg)	0.61	0.001
Adiponectin (ng/mL)	-0.47	0.013
Adiponectin (ng/mL)		
Beta CTX-collagen (ng/mL)	-0.45	0.03
Leptin (ng/mL)		
Body mass index (kg/m²)	0.50	0.009
Body fat mass (kg)	0.46	0.016
Final values		
Bone mineral content (g)		
Body fat mass (%)	-0.47	0.037
Body lean mass (%)	0.47	0.037
Body lean mass (kg)	0.51	0.020
Adiponectin/leptin (ng/mL)		
Subcutaneous fat (cm)	-0.53	0.01
Osteocalcin (ng/mL)		
Leptin (ng/mL)	-0.52	0.020

DISCUSSION

The first aim of the present investigation was to analyze the role of inflammatory biomarkers in bone turnover. The most important findings were the negative association with leptin concentration; and the positive correlation between the adiponectin/leptin ratio and osteocalcin. Therefore, we were able to confirm the hypothesis that pro/anti-inflammatory adipokine is a key mediator of bone turnover markers in obese adolescents.

According to our understanding, our group was the first to demonstrate the positive correlation between the adiponectin/leptin ratio and osteocalcin in obese adolescents, showing the beneficial effect of an improved adiponectin/leptin ratio on bone metabolism. Osteocalcin is a biomarker only secreted by osteoblasts, which enables the recognition of cell turnover in the skeletal system (7). Leptin concentration has an important influence on bone metabolism. In an experimental study leptin-deficient ob/ob and leptin-

resistant db/db showed increased osteocalcin levels (22), indicating that leptin is an inhibitor of osteoblastic bone formation.

Corroborating with this data, we were able to show a negative correlation between leptin and osteocalcin. In accordance, recently, investigations have shown that a reduction in leptin concentration correlated with an improvement of osteocalcin levels in obese adults (7). Additionally, weight loss promotes an increase in the adiponectin concentration, which plays an important role in bone mass. Another investigation showed that an increase in adiponectin concentration was associated with an improvement in the osteoblastic activity, suggesting an increase in osteocalcin concentration only in the experimental study. However, these authors suggest that adiponectin exerts an activity that increases bone mass by suppressing osteoclastogenesis and by activating osteoblastogenesis, indicating that adiponectin manipulation could be therapeutically beneficial for patients with osteopenia (8).

It is relevant to observed that, in our results a positive correlation was demonstrated between the adiponectin/leptin ratio and osteocalcin in obese adolescents, considering the baseline values. Additionally, at the end of treatment an increase in the adiponectin/leptin ratio without significant statistical changes in osteocalcin was observed. However, it is important to note a discreet change in the osteocalcin concentration was observed in the median baseline values compared with the final value (increase of 12%). In this way, it is possible to suggest that a positive change in the adiponectin/leptin ratio could promote benefits in osteocalcin concentration in obese adolescents. Moreover, a previous study considered the adiponectin/leptin ratio to be a better inflammatory marker for the metabolic syndrome population. This ratio has high sensitivity and specificity for the diagnosis of metabolic syndrome (11).

In fact, in the present study adiponectin was negatively correlated with visceral fat; and adiponectin/leptin correlated negatively with subcutaneous fat. It is likely that the impaired actions of adiponectin are clinically important in obese patients because adiponectin is the most abundant adipocyte-derived hormone with established anti-inflammatory effect (1).

Additionally, in the present investigation, it was found that both lean and body fat mass are predictors of osteocalcin. Concomitant to this, negative and positive correlations were observed between bone mineral content and body fat and lean body mass, respectively.

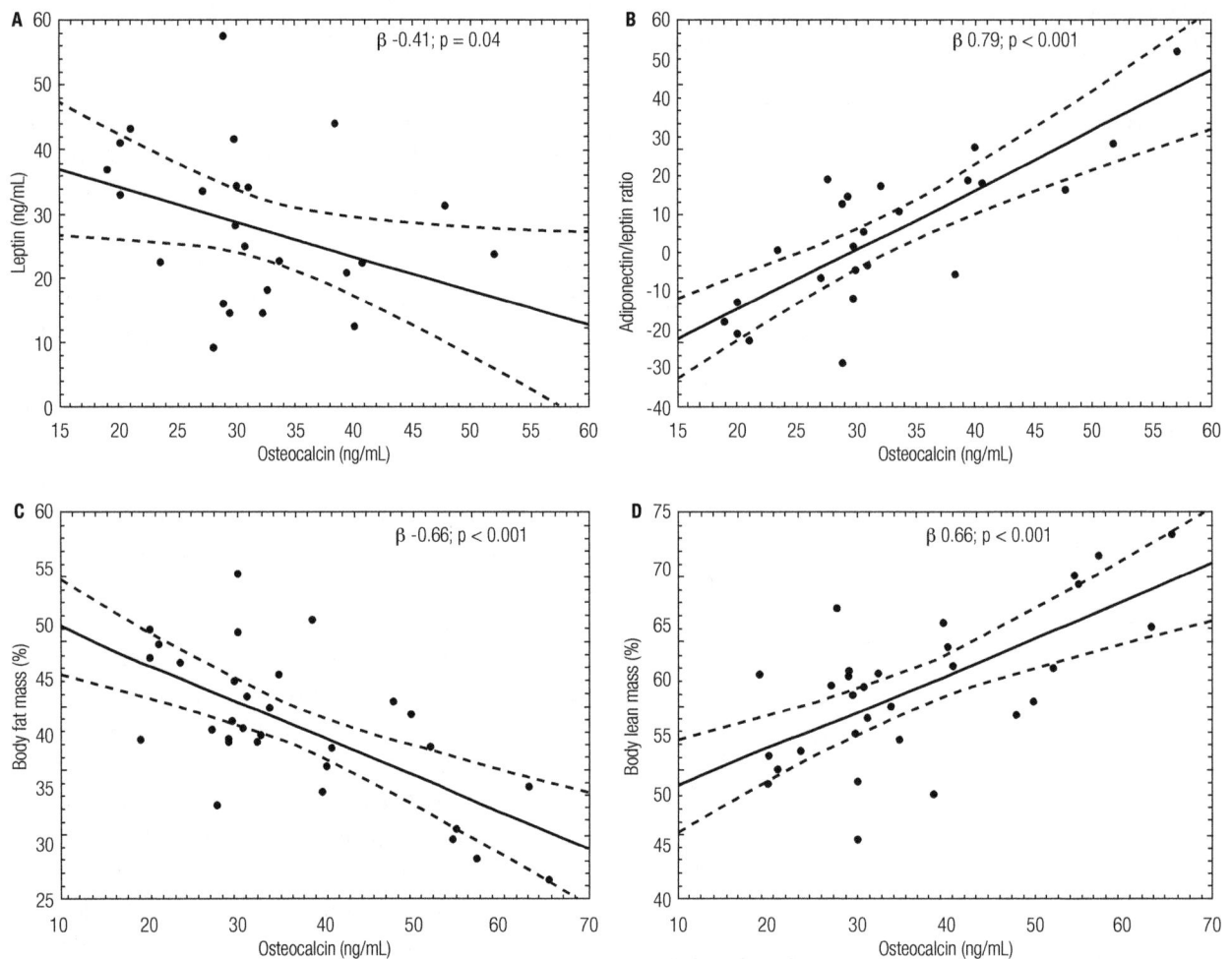

Figure 2. Simple linear regression established between osteocalcin (ng/mL) with: A) leptin (ng/mL); B) adiponectin/leptin ratio; C) body fat mass (%) and D) body lean mass (%).

In a previous investigation, it was demonstrated that the serum level of total osteocalcin was positively associated with fat-free mass independent of age, fat mass, leptin, and other confounders in premenopausal women. The hypothesis suggested to explain this association is based on the fact that fat-free mass could indirectly reflect the mechanical load on the bone, which can further stimulate bone formation, whereas low skeletal muscle mass is considered a risk factor for low bone mineral density (23). Moreover, corroborating with our findings, an inverse association was observed between osteocalcin and body fat mass in men with type 2 diabetes and in the elderly population. It is suggested that body fat mass accumulation is closely linked to bone turnover. Adipocytes are responsible for secreting many pro/anti-inflammatory cytokines such as TNF-alpha, interleukin-6, interleukin-10, leptin and

adiponectin, which are capable of modulating bone metabolism (24,25).

Notably, Beta-CTx collagen correlates negatively with adiponectin and positively with visceral fat. Adiponectin, an anti-inflammatory adipokine, could promote the acceleration of osteogenesis (26). Beta-CTx collagen is the C-terminal telopeptide of type I collagen, the main component (approximately 90%) of the protein matrix of bone. Beta-CTx collagen is released into the bloodstream during bone resorption and is almost entirely excreted by the kidneys. Its quantification serves as a specific marker for the degradation of mature type I collagen from the bone (5).

In addition, visceral fat promotes a secretion of many pro-inflammatory adipokines that are associated with an increase in the bone reabsorption and a decrease in bone formation (26). In this regard, our results showed that the pro-inflammatory profile present in obese adolescents is associated with an increase in Beta CTX-collagen and weight loss. A reduction in visceral fat, specifically, is associated with an increase in the adiponectin concentration and a reduction in the bone reabsorption biomarker as shown in the correlation analysis.

The second objective was to analyze the effects of interdisciplinary weight loss treatments on pro/anti-inflammatory adipokines and their role in bone turnover markers in obese adolescents. Therefore, another important finding from the present investigation is that weight loss therapy promotes a significant reduction in visceral fat (cm), subcutaneous fat (cm), visceral/subcutaneous ratio, total body fat mass and an increase in the lean body mass enhanced by nutritional counseling and physical exercise training. These results are important since it is well-established in the literature that fat deposition in the visceral compartment is related to the development of some diseases (1,27).

In fact, visceral fat plays a pathological role, due to the secretion of certain pro-inflammatory adipokines also related to the deterioration of bone mass and is associated with development of many comorbidities, such as metabolic syndrome, dyslipidemia, and cardiovascular complications. A prior study showed that an increase of 1 cm in visceral fat was associated with a 1.97 fold (95% CI 1.06–3.66) in boys and 2.08 fold (95% CI 1.38–3.13) in girls increased risk of developing nonalcoholic fatty liver disease (27).

In addition to these results, an increase in the IL-15 concentration after weight loss therapy was observed. IL-15 is considered an important fat mass regulator. In a prior investigation, a negative association between plasma IL-15 and fat mass was found, independent of the diagnosis of type 2 diabetes, which suggests that IL-15 may be involved in the regulation of body fat mass (28). In experimental research, it was found that the administration of IL-15 seems to decrease circulating triglycerides by decreasing both the liver lipogenic rate and very-low-density lipoprotein (VLDL). Moreover, IL-15 decreases lipoprotein lipase activity and the lipogenic rate in adipose tissue. Experimental studies showed a significant decrease in the intestinal lipid absorption, which may in part explain the anti-obesity effects of IL-15. Finally, it has been shown that lipoaspirate-derived human adipocytes treated with IL-15 inhibited pre-adipocyte differentiation.

The mechanism of IL-15 signaling in adipocytes however, is currently unknown (29). Together, these findings suggest that IL-15 treatment could result in weight loss and decreased visceral fat, corroborating with the control of the inflammatory state related to obesity (30).

Corroborating with our findings, Brunelli and cols. (31), showed that 24 weeks of moderate-high-intensity combined training (including aerobic and resistance exercises), in obese middle-aged men promotes an increase in the IL-15, concomitant with an improvement in the adiponectin concentration; and a decrease in the body fat. Also, it is suggested that the increase in the fat free mass and decreased body fat mass, may have contributed to the in IL-15 concentration in humans has a relevant anti-inflammatory function in the metabolic profile and may enhance energy expenditure to protect the body from obesity and type 2 diabetes (32).

Additionally, an increase in adiponectin concentration and adiponectin/leptin ratio was observed after interdisciplinary weight loss therapy. Adiponectin is a potent anti-inflammatory adipokine that possesses multiple beneficial effects on obesity-related medical complications (33). It may also have anti-atherogenic and anti-inflammatory properties, and high levels of circulating adiponectin have been related to a lower risk of coronary heart disease (34). However, no statistical difference was observed in the leptin concentration, probably explained because at baseline the adolescents showed a normal leptin concentration as recommended for this population (22). Although, it is relevant to note that hyperleptinemia is consider an important condition that contribute to the pro-inflammatory state observed in obesity population, including adolescents, and associated with comorbidities development (35). Considering bone health, studies demonstrated a negatively association between leptin and bone turnover biomarkers, especially with osteocalcin (7,10,36,37).

Another important result was the increase in BMC. This finding is possibly associated with improvement in the inflammatory profile, a reduction in visceral fat and the benefits of physical exercise intervention combined with other therapies realized by volunteers during the development of the study. It has been previously demonstrated that physical exercise can improve osteogenesis, which consequently increases bone mineral density and content (38). Moreover, resistance physical exercise at moderate intensity is related to decreased bone resorption markers (39). We know that aerobic physical exercises are associated with weight loss, but the combination of two kinds of physical exercise in the same session (aerobic plus resistance training) could optimize weight loss with greater benefits such as improvement in bone turnover markers and lean body mass as previously shown (2,40) as well as in the present study.

Finally, we showed that interdisciplinary weight loss therapy improves pro/anti-inflammatory profile and was related to bone turnover. Together, our results suggest the importance of controlling the inflammatory state and the effects on bone turnover markers related to obesity in adolescence.

CONCLUSIONS AND FUTURES DIRECTIONS

In the present study, we were able to show that both leptin and adiponectin/leptin ratio were negatively and positively associated with osteocalcin, respectively, modulating bone turnover markers. Finally, the interdisciplinary weight loss treatments were seen to be effective at reducing body fat mass, visceral fat and at increasing lean body mass, bone mineral content, adiponectin and IL-15. Together, these results suggest that this kind of intervention is considered an interesting alternative to prevent and treat obesity and promote bone health.

Acknowledgements: Support Foundation of São Paulo Research – Fapesp (2013/041364; 2013/19046-0; 2013/08522-6; 2015/14309-9), National Council for Scientific and Technological Development – CNPq (573587/2008-6; 300654/2013-8; 150177/2014-3) and Coordination of Higher Education Personnel Training – Capes.

REFERENCES

1. Dâmaso AR, de Piano A, Campos RMS, Corgosinho FC, Siegfried W, Caranti DA, et al. Multidisciplinary approach to the treatment of obese adolescents: effects on cardiovascular risk factors, inflammatory profile, and neuroendocrine regulation of energy balance. Int J Endocrinol. 2013;2013:541032.

2. Campos RM, de Mello MT, Tock L, da Silva PL, Corgosinho FC, Carnier J, et al. Interaction of bone mineral density, adipokines and hormones in obese adolescents girls submitted in an interdisciplinary therapy. J Pediatr Endocrinol Metab. 2013;26(7-8):663-8.

3. Campos RM, Lazaretti-Castro M, Mello MT, Tock L, Silva PL, Corgosinho FC, et al. Influence of visceral and subcutaneous fat in

4. Lac G, Cavalie H, Ebal E, Michaux O. Effects of a high fat diet on bone of growing rats. Correlations between visceral fat, adiponectin and bone mass density. Lipids Health Dis. 2008;7:16.

5. Peichl P, Griesmacherb A, Marteau R, Hejc S, Kumpan W, Müller MM, et al. Serum crosslaps in comparison to serum osteocalcin and urinary bone resorption markers. Clin Biochem. 2001;34(2):131-9.

6. Alfadda AA, Masood A, Shaik SA, Dekhil H, Goran M. Association between osteocalcin, metabolic syndrome, and cardiovascular risk factors: role of total and undercarboxylated osteocalcin in patients with type 2 diabetes. Int J Endocrinol. 2013;2013:197519.

7. Suh HS, Hwang IC, Lee KS, Kim KK. Relationships between serum osteocalcin, leptin and the effect of weight loss by pharmacological treatment in healthy, nonsmoking Korean obese adults. Clin Chim Acta. 2013;418:17-21.

8. Oshima K, Nampei A, Matsuda M, Iwaki M, Fukuhara A, Hashimoto J, et al. Adiponectin increases bone mass by suppressing osteoclast and activating osteoblast. Biochem Biophys Res Commun. 2005;331(2):520-6.

9. Kanazawa I, Yamaguchi T, Yano S, Yamauchi M, Yamamoto M, Sugimoto T. Adiponectin and AMP kinase activator stimulate proliferation, differentiation, and mineralization of osteoblastic MC3T3-E1 cells. BMC Cell Biol. 2007;8:51.

10. Saleem U, MosleyTH Jr, Kullo IJ. Serum osteocalcin is associated with measures of insulin resistance, adipokine levels, and the presence of metabolic syndrome. Arterioscler Thromb Vasc Biol. 2010;30(7):1474-8.

11. Mirza S, Qu HQ, Li Q, Martinez PJ, Rentfro AR, McCormick JB, et al. Adiponectin/leptin ratio and metabolic syndrome in a Mexican American population. Clin Invest Med. 2011;34(5):E290.

12. Choi BC, Pak AW. Multidisciplinarity, interdisciplinarity and transdisciplinarity in health research, services, education and policy: 1. Definitions, objectives, and evidence of effectiveness. Clin Invest Med. 2006;29(6):351-64.

13. Tanner JM, Whitehouse RH. Clinical longitudinal standards for height, weight, height velocity, weight velocity, and stages of puberty. Arch Dis Child. 1976;51(3):170-9.

14. Centers for Disease Control and Prevention. Hyattsville: National Center for Health Statistics. (Updates on 11 January 2007). Prevalence of overweight among children and adolescents: United States 1999-2002. Disponível em: http://www.cdc.gov/ nchs/products/pubs/pubd/hestats/overwght99.htm. Acesso em: 11 ago. 2013.

15. Black E, Petersen L, Kreutzer M, Toubro S, Sørensen TI, Pedersen O, et al. Fat mass measured by DXA varies with scan velocity. Obes Res. 2002;10(2):69-77.

16. Dossus L, Becker S, Achaintre D, Kaaks R, Rinaldi S. Validity of multiplex-based assays for cytokine measurements in serum and plasma from "non-diseased" subjects: comparison with ELISA. J Immunol Methods. 2009;350(1-2):125-32.

17. Gutin B, Ramsey L, Barbeau P, Cannady W, Ferguson M, Litaker M, et al. Plasma leptin concentrations in obese children: changes during 4-mo periods with and without physical training. Am J Clin Nutr. 1999;69(3):388-94.

18. Ribeiro-Filho FF, Faria AN, Azjen S, Zanella MT, Ferreira SR. Methods of estimation of visceral fat: advantages of ultrasonography. Obes Res. 2003;11(12):1488-94.

19. Donnelly JE, Blair SN, Jakicic JM, Manore MM, Rankin JW, Smith BK; American College of Sports Medicine. American College of Sports Medicine Position Stand. Appropriate physical activity intervention strategies for weight loss and prevention of weight regain for adults. Med Sci Sports Exerc. 2009;41(2):459-71.

20. Kraemer WJ, Ratamess NA, French DN. Resistance training for health and performance. Curr Sports Med Rep. 2002;1(3):165-71.

21. National Academic Press. Dietary Reference Intake. Applications in Dietary Assessment. Washington, DC; 2001.

22. Ducy P, Amling M, Takeda S, Priemel M, Schilling AF, Beil FT, et al. Leptin inhibits bone formation through a hypothalamic relay: a central control of bone mass. Cell. 2000;100(2):197-207.

23. Wu CH, Yang KC, Chang HH, Yen JF, Tsai KS, Huang KC. Sarcopenia is related to increased risk for low bone mineral density. J Clin Densitom. 2013;16(1):98-103.

24. Kanazawa I, Yamaguchi T, Yamauchi M, Yamamoto M, Kurioka S, Yano S, et al. Serum undercarboxylated osteocalcin was inversely associated with plasma glucose level and fat mass in type 2 diabetes mellitus. Osteoporos Int. 2011;22(1):187-94.

25. Kindblom JM, Ohlsson C, Ljunggren O, Karlsson MK, Tivesten A, Smith U, et al. Plasma osteocalcin is inversely related to fat mass and plasma glucose in elderly Swedish men. J Bone Miner Res. 2009;24(5):785-91.

26. Lee HW, Kim SY, Kim AY, Lee EJ, Choi JY, Kim JB. Adiponectin stimulates osteoblast differentiation through induction of COX2 in mesenchymal progenitor cells. Stem Cells. 2009;27(9):2254-62.

27. Dâmaso AR, do Prado WL, de Piano A, Tock L, Caranti DA, Lofrano MC, et al. Relationship between nonalcoholic fatty liver disease prevalence and visceral fat in obese adolescents. Dig Liver Dis. 2008;40(2):132-9.

28. Nielsen AR, Hojman P, Erikstrup C, Fischer CP, Plomgaard P, Mounier R, et al. Association between interleukin-15 and obesity: interleukin-15 as a potential regulator of fat mass. J Clin Endocrinol Metab. 2008;93(11):4486-93.

29. Almendro V, Carbó N, Busquets S, López-Soriano J, Figueras M, Ametller E, et al. Interleukin-15 decreases lipid intestinal absorption. Int J Mol Med. 2005;15(6):963-7.

30. Carbó N, López-Soriano J, Costelli P, Alvarez B, Busquets S, Baccino FM, et al. Interleukin-15 mediates reciprocal regulation of adipose and muscle mass: a potential role in body weight control. Biochim Biophys Acta. 2001;1526(1):17-24.

31. Brunelli DT, Chacon-Mikahil MP, Gáspari AF, Lopes WA, Bonganha V, Bonfante IL, et al. Combined training reduces subclinical inflammation in obese middle-age men. Med Sci Sports Exerc. 2015;47(10):2207-15.

32. Ye J. Beneficial metabolic activities of inflammatory cytokine interleukin 15 in obesity and type 2 diabetes. Front Med. 2015;9(2):139-45.

33. Manigrasso MR, Ferroni P, Santilli F, Taraborelli T, Guagnano MT, Michetti N, et al. Association between circulating adiponectin and interleukin-10 levels in android obesity: effects of weight loss. J Clin Endocrinol Metab. 2005;90(10):5876-9.

34. Wang Y, Zhou M, Lam KS, Xu A. Protective roles of adiponectin in obesity-related fatty liver diseases: mechanisms and therapeutic implications. Arq Bras Endocrinol Metabol. 2009;53(2):201-12.

35. Dâmaso AR, de Piano A, Sanches PL, Corgosinho F, Tock L, Oyama LM, et al. Hyperleptinemia in obese adolescents deregulates neuropeptides during weight loss. Peptides. 2011;32(7):1384-91.

36. Giudici KV, Kindler JM, Martin BR, Laing EM, McCabe GP, McCabe LD, et al. Associations among osteocalcin, leptin and metabolic health in children ages 9-13 years in the United States. Nutr Metab (Lond). 2017;14:25.

37. Jürimäe J, Lätt E, Mäestu J, Saar M, Purge P, Maasalu K, et al. Osteocalcin is inversely associated with adiposity and leptin in adolescent boys. J Pediatr Endocrinol Metab. 2015;28(5-6):571-7.

38. Lanyon LE, Rubin CT. Static vs dynamic loads as an influence on bone remodelling. J Biomech. 1984;17(12):897-905.

39. Whipple TJ, Le BH, Demers LM, Chinchilli VM, Petit MA, Sharkey N, et al. Acute effects of moderate intensity resistance exercise on bone cell activity. Int J Sports Med. 2004;25(7):496-501.

40. Foschini D, Araújo RC, Bacurau RF, De Piano A, De Almeida SS, Carnier J, et al. Treatment of obese adolescents: the influence of periodization models and ACE genotype. Obesity (Silver Spring). 2010;18(4):766-72.

3

Preoperatively undiagnosed papillary thyroid carcinoma in patients thyroidectomized for benign multinodular goiter

Fausto Fama[1], Alessandro Sindoni[2], Marco Cicciu[1], Francesca Polito[3],
Arnaud Piquard[4], Olivier Saint-Marc[4], Maria Gioffre'-Florio[1],
Salvatore Benvenga[3,5,6]

ABSTRACT

Objective: Incidental thyroid cancers (ITCs) are often microcarcinomas; among them, the most frequent histotype is the papillary one. The purpose of this study was to evaluate the rate of papillary thyroid cancer (PTC) in patients thyroidectomized for benign multinodular goiter. Subject and methods: We retrospectively evaluated the histological incidence of PTC in 207 consecutive patients who, in a 1-year period, underwent thyroidectomy for benign multinodular goiter. All patients came from an iodine-deficient area (Orleans, France) with three nuclear power stations located in the neighboring areas of the county town. Results: Overall, 25 thyroids (12.1%) harbored 37 PTC, of which 31 were microcarcinomas. In these 25 PTC patients, mean age was 55 ± 10 years (range 30-75), female:male ratio 20:5 (4:1). In 10 patients (40% of 25 and 4.8% of 207), PTCs were bilateral, and in 7 (2 with microPTCs) the thyroid capsule was infiltrated. These 7 patients underwent central and lateral cervical lymph node dissections, which revealed lymph node metastases in one and two cases, respectively. Radioiodine treatment was performed in 7 cases. Neither mortality nor transient and permanent nerve injuries were observed. Four (16%) transient hypocalcaemias occurred as early complications. At last follow-up visit (mean length of follow-up 17.2 ± 3.4 months), all patients were doing well and free of any clinical local recurrence or distant metastases. Conclusion: With a 12% risk that multinodular goiter harbors preoperatively unsuspected PTCs, which can have already infiltrated the capsule and that can be accompanied by PTC foci contralaterally, an adequate surgical approach has to be considered. Arch Endocrinol Metab. 2018;62(2):139-48

Keywords

Incidental thyroid cancer; benign thyroid disease; multinodular goiter; total thyroidectomy; papillary thyroid cancer

[1] Department of Human Pathology in Adulthood and Childhood "G. Barresi", University Hospital of Messina, Messina, Italy
[2] Department of Biomedical and Dental Sciences and of Morphological and Functional Images, University Hospital of Messina, Messina, Italy
[3] Department of Clinical & Experimental Medicine, University Hospital of Messina, Messina, Italy
[4] Department of General, Endocrine and Thoracic Surgery, Regional Hospital of Orleans, Orléans, France
[5] Master Program on Childhood, Adolescent and Women's Endocrine Health, University Hospital of Messina, Messina, Italy
[6] Interdepartmental Program on Molecular & Clinical Endocrinology, and Women's Endocrine Health, University Hospital of Messina, Messina, Italy

Correspondence to:
Alessandro Sindoni
Sezione di Scienze Radiologiche,
Dipartimento di Scienze Biomediche,
Odontoiatriche e delle Immagini
Morfologiche e Funzionali,
Via Consolare Valeria, 1
98125 – Messina, Italy
alessandrosindoni@alice.it

INTRODUCTION

In the thyroid literature the term *incidental* has been used to indicate an unsuspected finding; nevertheless, the nature of the incidental finding depends on the clinical context in which the nodules are found. Considering thyroid gland, the identification of thyroid cancer may be classified into 3 broad categories: 1) clinically detected cancer (not incidentally detected), 2) radiologically detected cancer (clinically unsuspected), and 3) pathologically detected cancer (clinically and radiologically unsuspected) (1). Incidental thyroid cancers (ITCs) are often microcarcinomas, most frequently of the papillary histotype (2-6); the mean tumor size of ITCs decreased during the last decades

(3,6). Namely, Boucek and cols. (7) divided ITC diagnoses into four different categories: i) neoplasms found incidentally after thyroidectomy whereas preoperatively only benign pathology was known; ii) neoplasms that were diagnosed incidentally on imaging, mainly ultrasonography (US), and that were evaluated further and confirmed by fine-needle aspiration cytology (FNAC); iii) neoplasms that appeared clinically as lymph node metastases, with primary thyroid carcinoma detected only at histological specimen examination; iv) thyroid cancer that is localized in ectopic thyroid tissue with clinical symptoms or metastases present. Besides these four groups, Liu and cols. (8) proposed another ITC group including patients that presented, despite benign thyroid disease ascertained at imaging and definitive histology, regional or distant lymph node metastases from primary thyroid carcinoma not identified at thyroid pathological examination.

An ITC discovered at histology, after surgical removal of the thyroid for a benign pathology, is the most frequent event (9-12). In thyroidectomy specimens, ITC prevalence ranges up to 40% (2). In autopsy studies, the reported prevalence of ITC ranges from 0.01% in USA to 35.6% in Finland (7). Recently, a study from U.S.A. have documented that most counties with the highest thyroid cancer incidence are in a contiguous area of eastern Pennsylvania, New Jersey, and southern New York State; radioactive exposures from 16 nuclear power reactors within a 90-mile radius in this area have indicated that these emissions are a likely etiological factor in rising thyroid cancer incidence rates (13).

Over the last 30 years, there has been an increase in the overall incidence of thyroid cancer, from 3.6 (in 1973) to 8.7 (in 2002) per 100,000 inhabitants (14). The incidence rate of papillary thyroid cancer PTC rose up more than any other malignancy (15,16), up to 93% of all thyroid cancers in Japan and up to 85.3% in Western countries (7). PTC is the most common histotype and microPTC represents up to 30% of all forms of papillary cancer (17).

The very recently released American Thyroid Association guidelines on thyroid nodules and cancer underscore that "a recent population based study from Olmsted County reported the doubling of thyroid cancer incidence from 2000-2012 compared to the prior decade as entirely attributable to clinically occult cancers detected incidentally on imaging or pathology" (18-20). By 2019, one study predicts that papillary thyroid cancer (PTC) will become the third most common cancer in women (21).

The purpose of this study was to evaluate the rate of histologically detected PTC in consecutive patients who were thyroidectomized for benign multinodular goiter (MNG) throughout a 1-year period at a single endocrine surgery unit. Of note, this surgery unit and patients' residence is located near to three nuclear power units. Our data were compared with those of the English language literature on the ITCs.

SUBJECTS AND METHODS

All patients of this retrospective cohort were admitted on the same day of the surgical procedures,

performed by 3 experienced endocrine surgeons under general anesthesia. Preoperatively, patients were studied by means of neck US and routine blood test, including hormones levels. The American Society of Anesthesiologists (ASA) physical status was assessed in all patients. In order to obtain a more homogeneous cohort of patients, we excluded patients with suspicious characteristics of the thyroid nodule(s) (i.e. irregular margin and/or contour and/or shape, calcifications, hypoechogenicity, vascularity or local invasion/lymph node metastases) at US (n = 19), history of previous neck surgery (n = 7), history of malignancy in other organs (n = 5) and ASA score greater than 4 (n = 2).

Parathyroid glands and recurrent nerves were identified in all cases, and specimens sent to pathologists for the frozen section; no cervical drains were placed systematically. Patients were discharged, generally in the second post-operative day, with a prescription of a weight-adjusted thyroxine treatment. Patients were referred to our endocrinological outpatient surveillance program. We defined microcarcinoma or macrocarcinoma any cancerous nodule up to 10 mm or greater than in maximum diameter, respectively. When multifocality occurred, we considered the largest neoplasm and classified according to its anatomical site. For purpose of comparison with the international literature, we run a PubMed search entering the words "incidental thyroid cancer" or "incidental thyroid carcinoma". The search was updated until November 2016. The search was limited taking into consideration only original papers. The references of the retrieved articles were also checked so as not to miss important clinical studies. Original articles reporting data about patients who underwent surgery for suspicious or preoperatively documented disease, as well as editorials, commentaries, review articles and similar types of articles were excluded. Animal studies were also excluded. Two researchers (A.S., S.B.) independently reviewed the titles and disagreements were resolved in a consensus meeting.

Statistical analysis

Results are expressed as mean ± standard deviation (SD). Laboratory data without normal distribution were described using median and percentile values. Fisher's exact test was used to analyze categorical data. The level for statistical significance was set at $P < 0.05$. Statistical analysis was performed using Kyplot v2.0 beta 13 version.

RESULTS

In our study from a French endocrine surgery unit, we retrospectively reviewed 207 consecutive patients, 169 were females (mean age of 53.0 ± 12.6 years [range 18-79]) and 38 males (mean age of 54.9 ± 14.2 years [range 21-78]), who underwent total thyroidectomy (TT) for benign bilateral MNG from January to December 2014. All patients came from an iodine-deficient area (Orleans, France) (22) with three nuclear power stations located in the neighboring areas of the county town (Figure 1). Clinico-laboratory data of all patients are shown in Table 1.

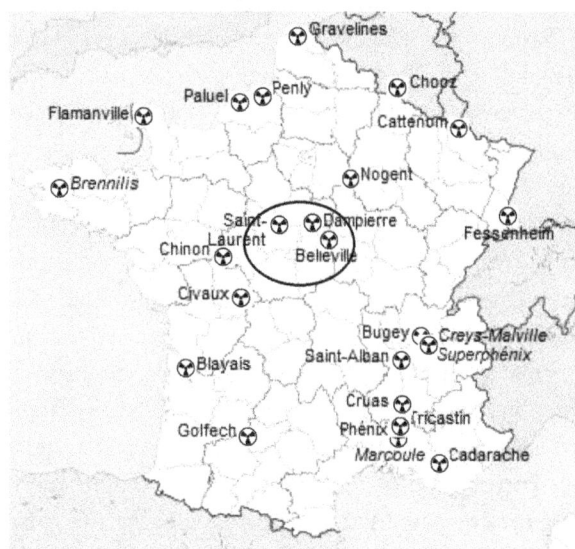

Figure 1. Topography of nuclear power plants in the neighboring areas of Orleans, France (ring).

Table 1. Demographic and clinico-laboratory characteristics of patients undergoing total thyroidectomy for benign multinodular goiter

	All patients (n = 207)
Age, years	
mean ± SD	53.9 ± 13.9
(range)	(18 – 79)
TSH, uUI/ml	
median	1.54
(interquartile range)	(1.07 – 2.27)
FT3, pmol/L	
median	5.6
(interquartile range)	(4.3 – 6.2)
FT4, pmol/L	
median	15.2
(interquartile range)	(12.8 – 16.9)
Tg, ng/ml	
median	24.2
(interquartile range)	(19.5 – 35.7)

SD: standard deviation; Tg: thyroglobulin.

Over the 12-month chronological window of our study, in 25/207 patients (12.1%) we discovered 37 preoperatively unsuspected, and therefore ITCs, all being PTCs. Their ASA score of these patients was ASA1 (n = 4), ASA2 (n = 18) and ASA3 (n = 3). Mean hospital stay was 1.1 ± 0.3 days; 23 (92%) were discharged on the 1st post-operative day and 2 on the 2nd post-operative day.

Of these 37 PTCs, 31 (86.1%) were microPTCs, with a maximum diameter ranging 1 to 6 mm, while 6 were macroPTCs (diameter range 12-16 mm). Overall, mean age of the 25 patients was 55 ± 10 years (range 30-75) with 20 being females (F:M ratio = 4:1). Patients with macroPTCs were 7 years older than patients with microPTCs (Table 2). Histopathological examination showed bilateral MNG in all cases (mean weight of the thyroid glands: 53.6 ± 45.7 g) and the additional presence of chronic lymphocytic thyroiditis or Hashimoto's thyroiditis (HT) in 6/25 patients (24%, all with positive thyroid peroxidase and thyroglobulin autoantibodies). Thyroid tumors were monofocal in 15 patients (all microPTCs; 15/37 tumors in 15 patients) and multifocal in 10. Of these multifocal PTCs, 16 were microcarcinomas and 6 macrocarciomas. In 5 of the 10 patients microPTCs and macroPTC coexisted.

Multifocal PTCs, including coexistence of micro (n = 16) and macroPTCs (n = 6), were always bilateral. Of the 15 monofocal microPTCs, 8 were right-sided, and 7 left-sided (Table 1). MicroPTCs and macroPTCs did not differ in distribution if we considered the right lobe-left lobe-isthmus location (P = 0.836 by Fisher's exact test) or the classification among the upper-middle-lower-isthmic localization in the thyroid (P = 0.334 by Fisher's exact test). Of the 6/207 patients with HT, 2/6 (33.3%) had 4 of the 37 PTCs, all 4 tumors being microPTCs.

Seven supplementary central and lateral cervical lymph node dissections were carried out, because 2 microPTCs and 5 PTCs were infiltrating the thyroid capsule at frozen sections. Lymph node metastases were found in one and two patients, respectively. Radioiodine treatment, with a dose of 100 mCi, was performed in 7 cases, because of the presence of poor prognostic factors such as capsular infiltration, macroPTC and/or multifocality.

Neither mortality nor transient and permanent nerve injuries were observed. Four (16%) transient hypocalcaemias occurred as early complications, and were successfully treated by a 6-week combined cholecalciferol and oral calcium supplementation.

Table 2. PTC patients and tumours characteristics

	Right lobe	Left lobe	Isthmus	Total
No. of nodules	17	16	4	37
(%)	(46.0%)	(43.2%)	(10.8%)	(100%)
No. of patients with multifocality	4	5	1	10/25
(%)	(16%)	(20%)	(4%)	(40.0%)
microPTC				
No. of nodules	14	14	3	31
(%)	(45.2%)	(45.2%)	(9.6%)	
Mean diameter (mm) ± SD	4.4 ± 2.7	3.9 ± 2.5	1	3.8 ± 2.6
Mean age (years) ± SD	55.9 ± 10.2	52.2 ± 7.7	57.0 ± 18.7	54.4 ± 9.9
F:M ratio	3.7:1	3.7:1	3:0	4.2:1
macroPTC				
No. of nodules	3	2	1	6
(%)	(50%)	(33.3%)	(16.7%)	
Mean diameter (mm) ± SD	13.0 ± 1.7	12.5 ± 0.7	30	15.7 ± 7.1
Mean age (years) ± SD	60.0 ± 13.5	67.5 ± 9.2	52	61.2 ± 11.1
F:M ratio	3:0	2:0	0:1	5:1

PTC: papillary thyroid carcinoma; SD: standard deviation; F: female; M, male.

At last follow-up visit (mean length of follow-up 17.2 ± 3.4 months), all patients were doing well and free of any clinical local recurrence or distant metastases.

An overview of the literature is summarized in Table 3 (23-68). Reported prevalence of ITC at surgery ranges between 2% and 40% (1,2,17,23-68): in Europe it varies from 2.2% to 27.4% and in the United States it varies from 3.3% to 33%. In some European countries, such as Romania, Czech Republic, Ukraine and Poland, the frequency of thyroid cancer showed a lower range (i.e. from 5 to 9.2%); in Turkey, excluding the study from Tasova and cols. (46), there has been a lower variation range in its reported incidence (7-10%). Rates from other European countries were: 12.5 % from Belgium, 10.4-11.1% from Italy and 12.0% from Greece.

Table 3. Summary of the literature on thyroid cancers that were discovered incidentally at thyroidectomy in patients underwent surgery for benign thyroid disease

Author (ref)	Years of study	Country	Patients studied	Surgical procedure	Rate of cancer	Comment
Fama' and cols., this study	One (2014)	France	207 pts	TT	In 25/207 (12.1%) pts, 37 PTC were detected (31 microPTCs and 6 PTCs)	10/25 (40.0%) pts had multifocal tumours; all pts underwent surgery for MNG
Daumerie and cols., 1998	1976 - 1995	Belgique	93 pts	TT in 16/47 (34.0%) pts with MNG (group I), PT in 39/46 (84.8%) pts with a solitary hot nodule (group II)	2/16 (12.5%) pts (group I) and 5/39 (12.8%) pts (group II) had microTC, with a total prevalence of 12.7%	
Dănilă and cols., 2008	2000 - 2006	Germany	92 pts	TT	2/92 (2.2%) pts had microPTC (tumour size ranged from 3 to 5 mm)	All pts had GD; multifocality and lymph node involvement were not detected
Pezzolla and cols., 2014	Jan 2010 - Jun 2013	Italy	256 pts	Surgical procedures in tumours pts 28/256): TT in 27/28, PT in 1/28 PT	In 28/256 (10.9%) pts, 40 TCs were detected (29 FV-PTC, 10 PTC and 1 FTC)	Pts underwent surgery for: 176 pts (MNG), 67 pts (GD), 12 pts (UNG) and 1 pt (PD)
Pezzolla and cols., 2010	n/a	Italy	165 pts	n/a	30/165 (18.2%) pts had TC (18 PTC, 6 FTC, 5 FV-PTC and 1 oncocytic carcinoma); 15/30 (50%) were microcarcinomas	Pts underwent surgery for: 132 pts (MNG), 30 pts (UNG), 2 pts (PD) and 1 pt (GD)

Author (ref)	Years of study	Country	Patients studied	Surgical procedure	Rate of cancer	Comment
Costamagna and cols., 2013	2001 - 2009	Italy	568 pts	TT in 499/568, PT in 69/568	53/568 (9.3%) pts had TC (24 FV-PTC, 20 PTC, 4 FTC, 4 MTC and 1 primitive thyroid paraganglioma); 32/53 (60.4%) had microPTCs	14/53 (26.4%) pts had multifocal tumours and in 12/53 (22.6%) were bilateral
Negro and cols., 2013*	2000 - 2010	Italy	970 pts	TT	84/ 970 (8.7%) pts had TC	
Botrugno and cols., 2011	2000 - 2008	Italy	462 pts	TT	41/462 (8.9%) pts had TC; the most common histotype was PTC	
Gelmini and cols., 2010	10 yrs	Italy	739 pts	TT in 503/739, PT in 239/739	82/739 (11.1%) pts had TC, mainly microPTC	Lymph-node metastases were found in the 3.6% of cases
Pisello and cols., 2007	Jan 2000 - Jan 2006	Italy	502 pts	TT in 458/502, PT in 44/502	17/502 (3.4%) pts had microPTC	In 34/502 (6.8%) pts, tumours were suspected preoperatively; 2/502 (0.4%) had multifocal microPTCs
Carlini and cols., 2006*	n/a	Italy	88 pts	TT	19/88 (21.6%) pts had TC	
Miccoli and cols., 2006	Feb 2002 - Nov 2003	Italy	998 pts	TT in 902/998 pts, PT in 96/998	104/998 (10.4%) pts had TC; the most common histotype was PTC (99/104)	Tumours were multifocal in 19.8% of the cases
Carlini and cols., 2005*	1-year	Italy	n/a	n/a	Incidence of microTC was 27.4%	
Pingitore and cols., 1993	1985 - 1991	Italy	2930 pts	n/a	132/2463 (5.4%) pts had TC	2463/2930 pts were considered clinically benign and 467/2930 pts malignant, preoperatively
Pascual Corrales and cols., 2012	n/a	Spain	372 pts	n/a	58/372 (15.6%) pts had TC	Pts underwent surgery for: 49 pts (EMNG), 8 pts (GD) and 1 pt (HMNG)
Slijepcevic and cols., 2015	2008-2013	Serbia	2466 pts	TT or PT	403/2466 (16.3%) pts had microPTC	
Zivaljević and cols., 2008	2004	Serbia	578 pts	n/a	53/578 (9.2%) pts had microTC	Pts underwent surgery for: 201 pts (MNG), 178 pts (thyroid adenoma), 89 pts (GD), 79 pts (PD) and 31 pts thyroiditis
Alecu and cols., 2014	2002 - 2012	Romania	145 pts	TT in 102/145 pts, PT in 43/145	10/145 (6.9%) pts had microPTC	
Muntean and cols., 2013	2002 - 2011	Romania	2168 pts	TT or PT	187/2168 (8.6%) pts had microPTC	In 66/187 (35.3%) pts had multifocal tumours, and in 31/187 (16.6%) were bilateral
Lukás and cols., 2010	2004 - 2008	Czech Republic	400 pts	TT or PT	34/400 (8.5%) pts had microTC; 32/34 (94.1%) were microPTCs	In 5/34 (14.7%) pts had multifocal tumours and in 4/34 (11.8%) were bilateral
Nechaĭ and cols., 2012*	2008 - 2009	Ukraine	608 pts	n/a	56/608 (9.2%) pts had TC; 43/56 (76.8%) were microPTCs	
Barczyński and cols., 2011*	1999 - 2009	Poland	8132 pts	TT in 2918/8132 pts, PT in 5214/8132	406/8132 (5.0%) pts had TC	
Vasileiadis and cols., 2013	2001 - 2009	Greece	2236 pts	TT	268/2236 (12.0%) pts had microPTC.	

Author (ref)	Years of study	Country	Patients studied	Surgical procedure	Rate of cancer	Comment
Siassakos and cols., 2008	Jan 1997 - Jul 2001	Greece	191 pts	TT	29/191 (15.2%) pts had microTC (18 microFTC, 10 microPTC and 1 microMTC)	In 8/29 (27.6%) pts had multifocal microcarcinomas
Sakorafas and cols., 2007	Feb 1990 - Feb 2002	Greece	380 pts	TT in 377/380 pts, PT in 3/380	27/380 (7.1%) pts had microPTC	In 11/27 (40.7%) pts had multifocal tumours
Yazici and cols., 2015	2010-2013	Turkey	86 pts	TT or PT	6/86 (7.0%) pts had TC (4 microPTC and 2 PTC)	
Tasova and cols., 2013	Mar 2007 - May 2011	Turkey	443 pts	TT in 401/443, PT in 42/443	66/443 (14.9%) pts had TC (56 PTC, 4 FTC and 6 indeterminate lesions)	
Karakoyun and cols., 2013	Jan 2010 - Aug 2011	Turkey	50 pts	TT	5/50 (10.0%) pts had microPTC.	
Berker and cols., 2011	Jan 2004 - Jan 2009	Turkey	337 pts	TT	18/337 (5.3%) pts had microTC	Pts underwent surgery for: 278 pts (MNG), 59 pts (GD)
Tezelman and cols., 2009	1988-2007	Turkey	2906 pts	PT in 1695/2906 (group 1), TT in 1211/2906 (group 2)	210/2906 (7.2%) pts had TC (81 in group 1 and 129 in group 2)	
Giles and cols., 2004	Sep 2001 - Dec 2002	Turkey	218 pts	TT in 109/218 (group 1), and PT in 109/218 (group 2)	18/218 (8.3%) pts had PTC (10 in group 1 and 8 in group 2)	All pts underwent surgery for MNG
Fernando and cols., 2009	2003 - 2005	Sri Lanka	68 pts	TT	6/68 (8.8%) pts had TC (2 PTC, 2 MTC and 2 FTC)	
John and cols., 2014	Jan 2005 - Jun 2012	India	1300 pts	TT or PT	94/1300 (7.2%) pts had microPTC	
Wu and cols., 1993*	1962 - 1991	China	135 pts	n/a	54/135 (40.0%) pts had TC	
Koh and cols., 1992	n/a	Malaysia	107 pts	n/a	8/107 (7.5%) pts had TC, mainly PTC	All pts underwent surgery for MNG
Preece and cols., 2014	Sep 1994 - Aug 2012	Australia	1508 pts	TT	96/1508 (6.4%) pts had TC	Pts underwent surgery for: 963 pts (MNG), 295 pts (TNG), 250 pts (GD)
Bron and cols., 2004	1998-2002	Australia	834 pts	TT	71/834 (8.5%) pts had TC (33 microPTC, 22 PTC, 11 FTC, 5 other)	74/834 had previously undergone PT
Bhuiyan and cols., 2015	2003-2008	South Africa	90 pts	TT	10/90 (11.1%) pts had TC (3 PTC and 7 FTC)	
Bombil and cols., 2014	2005-2010	South Africa	162 pts	TT	4/162 (2.5%) pts had PTC (3/4 were FV-PTC)	
Edino and cols., 2010	2000-2006	Nigeria	160 pts	n/a	24/160 (15.0%) pts had TC (13 FTC, 10 PTC, 1 MTC and 1 ATC)	In 6/25 (24.0%) pts tumours were detected preoperatively by FNAC
Choong and cols., 2015	1990-2014	USA	148 pts	TT (120 pts) or PT (28 pts)	7/148 (4.7%) pts had TC (5 PTC, 1 FTC and 1 MTC)	All pts underwent surgery for TNG
Ergin and cols., 2014	2005-2013	USA	493 pts	TT	69/248 (28%) pts in EG group and 64/245 (26%) pts in GD group had microPTC	Pts underwent surgery for: 248 pts (EG), 245 pts (GD)
Bahl and cols., 2014*	2003-2012	USA	2090 pts	n/a	680/2090 (33%) pts had TC	
Phitayakorn and cols., 2013	Dec 1985 - Mar 2010	USA	300 pts	TT or PT	31/300 (10.3%) pts had TC (22 microPTC, 8 PTC and 1 FTC)	
Phitayakorn and cols., 2008	1990-2007	USA	506 pts	TT, PT in 10 pts with GD	11/333 (3.3%) nonTNG pts had PTC, 2/92 (2.2%) GD pts had microPTC, 5/81 (6.2%) TNG pts had TC (3 PTC, 1 FTC and 1 MTC)	Pts underwent surgery for: 333 pts (nonTNG), 92 pts (GD), 81 pts (TNG)

Author (ref)	Years of study	Country	Patients studied	Surgical procedure	Rate of cancer	Comment
Smith and cols., 2013	2000-2011	USA	1523 pts	n/a	238/1523 (15.6%) pts had TC (175 PTC, 39 FV-PTC, 11 FTC and 13 other malignancies)	
Smith and cols., 2013*	2002-2011	USA	164 pts	n/a	30/164 (18.3%) pts had TC	All pts underwent surgery for TNG
Dunki-Jacobs and cols., 2012	2001-2007	USA	723 pts	TT or PT	194/723 (27%) pts had TC (PTC or microPTC)	In 137/194 (70.6%) pts, tumours were suspected preoperatively
Bradly and cols., 2009	Jan 2000 - May 2008	USA	678 pts	TT or PT	81/678 (12%) pts had PTC	
Lokey and cols., 2005*	Dec 1998 -Dec 2003	USA	738 pts	n/a	28/738 (3.8%) pts had TC (mainly microPTC)	

pts: patients; TT: total thyroidectomy; PT: partial thyroidectomy; TC: thyroid carcinoma; PTC: papillary thyroid carcinoma; FV-PTC: follicular variant of papillary thyroid carcinoma; FTC: follicular thyroid carcinoma; MTC: medullary thyroid carcinoma; ATC: anaplastic thyroid carcinoma; MNG: multinodular goiter; UNG: uninodular goiter; TNG: toxic nodular goiter; GD, Graves' disease; PD, Plummer's disease; HT, Hashimoto's thyroiditis; EG, euthyroid goiter; EMNG, euthyroid multinodular goiter; HMNG, hyperthyroid multinodular goiter, FNAC: fine-needle aspiration cytology; n/a: not available.

* Tabulated data taken from the abstracts written in English and/or illustrative material.

DISCUSSION

The increased incidence of thyroid carcinoma seems to be related to an improved diagnostic approach, given by a widespread use of US and cytology, but also by the employment of new imaging techniques, such as ^{18}F-fluoro-deoxyglucose positron emission tomogram/computed tomography (^{18}F-FDG-PET/CT) (69-71). Among patients who performed neck US for suspected parathyroid disease, incidental thyroid nodules were found in 46% of them (72). Similarly, thyroid incidentalomas discovered during CT or magnetic resonance imaging that had been carried out for other reasons have been reported with an incidence of 16% (73,74); moreover, 9% to 13% were discovered during carotid US (75,76), and 2% to 3% at ^{18}F-FDG-PET/CT scan (77-79). The prevalence of incidental thyroid nodules on US in the general population ranges between 42% and 67% (80,81). In thyroidectomy specimens, ITC prevalence ranges up to 40% (2). In autopsy studies, the reported prevalence of ITC ranges from 0.01% in USA to 35.6% in Finland (7).

The overview of the literature (Table 3, refs. 23-68), has shown that one-third (n = 16) of the studies are on cohorts of thyroidectomized patients smaller than ours (n = 50 to 191, compared to 207), and one-seventh of the studies (n = 7) are on cohorts slightly greater than ours (256 to 8,132). Prevalence of ITC at surgery ranges between 2% and 40% (1,2,17,23-68). In Europe, the frequency of ITC varies from 2.2% to 27.4%, and a similar wide range (3.3% to 33%) is observed in the United States. Interestingly, in Eastern Europe (Romania, Czech Republic, Ukraine, Poland), the frequency of thyroid cancer is relatively low (range 5-9.2%). In Turkey, excluding the study from Tasova and cols. (46), there is a lower variation range in the reported incidence of thyroid cancer (7-10%).

One comment deserves the coexistence of ITCs with HT. We found a 33% rate of ITCs (always microPTCs) in patients with histologically confirmed HT. This rate is greater than that reported in one recent retrospective study from Serbia (37). Slijepcevic and cols. (37) also investigated the prevalence of microPTC in patients operated for benign thyroid diseases in a retrospective study of 2,466 patients who underwent thyroid surgery from 2008 to 2013. The overall prevalence of microPTC was 16.3%, the highest being in HT. Smith and cols. (63) examined cancer frequency in patients referred for removal of benign thyroid disease in a multi-institutional series of 2,551 patients. Indeterminate/malignant FNA diagnoses were excluded (n = 1,028). Overall, 238 (15.6%) cancers were found, and 275 patients had thyroiditis (18%). Presence of thyroiditis was not associated with cancer, because there were 47 ITCs in the 275 patients compared with 191 ITCs in 1,247 patients without thyroiditis (17.1% vs 15.3%). Our rate of 33.3% was highly significant as well as the 22.7% (χ^2 = 10.80, P < 0.001) of Slijepcevic and cols. (37), whereas the rate of 17.1% (χ^2 = 0.388, P = 0.533) reported by Smith and cols. did not reach statistical significance.

The limitations of this study are due to its retrospective nature. Another limitation is the natural history of thyroid cancer, which is a slow growing tumor, so that extended follow-up is needed to evaluate the long-term outcomes. The strength of the study lies in its short course, avoiding that a variable number of pathologists histologically examined the specimens using different methods of evaluation.

Our 12.1% rate is comparable to rates from other European countries, including Belgium, Italy (25,30,33) and Greece (17). Because Italy and Greece have no nuclear plants, we tend to exclude that our rate was influenced by the relative vicinity of our medical center and residence of patients to three nuclear plant units (82). A systematic review and meta-analysis on this issue does not support an association between living near nuclear power plants and risk of thyroid cancer. However, sensitivity analysis by exposure definition demonstrated that living less than 20 km from nuclear power plants was associated with a significant increase in the risk of thyroid cancer (83). Additionally, with a 12% risk that MNG harbors preoperatively unsuspected PTCs which can have already infiltrated the capsule and that are accompanied frequently by other PTC foci contralaterally, an adequate surgical approach has to be considered.

The operative management of benign thyroid diseases includes partial and total thyroidectomy: the first one preserves thyroid function, sparing patients the need for lifelong thyroid hormone replacement (84); moreover, microPTCs can have an excellent prognosis not requiring completion thyroidectomy. On the other hand, total thyroidectomy may present complications, such as hypoparathyroidism (often transient) (85) and recurrent laryngeal nerve injury (84), which occurs in 6% and 1% of patients, respectively (84). However, reoperation after partial thyroidectomy can be needed in cases with multifocal thyroid cancer or for radioactive iodine ablation.

In our experience, total thyroidectomy showed neither mortality nor transient and permanent nerve injuries, avoiding the risk of recurrence and necessity of completion thyroidectomy, with its known technical difficulties and increased risk of complications, and also avoiding the risk of ITC presence in remnant tissue.

REFERENCES

1. Bahl M, Sosa JA, Nelson RC, Esclamado RM, Choudhury KR, Hoang JK. Trends in incidentally identified thyroid cancers over a decade: a retrospective analysis of 2,090 surgical patients. World J Surg. 2014; 38:1312-17.

2. Siassakos D, Gourgiottis S, Moustafellos P, Dimopoulos N, Hadjiyannakis E. Thyroid microcarcinoma during thyroidectomy. Singapore Med J. 2008;49:23-5.

3. Trimboli P, Ulisse S, Graziano FM, Marzullo A, Ruggieri M, Calvanese A, et al. Trend in thyroid carcinoma size, age at diagnosis, and histology in a retrospective study of 500 cases diagnosed over 20 years. Thyroid. 2006;16:1151-5.

4. Ahn HS, Welch HG. South Korea's Thyroid-Cancer "Epidemic"--Turning the Tide. N Engl J Med. 2015;373:2389-90.

5. Lin JD, Chao TC, Weng HF, Huang HS, Ho YS. Clinical presentations and treatment for 74 occult thyroid carcinoma. Comparison with nonoccult thyroid carcinoma in Taiwan. Am J Clin Oncol. 1996;19:504-8.

6. Ahmed SR, Ball DW. Clinical review: incidentally discovered medullary thyroid cancer: diagnostic strategies and treatment. J Clin Endocrinol Metab. 2011;96:1237-45.

7. Boucek J, Kastner J, Skrivan J, Grosso E, Gibelli B, Giugliano G, et al. Occult thyroid carcinoma. Acta Otorhinolaryngol Ital. 2009;29:296-304.

8. Liu H, Lv L, Yang K. Occult thyroid carcinoma: a rare case report and review of literature. Int J Clin Exp Pathol. 2014;7:5210-4.

9. Saint Marc O, Cogliandolo A, Piquard A, Famà F, Pidoto RR. LigaSure vs clamp-and-tie technique to achieve hemostasis in total thyroidectomy for benign multinodular goiter: a prospective randomized study. Arch Surg. 2007;142:150-6.

10. Lasithiotakis K, Grisbolaki E, Koutsomanolis D, Venianaki M, Petrakis I, Vrachassotakis N, et al. Indications for surgery and significance of unrecognized cancer in endemic multinodular goiter. World J Surg. 2012;36:1286-92.

11. Ito Y, Higashiyama T, Takamura Y, Miya A, Kobayashi K, Matsuzuka F, et al. Prognosis of patients with benign thyroid diseases accompanied by incidental papillary carcinoma undetectable on preoperative imaging tests. World J Surg. 2007;31:1672-6.

12. Lin J, Kuo S, Chao T, Hsueh C. Incidental and nonincidental papillary thyroid microcarcinoma. Ann Surg Oncol. 2008;15:2287-92.

13. Mangano JJ. Geographic variation in U.S. thyroid cancer incidence and a cluster near nuclear reactors in New Jersey, New York, and Pennsylvania. Int J Health Serv. 2009;39:643-61.

14. Davies L. Welch H. Increasing incidence of thyroid cancer in the United States, 1973-2002. JAMA. 2006;295:2164-7.

15. Rizzo M, Sindoni A, Talamo Rossi R, Bonaffini O, Panetta S, Scisca C, et al. Annual increase in the frequency of papillary thyroid carcinoma as diagnosed by fine-needle aspiration at a cytology unit in Sicily. Hormones (Athens). 2013;12:46-57.

16. Mazzaferri EL. Managing thyroid microcarcinomas. Yonsei Med J. 2012;53:1-14.

17. Vasileiadis I, Karatzas T, Vasileiadis D, Kapetanakis S, Charitoudis G, Karakostas E, et al. Clinical and pathological characteristics of incidental and nonincidental papillary thyroid microcarcinoma in 339 patients. Head Neck. 2014;36:564-70.

18. Brito JP, Al Nofal A, Montori VM, Hay ID, Morris JC. The Impact of Subclinical Disease and Mechanism of Detection on the Rise in Thyroid Cancer Incidence: A Population-Based Study in Olmsted County, Minnesota During 1935 Through 2012. Thyroid. 2015;25:999-1007.

19. Haugen BR, Alexander EK, Bible KC, Doherty GM, Mandel SJ, Nikiforov YE, et al. 2015 American Thyroid Association Management Guidelines for Adult Patients with Thyroid Nodules and Differen-

tiated Thyroid Cancer: The American Thyroid Association Guidelines Task Force on Thyroid Nodules and Differentiated Thyroid Cancer. Thyroid. 2016;26:1-133.

20. Francis GL, Waguespack SG, Bauer AJ, Angelos P, Benvenga S, Cerutti JM, et al.; American Thyroid Association Guidelines Task Force. Management Guidelines for Children with Thyroid Nodules and Differentiated Thyroid Cancer. Thyroid. 2015;25:716-59.

21. Aschebrook-Kilfoy B, Schechter RB, Shih YC, Kaplan EL, Chiu BC, Angelos P, et al. The clinical and economic burden of a sustained increase in thyroid cancer incidence. Cancer Epidemiol Biomarkers Prev. 2013;22:1252-9.

22. Valeix P, Zarebska M, Preziosi P, Galan P, Pelletier B, Hercberg S. Iodine deficiency in France. Lancet. 1999;353:1766-7.

23. Daumerie C, Ayoubi S, Rahier J, Buysschaert M, Squifflet JP. Prevalence of thyroid cancer in hot nodules. Ann Chir. 1998;52:444-8.

24. Dănilă R, Karakas E, Osei-Agyemang T, Hassan I. Outcome of incidental thyroid carcinoma in patients undergoing surgery for Graves' disease. Rev Med Chir Soc Med Nat Iasi. 2008;112:115-8.

25. Pezzolla A, Marzaioli R, Lattarulo S, Docimo G, Conzo G, Ciampolillo A, et al. Incidental carcinoma of the thyroid. Int J Surg. 2014;12 Suppl 1:S98-102.

26. Pezzolla A, Lattarulo S, Milella M, Barile G, Pascazio B, Ciampolillo A, et al. Incidental carcinoma in thyroid pathology: our experience and review of the literature. Ann Ital Chir. 2010;81:165-9.

27. Costamagna D, Pagano L, Caputo M, Leutner M, Mercalli F, Alonzo A. Incidental cancer in patients surgically treated for benign thyroid disease. Our experience at a single institution. G Chir. 2013;34:21-6.

28. Negro R, Piana S, Ferrari M, Ragazzi M, Gardini G, Asioli S, et al. Assessing the risk of false-negative fine-needle aspiration cytology and of incidental cancer in nodular goiter. Endocr Pract. 2013;19:444-50.

29. Botrugno I, Lovisetto F, Cobianchi L, Zonta S, Klersy C, Vailati A, et al. Incidental carcinoma in multinodular goiter: risk factors. Am Surg. 2011; 77:1553-8.

30. Gelmini R, Franzoni C, Pavesi E, Cabry F, Saviano M. Incidental thyroid carcinoma (ITC): a retrospective study in a series of 737 patients treated for benign disease. Ann Ital Chir. 2010;81:421-7.

31. Pisello F, Geraci G, Sciumè C, Li Volsi F, Modica G. Total thyroidectomy of choice in papillary microcarcinoma. G Chir. 2007;28:13-9.

32. Carlini M, Giovannini C, Mercadante E, Castaldi F, Dell'Avanzato R, Zazza S. Incidental thyroid microcarcinoma in benign thyroid disease. Incidence in a total of 100 consecutive thyroidectomies. Chir Ital. 2006;58:441-7.

33. Miccoli P, Minuto MN, Galleri D, D'Agostino J, Basolo F, Antonangeli L, et al. Incidental thyroid carcinoma in a large series of consecutive patients operated on for benign thyroid disease. ANZ J Surg. 2006;76:123-6.

34. Carlini M, Giovannini C, Castaldi F, Mercadante E, Dell'Avanzato R, Zazza S, et al. High risk for microcarcinoma in thyroid benign diseases. Incidence in a one year period of total thyroidectomies. J Exp Clin Cancer Res. 2005;24:231-6.

35. Pingitore R, Vignati S, Bigini D, Ciancia EM. Post-operative examination of 2930 thyroid glands: observations on primary carcinoma. Incidental carcinoma and the preoperative diagnostic assessment of thyroidectomy for cancer. Pathologica. 1993;85:591-605.

36. Pascual Corrales E, Príncipe RM, Laguna Muro S, Martínez Regueira F, Alcalde Navarrete JM, Guillén Grima F, et al. Incidental differentiated thyroid carcinoma is less prevalent in Graves' disease than in multinodular goiter. Endocrinol Nutr. 2012;59:169-73.

37. Slijepcevic N, Zivaljevic V, Marinkovic J, Sipetic S, Diklic A, Paunovic I. Retrospective evaluation of the incidental finding of 403 papillary thyroid microcarcinomas in 2466 patients undergoing thyroid surgery for presumed benign thyroid disease. BMC Cancer. 2015;15:330.

38. Zivaljević VR, Diklić AD, Krgović KLj, Zorić GV, Zivić RV, Kalezić NK, et al. The incidence rate of thyroid microcarcinoma during surgery benign disease. Acta Chir Iugosl. 2008;55:69-73.

39. Alecu L, Alecu L, Bărbulescu M, Ursuţ B, Enciu O, Slavu I, et al. Occult thyroid carcinoma in our experience – should we reconsider total thyroidectomy for benign thyroid pathology? Chirurgia (Bucur). 2014 ;109:191-7.

40. Muntean V, Domsa I, Zolog A, Piciu D, Fabian O, Bosu R, et al. Incidental papillary thyroid microcarcinoma: is completion surgery required? Chirurgia (Bucur). 2013;108:490-7.

41. Lukás J, Paska J, Hintnausová B, Lukás D, Syrůcek M, Sýkorová P. The occurrence of microcarcinomas in the patients after thyroidectomy--retrospective analysis. Cas Lek Cesk. 2010;149:378-80.

42. Nechaĭ OP, Larin OS, Cheren'ko SM, Sheptukha SA, Smoliar VA, Zolotar'ov PO. "Incidental" thyroid carcinoma among patients in surgical treatment for nontumors thyroid desease. Klin Khir. 2012;7:9-11.

43. Barczyński M, Konturek A, Stopa M, Cichoń S, Richter P, Nowak W. Total thyroidectomy for benign thyroid disease: is it really worthwhile? Ann Surg. 2011;254:724-9.

44. Sakorafas GH, Stafyla V, Kolettis T, Tolumis G, Kassaras G, Peros G. Microscopic papillary thyroid cancer as an incidental finding in patients treated surgically for presumably benign thyroid disease. J Postgrad Med. 2007;53:23-6.

45. Yazici P, Mihmanli M, Bozdag E, Aygun N, Uludag M. Incidental Finding of Papillary Thyroid Carcinoma in the Patients with Primary Hyperparathyroidism. Eurasian J Med. 2015;47:194-8.

46. Tasova V, Kilicoglu B, Tuncal S, Uysal E, Sabuncuoglu MZ, Tanrikulu Y, et al. Evaluation of incidental thyroid cancer in patients with thyroidectomy. West Indian Med J. 2013;62:844-8.

47. Karakoyun R, Bülbüller N, Koçak S, Habibi M, Gündüz U, Erol B, et al. What do we leave behind after neartotal and subtotal thyroidectomy: just the tissue or the disease? Int J Clin Exp Med. 2013;6:922-9.

48. Berker D, Isik S, Ozuguz U, Tutuncu YA, Kucukler K, Akbaba G, et al. Prevalence of incidental thyroid cancer and its ultrasonographic features in subcentimeter thyroid nodules of patients with hyperthyroidism. Endocrine. 2011;39:13-20.

49. Tezelman S, Borucu I, Senyurek Giles Y, Tunca F, Terzioglu T. The change in surgical practice from subtotal to near-total or total thyroidectomy in the treatment of patients with benign multinodular goiter. World J Surg. 2009;33:400-5.

50. Giles Y, Boztepe H, Terzioglu T, Tezelman S. The advantage of total thyroidectomy to avoid reoperation for incidental thyroid cancer in multinodular goiter. Arch Surg. 2004;139:179-82.

51. Fernando R, Mettananda DS, Kariyakarawana L. Incidental occult carcinomas in total thyroidectomy for benign diseases of the thyroid. Ceylon Med J. 2009;54:4-6.

52. John AM, Jacob PM, Oommen R, Nair S, Nair A, Rajaratnam S. Our experience with papillary thyroid microcancer. Indian J Endocrinol Metab. 2014;18:410-3.

53. Wu Y. Occult carcinoma of the thyroid. Zhonghua Wai Ke Za Zhi. 1993;31:609-11.

54. Koh KB, Chang KW. Carcinoma in multinodular goitre. Br J Surg. 1992;79:266-7.

55. Preece J, Grodski S, Yeung M, Bailey M, Serpell J. Thyrotoxicosis does not protect against incidental papillary thyroid cancer. Surgery. 2014;156:1153-6.

56. Bron LP, O'Brien CJ. Total thyroidectomy for clinically benign disease of the thyroid gland. Br J Surg. 2004;91:569-74.

57. Bhuiyan MM, Machowski A. Nodular thyroid disease and thyroid malignancy: Experience at Polokwane Mankweng Hospital Complex, Limpopo Province, South Africa. S Afr Med J. 2015;105:570-2.

58. Bombil I, Bentley A, Kruger D, Luvhengo TE. Incidental cancer in multinodular goitre post thyroidectomy. S Afr J Surg. 2014;52:5-9.

59. Edino ST, Mohammed AZ, Ochicha O, Malami SA, Yakubu AA. Thyroid cancers in nodular goiters in Kano, Nigeria. Niger J Clin Pract. 2010;13:298-300.

60. Choong KC, McHenry CR. Thyroid cancer in patients with toxic nodular goiter--is the incidence increasing? Am J Surg. 2015;209:974-6.

61. Ergin AB, Saralaya S, Olansky L. Incidental papillary thyroid carcinoma: clinical characteristics and prognostic factors among patients with Graves' disease and euthyroid goiter, Cleveland Clinic experience. Am J Otolaryngol. 2014;35:784-90.

62. Phitayakorn R, Morales-Garcia D, Wanderer J, Lubitz CC, Gaz RD, Stephen AE, et al. Surgery for Graves' disease: a 25-year perspective. Am J Surg. 2013;206:669-73.

63. Smith JJ, Chen X, Schneider DF, Broome JT, Sippel RS, Chen H, et al. Cancer after thyroidectomy: a multi-institutional experience with 1,523 patients. J Am Coll Surg. 2013;216:571-7.

64. Smith JJ, Chen X, Schneider DF, Nookala R, Broome JT, Sippel RS, et al. Toxic nodular goiter and cancer: a compelling case for thyroidectomy. Ann Surg Oncol. 2013;20:1336-40.

65. Dunki-Jacobs E, Grannan K, McDonough S, Engel AM. Clinically unsuspected papillary microcarcinomas of the thyroid: a common finding with favourable biology? Am J Surg. 2012;203:140-4.

66. Bradly DP, Reddy V, Prinz RA, Gattuso P. Incidental papillary carcinoma in patients treated surgically for benign thyroid diseases. Surgery. 2009;146:1099-104.

67. Phitayakorn R, McHenry CR. Incidental thyroid carcinoma in patients with Graves' disease. Am J Surg. 2008;195:292-7.

68. Lokey JS, Palmer RM, Macfie JA. Unexpected findings during thyroid surgery in a regional community hospital: a 5-year experience of 738 consecutive cases. Am Surg. 2005;71:911-3.

69. Roti E, Rossi R, Trasforini G, Bertelli F, Ambrosio MR, Busutti L, et al. Clinical and histological characteristics of papillary thyroid microcarcinoma: results of a retrospective study in 243 patients. J Clin Endocrinol Metab. 2006;91:2171-8.

70. Besic N, Zgajnar J, Hocevar M, Petric R. Extent of thyroidectomy and lymphadenectomy in 254 patients with papillary thyroid microcarcinoma: a single-institution experience. Ann Surg Oncol. 2009;16:920-8.

71. Bae JS, Chae BJ, Park WC, Kim JS, Kim SH, Jung SS, et al. Incidental thyroid lesions detected by FDG-PET/CT: prevalence and risk of thyroid cancer. World J Surg Oncol. 2009;7:63.

72. Horlocker TT, Hay JE, James EM. Prevalence of incidental nodular thyroid disease detected during high-resolution parathyroid ultrasonography. In: G. Medeiros-Neto, E. Gaitan, editors. Fron-tiers in Thyroidology, Vol 2. New York: Plenum Medical; 1985. p. 1309-12.

73. Shetty SK, Maher MM, Hahn PF, Halpern EF, Aquino SL. Significance of incidental thyroid lesions detected on CT: correlation among CT, sonography, and pathology. AJR Am J Roentgenol. 2006;187:1349-56.

74. Youserm DM, Huang T, Loevner LA, Langlotz CP. Clinical and economic impact of incidental thyroid lesions found with CT and MR. AJNR Am J Neuroradiol. 1997;18:1423-8.

75. Steele SR, Martin MJ, Mullenix PS, Azarow KS, Andersen CA. The significance of incidental thyroid abnormalities identified during carotid duplex ultrasonography. Arch Surg. 2005;140:981-5.

76. Carroll BA. Asymptomatic thyroid nodules: incidental sonographic detection. AJR Am J Roentgenol . 1982;138:499-501.

77. Cohen MS, Arslan N, Dehdashti F, Doherty GM, Lairmore TC, Brunt LM, et al. Risk of malignancy in thyroid incidentalomas identified by fluorodeoxyglucose-positron emission tomography. Surgery. 2001;130:941-6.

78. Are C, Hsu JF, Schoder H, Shah JP, Larson SM, Shaha AR. FDG-PET detected thyroid incidentalomas: need for further investigation? Ann Surg Oncol. 2007;14:239-47.

79. Kim TY, Kim WB, Ryu JS, Gong G, Hong SJ, Shong YK. 18F-fluoro-deoxyglucose uptake in thyroid from positron emission tomogram (PET) for evaluation in cancer patients: high prevalence of malignancy in thyroid PET incidentaloma. Laryngoscope. 2005;115:1074-8.

80. Brander A, Viikinkowski P, Nickels J, Kivisaari L. Thyroid gland: US screening in a random adult population. Radiology. 1991;181:683-7.

81. Ezzat S, Sarti DA, Cain DR, Braunstein GD. Thyroid incidentalomas. Prevalence by palpation and ultrasonography. Ann Intern Med. 1994;154:1838-40.

82. Fama' F, Cicciu' M, Lo Giudice G, Sindoni A, Palella J, Piquard A, et al. Pattern of nodal involvement in papillary thyroid cancer: a challenge of quantitative analysis. Int J Clin Exp Pathol. 2015;8:11629-34.

83. Kim J, Bang Y, Lee WJ. Living near nuclear power plants and thyroid cancer risk: A systematic review and meta-analysis. Environ Int. 2016;87:42-8.

84. Pearce EN, Braverman LE. Papillary thyroid microcarcinoma outcomes and implications for treatment. J Clin Endocrinol Metab. 2004;89:3710-2.

85. Famà F, Cicciù M, Polito F, Cascio A, Gioffré-Florio M, Piquard A, et al. Parathyroid Autotransplantation During Thyroid Surgery: A Novel Technique Using a Cell Culture Nutrient Solution. World J Surg. 2016. In press.

4

Progranulin concentration in relation to bone mineral density among obese individuals

Alireza Milajerdi[1,2], Zhila Maghbooli[1], Farzad Mohammadi[2],
Banafsheh Hosseini[2], Khadijeh Mirzaei[2]

ABSTRACT

Objective: Adipose tissue, particularly visceral adipose tissue, secretes a variety of cytokines, among which progranulin is a glycoprotein related to the immune system. Along with other secreted proteins, progranulin may be associated with bone mineral density. The aim of this study was to find out whether there are associations between the progranulin and bone mineral density among obese people. Subjects and methods: This cross-sectional study was conducted on 244 obese participants (aged 22-52). Serum progranulin, high sensitive C-reactive protein, oxidised-low dencity lipoprotein, tumor necrosis factor-α, parathormone, vitamin D, and interleukins of 1 β, 4, 6, 10, 13, and 17 concentrations were measured. Anthropometric measurements, body composition and bone mineral density were also assessed. Results: Serum progranulin was directly associated with interleukin-6 and interleukin-1β, while it had a negative association with interleukin-17 and tumor necrosis factor-α. We also observed a statistically significant direct association between progranulin concentration and visceral fat, abdominal fat, waist, abdominal and hip circumferences, hip T-score, and Z-score and T-score for the lumbar region. A partial correlation test has also shown a significant positive correlation regarding serum progranulin and the hip Z-score. Moreover, progranulin level is inversely associated with ospteopenia (P = 0.04 and CI: 0.17,0.96). Conclusion: Our study revealed that central obesity may be related to increased progranulin concentration. In addition, progranulin concentration was directly related to bone formation parameters, which indicates the protective effects of progranulin on bone density. Further studies are needed to clarify the exact mechanisms underlying these associations. Arch Endocrinol Metab. 2018;62(2):179-86

Keywords
Bone mineral density; progranulin; obesity; osteopenia; cytokine

[1] Endocrinology and Metabolism Clinical Sciences Institute, Tehran University of Medical Sciences, Tehran, Iran
[2] Department of Community Nutrition, School of Nutritional Sciences and Dietetics, Tehran University of Medical Sciences (TUMS), Tehran, Iran

Correspondence to:
Khadijeh Mirzaei
Department of Community Nutrition, School of Nutritional Sciences and Dietetics, Tehran University of Medical Sciences (TUMS), Tehran, Iran
P.O. Box: 14155-6117 – Tehran, Iran
mirzaei_kh@tums.ac.ir

INTRODUCTION

Compelling evidence indicates that obesity is associated with inflammation and immune system function (1,2). Due to the function of adipose tissue as an endocrine gland which secretes several cytokines, this association has frequently been attributed to central obesity (3). Indeed, some studies have regarded inflammation as a risk factor for osteoporosis (4,5). However, the precise mechanism underlying the role of inflammation as well as the association between obesity, inflammation and osteoporosis has not yet been clarified. Some data suggest that cytokines secreted from adipose tissue may play a major role in osteoporosis (6). Osteoporosis is considered as one of the most serious chronic diseases in the present century (7). According to the international definition, osteoporosis defined as a 2.5 Standard Deviation (SD) reduction in Bone Mineral Density (BMD) (8,9).

Progranulin (PGRN) is a cytokine that is secreted from adipose tissue, and also, is a secretory 593-amino acid glycoprotein with a widespread expression in different cells, such as immune system cells (10). PGRN is also regarded as a growth factor, similar to IGF-1, with inflammatory properties (11). There are some studies that suggested PGRN concentration is associated with the extent of visceral adiposity (12,13). It seems that PGRN can activate some inflammatory pathways (14) and, as mentioned, this can affect BMD (15) and facilitate the development of osteoporosis. Furthermore, a recent study by Romanello and cols. has suggested a proliferative and pro-survival effect of PGRN on osteocyte-like cells. The research demonstrated that PGRN can induce phosphorylation of mitogen-activated protein kinase in both HOBIT and osteocytic cells. Moreover, the authors reported that Risedronate, a bisphosphonate drug which has been widely used in the treatment of osteoporosis, induces the expression as well as the secretion of PRGN in the HOBIT secretome. These findings suggested the possible role of PGRN in osteoblast/osteocyte biology (16).

The aim of this study was to find out whether there are associations between progranulin and bone mineral density among obese people.

MATERIALS AND METHODS

Study population

In this cross sectional study, 244 class I and II obese ($30 \leq$ BMI < 40 kg/m^2) participants (22 to 52 years old) were recruited from Shariati hospital. The study protocol was approved by the ethics committee of the Endocrinology and Metabolism Research Center of Tehran University of Medical Sciences (TUMS) with the following identification: 90-03-27-14619. The inclusion criteria namely were having a BMI in the range of 30-39.99kg/m^2, and being aged from 22-52. Exclusion criteria were defined as having any history of inflammatory conditions or inflammatory diseases, cardiovascular disease, diabetes mellitus, thyroid diseases, cancer or malignancies, hypertension or hypotensive drug abuse, hepatic, heart, or renal disease, chronic or acute infections, smoking, drug or alcohol abuse, and pregnancy. Each participant was completely informed regarding the study protocol and provided a written and informed consent form before taking part in the study.

Laboratory measurements

All blood samples were collected from 8:00 to 10:00 a.m. after an 8-12 hours fast at the EMRC laboratory in Shariati hospital of TUMS. To collect serums, blood samples were centrifuged for 10 minutes at 3000 rpm. Serum samples were aliquoted and stored at -80°C until they were analyzed. Serum high sensitive C-reactive protein (hsCRP), as a sensitive marker of inflammation, was measured by an imonoturbidimetric assay (Randox laboratories kit, Hitachi 902). Serum concentrations of adipokines (including interleukins of 1 β, 4, 6, 10, 13, and 17) were measured in triplicate and 10 replicates per EIA plate under internal quality controls. Serum concentration of interleukin 6 (IL-6) was analyzed by EIA kit (Enzo Life Sciences, Inc. Sensitivity: 3.75 pg/mL; inter-assay variability: 3.7%; intra-assay variability: 3.9%). Serum concentration of interlukin 4 (IL-4) was also assessed by EIA kit (Enzo Life Sciences, Inc. Sensitivity: < 2 pg/mL; in intra CV was 4.3% and interCV was 4.7%). TNF-α concentration was determined by EIA kit (Enzo Life Sciences, Inc. Sensitivity: 8.43 pg/mL;

inter-assay variability: 6%; intra-assay variability: 3.6%). Serum PGRN concentration was measured by ELISA kit (AdipoGen; Seoul, South Korea. Sensitivity: 32 pg/mL; inter-assay variability: 4.7%; intra-assay variability: 3.79%) under internal quality controls (17).

Anthropometric measurement

Weights and heights were measured with participants wearing light clothes and without shoes. Weight was measured using a digital scale (Sega 707, Hamburg, Germany) to the nearest 0.1 kg. Height was measured using a stadiometer (Seca, Hamburg, Germany) to the nearest 0.1 cm. Body mass index (BMI) was calculated using the "weight(kg)/height^2(m^2)" equation. Waist circumference (WC) was measured in the middle point of the iliac crest and ribcage.

Body composition analysis

Participant body composition was assessed by *Body Composition Analyzer BC-418MA – Tanita (United Kingdom)*. This Bioelectrical Impedance Analyzer (BIA) sends out a very weak electric current across the body to measure its electrical resistance. Before assessing body composition, the manufacturer's instructions were followed to ensure accurate assessment. Participants were asked not to exercise vigorously, put aside any electrical device (mobile phone, etc.), or to intake excessive fluid or food. As changes in body-water distribution and body temperature can have a major impact on measurements, they were performed in the morning in a fasting condition (always urinating before taking measurements, etc.) to get a more accurate measurement every single time. To prevent inaccurately low body fat percentage measurements and other measurement errors, both arms were always held straight down when taking measurements. The device calculates the body fat percentage, fat mass and fat-free mass, and predicts the muscle mass on the basis of data obtained by dual-energy X-ray absorptiometry using bioelectrical impedance analysis (18).

BMD measurement

In this study, BMD was measured by the Dual Energy X-ray Absorptiometery (DEXA) method at the hip and lumbar spine (vertebra L2-L4). The average coefficient of variation (CV) for measuring BMD in our device was 1.04%. According to the World Health Organization (WHO) standard, normal bone mass was defined as

BMD ≥ -1 standard deviation (SD), osteopenia as -1 < BMD <-2.5 SD, and osteoporosis as BMD ≤ -2.5 SD. Osteoporosis was diagnosised based on the T-score (19).

Statistical analysis

The study population was divided into two groups based on median PGRN concentration (< 113.30 and ≥ 113.30 pg/mL), then the study variables were compared among the two groups using an independent T-test. The association between serum PGRN concentration and BMD measurements was examined through a partial correlation test after adjusting for weight and fat mass. The level of statistical significance was set to < 0.05 All statistical analysis was performed using SPSS version 16.0 (Chicago, IL).

RESULTS

The particpants' mean (±SD) of age, height, BMI, and weight were 39.12 ± 11.90 years, 162.42 ± 8.80 cm, 35.32 ± 3.98 kg/m², and 93.68 ± 14.75 kg, respectively. The mentioned variables were 37.10 ± 12.77 years, 176.44 ± 6.89 cm, 35.30 ± 3.49 kg/m², and 108.42 ± 15.74 kg respectively, in men, and 39.60 ± 11.68 years, 159.87 ± 6.38 cm, 35.33 ± 4.10 kg/m², and 90.15 ± 12.14 kg, respectively in women. From 244 participants, 68 subjects (27.86%) were osteopenic and 176 individuals (72.14%) had normal BMD. The population characteristics, body composition, BMD, and laboratory measurements of participants are summarized in Table 1. As shown in the table, mean serum parathyroid hormone (PTH) and vitamin D (VitD) concentrations of participants were above and within the normal ranges respectively (10-55 pg/mL for PTH and 30-74 ng/mL for VitD). The visceral fat rating showed that central obesity may be more serious in men compared to women (Table 1). Additionally, the DEXA assay showed an osteopenic condition only in the lumbar spine (L2-L4) of women, when BMD was expressed as mean ± (SD) T-score (T-score < -1).

Association between PGRN, anthropometric measures, and body composition

Our analysis revealed that mean BMI, fat percentage, fat mass, fat free mass, visceral fat, trunk fat, waist circumference, abdominal and hip circumferences were greater in the high serum PGRN concentration group compared to the low serum PGRN concentration one

(Table 2). However, the association was statistically significant for visceral fat, trunk fat, waist, abdominal and hip circumferences (p < 0.05). We also found a higher mean of age (p = 0.17) and total body water (p = 0.28) in the high serum PGRN concentration group, which were not significant. In addition, a difference in the Central Adiposity Index (CAI) lower than 25 and above 75 centile value was seen in participants, with the following results reported: waist circumference was 95.83 cm ± 3.64 SE and 98.16 ± 1.97 in participants in

Table 1. Population characteristics, body composition, bone mineral density and laboratory measurements of the participants

Variables	Men (n = 57)	Women (n = 187)
Anthropometry:		
Age (years)	37.10 ± 12.77	39.60 ± 11.68
Weight (kg)	108.42 ± 15.74	90.15 ± 12.14
Height (21)	176.44 ± 6.89	159.87 ± 6.38
BMI (kg/cm²)	35.30 ± 3.49	35.33 ± 4.10
Fat percent (%)	30.11 ± 4.23	42.43 ± 4.75
Fat mass (kg)	32.98 ± 8.22	38.48 ± 8.21
Fat-free mass (kg)	75.41 ± 9.53	51.66 ± 6.57
Visceral fat rating (kg)	14.24 ± 4.05	9.99 ± 2.46
Trunk fat percent (%)	20.80 ± 4.67	18.75 ± 4.37
Biochemistry characteristics:		
Progranulin (pg/mL)	119.22 ± 30.13	120.86 ± 44.02
Vitamin D (ng/mL)	32.43 ± 4.50	38.28 ± 36.39
Hs-CRP (mg/L)	2.35 ± 2.32	4.75 ± 5.86
Ox-LDL (U/dL)	556.31 ± 58.85	583.02 ± 85.54
TNF-α (pg/mL)	13.68 ± 30.92	7.67 ± 14.01
PTH (pg/mL)	84.74 ± 54.19	89.89 ± 49.90
IL-1β (pg/mL)	0.01 ± 0.00	0.01 ± 0.00
IL-4 (pg/mL)	1.47 ± 0.86	1.81 ± 1.07
IL-6 (pg/mL)	30.28 ± 18.99	24.09 ± 20.66
IL-10 (pg/mL)	31.85 ± 38.65	14.12 ± 15.44
IL-13 (pg/mL)	32.35 ± 33.60	41.61 ± 30.41
IL-17 (pg/mL)	0.28 ± 0.13	0.95 ± 1.33
Bone densitometry:		
Hip BMD	1.17 ± 0.16	1.08 ± 0.16
Hip T-score	0.64 ± 1.27	0.58 ± 1.10
Hip Z-score	0.18 ± 1.03	0.22 ± 0.99
Lumbar BMD	1.24 ± 0.18	1.19 ± 0.16
Lumbar T-score	0.24 ± 1.58	-0.10 ± 1.17
Lumbar Z-score	-0.48 ± 1.45	-0.68 ± 1.13

BMI: body mass index; Hs-CRP: high sensitive C-reactive protein; TNF-α: tumor necrosis factor-α; IL: interleukin; Ox-LDL: oxidized-low density lipoprotein; PTH: parathormone; BMD: bone mineral density.

the lower than 25 and above 75 centile for progranulin value, respectively, which was not significant (P-value = 0.12). Results also highlighted values of WHR (0.86 ± 0.01 and 0.87 ± 0.01 and P-value = 0.75), visceral fat (6.30 ± 0.66 and 7.88 ± 0.41 and P-value < 0.0001) and BMI (27.85 ± 1.12 and 31.06 ± 0.65 and P-value = 0.001) in lower than 25 and above 75 centile for progranulin value, respectively.

Table 2. Anthropometric measures and body composition between groups with low and high concentrations of PGRN

Variables	Relative PGRN concentration (n = 244)		P value
	Low concentration (n = 122)	High concentration (n = 122)	
Age (years)	38.08 ± 12.86	40.16 ± 11.22	0.17
BMI (kg/cm²)	34.54 ± 3.85	35.12 ± 4.44	0.27
Fat percent (%)	40.79 ± 6.56	40.86 ± 6.32	0.93
Fat mass (kg)	36.32 ± 8.86	37.40 ± 9.00	0.34
Fat-free mass (kg)	52.50 ± 9.53	53.76 ± 8.98	0.28
Visceral fat rating (kg)	9.56 ± 2.94	10.45 ± 2.71	**0.01**
Trunk fat percent (%)	17.57 ± 5.42	19.13 ± 4.39	**0.01**
Waist circumference (21)	97.00 ± 9.99	101.56 ± 9.46	**< 0.001**
Abdominal circumference (21)	111.42 ± 8.88	116.45 ± 10.56	**< 0.001**
Hip circumference (21)	114.00 ± 7.09	118.38 ± 11.55	**< 0.001**
TBW (%)	38.42 ± 6.99	39.36 ± 6.57	0.28

BMI: body mass index; TBW: total body water.

Association between PGRN and other cytokines

According to an independent T-test, mean serum concentrations of IL-1β, IL-13, Il-10, Il-6, and Il-4 were greater in those in the high serum PGRN concentration group (Table 3), while mean serum levels of IL-17, TNF-α, and hs-CRP were lower in the high PGRN concentration group compared to the low serum PGRN concentration one. However, it should be noted that these associations were statistically significant only for IL-1β, IL-17, IL-6, and TNF-α (p < 0.05).

Association between PGRN and bone health variables

According to an independent T-test, mean hip BMD and hip T-score and Z-score, as well as T-score and Z-score for the lumbar spine (L2-L4 vertebra) were greater in the high serum PGRN concentration group (Table 4). However, it should be noted that these associations were statistically significant only for hip

T-score and Z-score and the lumbar T-score (p < 0.05) and was marginally significant considering total BMD (p = 0.05). Moreover, a partial correlation between serum PGRN concentration and BMD measurements adjusted for fat mass, indicated a significant positive correlation with hip Z-score (r = 0.35, p < 0.05). However, after factoring in weight, none of the observed correlations were significant (Table 5, part A). Additionally, a binary regression analysis was done to strengthen our findings, (as shown in Table 5, part B). After adjustment for age and BMI, the PGRN level was strongly and inversely associated with osteopenia (P = 0.04 and CI: 0.17,0.96). Figure 1 demonstrates that there was a significantly lower number of osteopenic patients in the high serum PGRN concentration group.

Table 3. Cytokine concentrations between groups with low and high concentrations of PGRN

Variables	Relative PGRN concentration (n = 244)		P value
	Low concentration (n = 122)	High concentration (n = 122)	
Hs-CRP (mg/L)	4.91 ± 4.98	4.73 ± 6.99	0.81
TNF-α (pg/mL)	10.67 ± 19.68	3.53 ± 2.09	**< 0.001**
IL-1β (pg/mL)	0.01 ± 0.00	0.02 ± 0.01	**< 0.001**
IL-4 (pg/mL)	2.02 ± 1.35	2.21 ± 0.79	0.18
IL-6 (pg/mL)	16.68 ± 11.80	28.29 ± 28.15	**< 0.001**
IL-10 (pg/mL)	12.43 ± 12.21	15.51 ± 22.45	0.18
IL-13 (pg/mL)	41.83 ± 29.24	47.01 ± 31.44	0.18
IL-17 (pg/mL)	1.31 ± 1.55	0.45 ± 0.61	**< 0.001**

Hs-CRP: high sensitive C-reactive protein; TNF-α: tumor necrosis factor-α; IL: interleukin.

Table 4. Bone mineral density measurements between groups with low and high concentrations of PGRN

Variables	Relative PGRN concentration (n = 244)		P value
	Low concentration (n = 122)	High concentration (n = 122)	
Vitamin D (ng/mL)	32.76 ± 35.92	28.69 ± 13.99	0.24
PTH (pg/mL)	92.00 ± 56.76	105.74 ± 63.04	0.09
Hip BMD	1.07 ± 0.23	1.12 ± 0.17	**0.05**
Hip T-score	0.18 ± 0.79	1.05 ± 1.50	**< 0.001**
Hip Z-score	-0.13 ± 0.89	0.68 ± 1.30	**< 0.001**
Lumbar BMD	1.15 ± 0.13	1.18 ± 0.16	0.10
Lumbar T-score	-0.41 ± 1.16	-0.08 ± 1.36	**0.04**
Lumbar Z-score	-0.85 ± 1.07	-0.61 ± 1.38	0.13

BMD: bone mineral density; PTH: parathormone.

Table 5. A: Partial correlation between PGRN concentration and bone mineral density measurements

	Adjusted for	Hip BMD	Hip T-score	Hip Z-score	Lumbar BMD	Lumbar T-score	Lumbar Z-score
Progranulin concentration (pg/mL)	Weight r	0.21	0.32	0.33	0.24	0.24	0.26
	P value	0.25	0.75	0.65	0.19	0.18	0.15
	Fat mass r	0.19	0.33	0.35	0.22	0.23	0.26
	P value	0.30	0.06	**0.04**	0.22	0.21	0.14

BMD: bone mineral density.

B: Binary regression model for analyzing the relationship between Progranulin Concentration and risk of osteopenia in obese people

PGRN	Crude model			Model 1			Model 2			Model 3		
	B ± SE	CI	P	B ± SE	CI	P	B ± SE	CI	P	B ± SE	CI	P
	-0.47 ± 0.32	0.33, 1.69	0.14	-0.52 ± 0.33	0.30, 1.30	0.11	-0.90 ± 0.99	0.17, 0.96	**0.04**	-0.81 ± 0.44	0.18, 1.07	0.07

Model 1: Adjusted for age; Model 2: Adjusted for age and BMI; Model 3: Adjusted for age, BMI and gender; PGRN: Progranulin

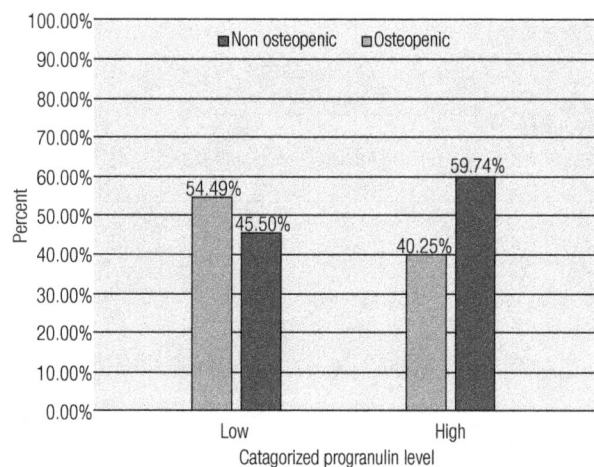

Figure 1. Variety of osteopenia by categorized progranulin level.

Additionally, we found that serum PTH was greater in the high serum PGRN concentration group (p = 0.09), while vitamin D was lower in this group, in comparision with those who had lower serum concentrations of PGRN (p = 0.24). However, none of them were statistically significant.

Meanwhile, comparing the prevalence of osteopenia among these two groups indicated that the osteopenic patients had considerably lower serum PRGN concentrations (Figure 1).

DISCUSSION

In the current study, a significant association was found between PGRN concentration and the serum levels of some cytokines, which can be explained by the regulatory roles of PGRN on signaling pathways. To illustrate this, it can be observed that serum PGRN was directly associated with the levels of serum IL-1β and Il-6, while it was inversely related to IL-17 and TNF-α serum levels. Results also showed significant associations between PGRN concentration and visceral and trunk fat. Increased hip, waist and abdominal circumferences were also observed in the higher concentration PGRN group. Furthermore, high PGRN was related to higher hip T- and Z-score and also lumbar T-score.

These findings agreed with Zhang and cols.'s study, which found a significant linear correlation between PGRN concentration and IL-6 serum levels in patients with primary Sjögren's syndrome (20). Frampton and cols. also have reported that Il-6 can activate the ERK1/2/RSK1/C/EBPβ pathway and PGRN synthesis as a consequence (21). Furthermore, several studies have shown that PGRN may antagonize TNF-α by the activation of its receptors, therefore PGRN may have some anti-inflammatory properties (22). Studies have also regarded TNF-α as an inhibitor of osteoblast differentiation, as well as an activator of osteoclastogenesis (23).

According to previous studies, IL-6 and IL-1β induce bone resorption and inhibit bone formation (24). Although it has been widely reported that IL-17 mediates diverse inflammatory processes, its effects on bone resorption has recently been documented (25). It seems that IL-17 and TNF-α synergically stimulate bone resorption (26).

This study demonstrated a significant linear association between PGRN concentration and central obesity parameters including visceral fat, abdominal fat, waist, abdominal and hip circumferences. Along the same lines as these findings, previous studies have found that the PGRN gene expresses in macrophages existing in fat tissues, especially visceral fat (12,13). Youn and cols. reported that PGRN concentration was significantly associated with central and general obesity parameters, which can be described by stimulating omental adipose tissue macrophage infiltration by PGRN (13). Pradeep and cols. measured PGRN concentrations in serum and gingival crevicular fluid of 40 patients suffering from chronic periodentitis with and without obesity. The authors reported that the serum PGRN concentration was higher in both serum and gingival crevicular fluid in obese periodentitic patients; which can indicate that inflammation related to periodentitis and obesity may also be associated with PGRN concentration (27). In agreement with these findings, Hossein-Nezhad and cols. demonstrated an association between BMI and central obesity with PGRN gene expression and circulation levels, which revealed that PGRN is related to obesity through *glucose homeostasis* and metabolism regulation (28).

Since we observed a linear association between PGRN concentration and central obesity parameters, changes in the secretion of cytokines may be attributed to adipose tissue expansion. Similarly, Zizza and cols.'s study found a negative association between IL-17 and visceral obesity (29). Furthermore, Mohamed-Ali's study showed that subcutaneous fat was associated with IL-6 but not with TNF-α (30).

Results from previous studies have indicated that visceral fat, as well as subcutaneous fat, as measured by computer tomography scan, and BMI have a negative association with bone density. More importantly, correlations regarding visceral fat and decreased bone density remained statistically significant even after adjustment for age, sex, and BMI (31). This study's findings demonstrate PGRN's effect on osteogenesis, as can be seen in the hip T-score and Z-score and T-score for the lumbar vertebra, which were significantly associated with PGRN concentration. Similarly to this study, Romanello and cols. demonstrated the proliferative and pro-survival effects of PRGN on osteocyte-like cells (16). Likewise, a recent study by Oh and cols. indicated a new regulatory axis by which PGRN may induce osteoclastogenesis. This axis is regarded as the (RANKL)/RANK axis, and PGRN may induce this pathway by stimulating PIRO expression (32). Documented results showed that recombinant

human PGRN can induce phosphorylation of mitogen-activated protein kinase in both HOBIT and osteocytic cells and induce cell proliferation and survival. Moreover, they found that Risedronate, a widely used bisphosphonate drug in the treatment of osteoporosis, can induce the expression and secretion of PGRN in the HOBIT secretome (16). These findings have shown the probable preventive effects of PGRN on osteoporosis by modulating bone loss. In addition, results from previous studies reported that PGRN growth factor enhances chondrocyte differentiation and endochondral ossification by regulating BMP-2 and TNF signaling, therefore PGRN injections may play an important role in bone healing, particularly in fracture conditions (33). A disadvantage of the present cross-sectional study is that it does not allow definite conclusions to be made regarding cause and effect. PGRN might affect BMD or vice versa.

In conclusion, the findings of this study showed that central obesity expansion is associated with increased PGRN concentration. PGRN has some paradoxical relation with the levels of cytokine secretion, in that it has a direct association with the secretion of IL-1β and IL-6, while it inhibits the secretion of IL-17 and TNF-α. According to the aforementioned mechanisms, these changes in cytokine secretion have both degenerative and protective effects on bone structure and BMD. Aditionally, the association between obesity and bone mineral density has been demonstrated by several studies, though its effects depend on the definition of obesity; if obesity is regarded as increased body fat levels, it can be considered as a risk factor for a lower BMD, which can be affected by increased adipokines, subsequently causing a lower BMD (34). However, obesity seems to play its role as a protective factor against osteoporosis if it is defined as an increase in body weight, which can be explained by a higher level of circulating estradiol, increased peak bone mass and greater gravitational load (35). The direct observed association between PGRN concentration and bone formation parameters indicates that PGRN may have some bone-protective effects through various mechanisms other than cytokine secretion regulation. Further studies are needed to address the cellular and molecular mechanisms of both general and central obesity, as well as PGRN's effects on bone formation and absorption.

Authors' contributions: study concept and design: Khadijeh Mirzaei; acquisition of data: Khadijeh Mirzaei and Alireza Milajerdi;

analysis and interpretation of data: Khadijeh Mirzaei and Alireza Milajerdi; drafting of the manuscript: Alireza Milajerdi, Banafshe Hosseini and Farzad Mohammadi; critical revision of the manuscript for important intellectual content: Khadijeh Mirzaei, Alireza Milajerdi and Farzad Mohammadi; statistical analysis: Khadijeh Mirzaei; administrative, technical, and material support: Khadijeh Mirzaei and Zhila Maghbooli; study supervision: Khadijeh Mirzaei.

Acknowledgment: we are particularly grateful to all participants in the study for their dedication and contribution to the research. This study was supported by Tehran University of Medical Sciences Grant for research (ID: 14619, 31818).

REFERENCES

1. Bastard JP, Maachi M, Lagathu C, Kim MJ, Caron M, Vidal H, et al. Recent advances in the relationship between obesity, inflammation, and insulin resistance. Eur Cytokine Netw. 2006;17(1):4-12.

2. de Heredia FP, Gómez-Martínez S, Marcos A. Obesity, inflammation and the immune system. Proc Nutr Soc. 2012;71(2):332-8.

3. Panagiotakos DB, Pitsavos C, Yannakoulia M, Chrysohoou C, Stefanadis C. The implication of obesity and central fat on markers of chronic inflammation: The ATTICA study. Atherosclerosis. 2005 Dec;183(2):308-15.

4. Al-Daghri NM, Yakout S, Al-Shehri E, Al-Fawaz HA, Aljohani N, Al-Saleh Y. Inflammatory and bone turnover markers in relation to PTH and vitamin D status among saudi postmenopausal women with and without osteoporosis. Int J Clin Exp Med. 2014;7(10):3528-35.

5. Zhang J, Fu Q, Ren Z, Wang Y, Wang C, Shen T, et al. Changes of serum cytokines-related Th1/Th2/Th17 concentration in patients with postmenopausal osteoporosis. Gynecol Endocrinol. 2015;31(3):183-90.

6. Gonnelli S, Caffarelli C, Nuti R. Obesity and fracture risk. Clin Cases Miner Bone Metab. 2014;11(1):9-14.

7. Kehler T. Epidemiology of osteoporosis and osteoporotic fractures. Reumatizam. 2014;61(2):60-4.

8. World Health Organization. Assessment of Fracture Risk and Its Application to Screening for Postmenopausal Osteoporosis. Technical Report Series 843. Geneva: WHO, 1994.

9. Mahan L, Escott-Stump S, Raymond JL, Krause MV. Krause's Food & the Nutrition Care Process, (Krause's Food & Nutrition Therapy). Philadelphia: WB Saunders. Elsevier; 2012.

10. Luo L, Lü L, Lu Y, Zhang L, Li B, Guo K, et al. Effects of hypoxia on progranulin expression in HT22 mouse hippocampal cells. Mol Med Rep. 2014;9(5):1675-80.

11. Wei Z, Huang Y, Xie N, Ma Q. Elevated expression of secreted autocrine growth factor progranulin increases cervical cancer growth. Cell Biochem Biophys. 2015;71(1):189-93.

12. Tanaka Y, Takahashi T, Tamori Y. Circulating progranulin level is associated with visceral fat and elevated liver enzymes: significance of serum progranulin as a useful marker for liver dysfunction. Endocr J. 2014;61(12):1191-6.

13. Youn BS, Bang SI, Klöting N, Park JW, Lee N, Oh JE, et al. Serum progranulin concentrations may be associated with macrophage infiltration into omental adipose tissue. Diabetes. 2009;58(3):627-36.

14. Ong CHP, Zhiheng H, Kriazhev L, Shan X, Palfree RGE, Bateman A. Regulation of progranulin expression in myeloid cells. Am J Physiol Regul Integr Comp Physiol. 2006;291(6): R1602-R12.

15. Katsuyama E, Miyamoto H, Kobayashi T, Sato Y, Hao W, Kanagawa H, et al. Interleukin-1 receptor-associated kinase-4 (IRAK4) promotes inflammatory osteolysis by activating osteoclasts and inhibiting formation of foreign body giant cells. J Biol Chem. 2015;290(2):716-26.

16. Romanello M, Piatkowska E, Antoniali G, Cesaratto L, Vascotto C, Iozzo RV, et al. Osteoblastic cell secretome: a novel role for progranulin during risedronate treatment. Bone. 2014;58:81-91.

17. Hossein-Nezhad A, Mirzaei K, Ansar H, Khooshechin G, Ahmadivand Z, Keshavarz SA. Mutual role of PGRN/TNF-α on osteopenia developing in obesity's inflammation state. Minerva Med. 2012;103(3):165-75.

18. Mirzaei K, Hossein-Nezhad A, Emamgholipour S, Ansar H, Khosrofar M, Tootee A, et al. An exonic peroxisome proliferator-activated receptor-γ coactivator-1α variation may mediate the resting energy expenditure through a potential regulatory role on important gene expression in this pathway. J Nutrigenet Nutrigenomics. 2012;5(2):59-71.

19. Hossein-Nezhad A, Khoshniat Nikoo M, Mirzaei K, Mokhtarei F, Aghaei Meybodi HR. Comparison of the bone turn-over markers in patients with multiple sclerosis and healthy control subjects. Eur J Inflamm. 2010;8(2):67-73.

20. Zhang N, Yang N, Chen Q, Qiu F, Li X. Upregulated expression level of the growth factor, progranulin, is associated with the development of primary Sjögren's syndrome. Experimental and therapeutic medicine. 2014;8(5):1643-7.

21. Frampton G, Invernizzi P, Bernuzzi F, Pae HY, Quinn M, Horvat D, et al. Interleukin-6-driven progranulin expression increases cholangiocarcinoma growth by an Akt-dependent mechanism. Gut. 2012;61(2):268-77.

22. Tian Q, Zhao S, Liu C. A solid-phase assay for studying direct binding of progranulin to TNFR and progranulin antagonism of TNF/TNFR interactions. Methods Mol Biol. 2014;1155:163-72.

23. Lam J, Takeshita S, Barker JE, Kanagawa O, Ross FP, Teitelbaum SL. TNF-alpha induces osteoclastogenesis by direct stimulation of macrophages exposed to permissive levels of RANK ligand. J Clin Invest. 2000;106(12):1481-8.

24. Ishimi Y, Miyaura C, Jin CH, Akatsu T, Abe E, Nakamura Y, et al. IL-6 is produced by osteoblasts and induces bone resorption. J Immunol. 1990;145(10):3297-303.

25. Boroń D, Agnieszka SM, Daniel K, Anna B, Adam K. Polymorphism of interleukin-17 and its relation to mineral density of bones in perimenopausal women. Eur J Med Res. 2014;19:69.

26. Shen F, Ruddy MJ, Plamondon P, Gaffen SL. Cytokines link osteoblasts and inflammation: microarray analysis of interleukin-17- and TNF-alpha-induced genes in bone cells. J Leukoc Biol. 2005;77(3):388-99.

27. Pradeep AR, Priyanka N, Prasad MV, Kalra N, Kumari M. Association of progranulin and high sensitivity CRP concentrations in gingival crevicular fluid and serum in chronic periodontitis subjects with and without obesity. Dis Markers. 2012;33(4):207-13.

28. Hossein-Nezhad A, Mirzaei K, Ansar H, Emam-Gholipour S, Tootee A, Keshavarz SA, et al. Obesity, inflammation and resting energy expenditure: possible mechanism of progranulin in this pathway. Minerva Endocrinol. 2012;37(3):255-66.

29. Zizza A, Guido M, Grima P. Interleukin-17 regulates visceral obesity in HIV-1-infected patients. HIV Med. 2012;13(9):574-7.

30. Mohamed-Ali V, Goodrick S, Rawesh A, Katz DR, Miles JM, Yudkin JS, et al. Subcutaneous adipose tissue releases interleukin-6, but not tumor necrosis factor-alpha, in vivo. J Clin Endocrinol Metab. 1997;82(12):4196-200.

31. Zhang P, Peterson M, Su GL, Wang SC. Visceral adiposity is negatively associated with bone density and muscle attenuation. Am J Clin Nutr. 2015;101(2):337-43.

32. Oh J, Kim JY, Kim HS, Oh JC, Cheon YH, Park J, et al. Progranulin and a five transmembrane domain-containing receptor-like gene are the key components in receptor activator of nuclear factor κB (RANK)-dependent formation of multinucleated osteoclasts. J Biol Chem. 2015;290(4):2042-52.

33. Zhao YP, Tian QY, Frenkel S, Liu CJ. The promotion of bone healing by progranulin, a downstream molecule of BMP-2, through inter-acting with TNF/TNFR signaling. Biomaterials. 2013;34(27):6412-21.

34. Aguirre L, Napoli N, Waters D, Qualls C, Villareal DT, Armamento-Villareal R. Increasing adiposity is associated with higher adipo-kine levels and lower bone mineral density in obese older adults. J Clin Endocrinol Metab. 2014;99(9):3290-7.

35. Shetty S, Kapoor N, Naik D, Asha HS, Prabu S, Thomas N. Os-teoporosis in healthy South Indian males and the influence of life style factors and vitamin D status on bone mineral density. J Osteoporosis. 2014;2014: ID 723238.

5

Clinical outcomes of low and intermediate risk differentiated thyroid cancer patients treated with 30mCi for ablation or without radioactive iodine therapy

Shirlei Kugler Aiçar Súss[1,2], Cleo Otaviano Mesa Jr.[2],
Gisah Amaral de Carvalho[2], Fabíola Yukiko Miasaki[2],
Carolina Perez Chaves[3], Dominique Cochat Fuser[3], Rossana Corbo[1],
Denise Momesso[1], Daniel A. Bulzico[1], Hans Graf[2], Fernanda Vaisman[1]

ABSTRACT

Objective: To retrospectively evaluate the outcomes of patients with low and intermediate risk thyroid carcinoma treated with total thyroidectomy (TT) and who did not undergo radioiodine remnant ablation (RRA) and to compare them to patients receiving low dose of iodine (30 mCi). Subjects and methods: A total of 189 differentiated thyroid cancer (DTC) patients treated with TT followed by 30mCi for RRA or not, followed in two referral centers in Brazil were analyzed. Results: From the 189 patients, 68.8% was ATA low-risk, 30.6% intermediate and 0.6% high risk. Eighty-seven patients underwent RRA and 102 did not. The RRA groups tended to be younger and had a higher frequency of extra-thyroidal extension (ETE). RRA did not have and impact on response to initial therapy neither in low ($p = 0.24$) nor in intermediate risk patients ($p = 0.66$). It also had no impact on final outcome and most patients had no evidence of disease (NED) at final follow-up. Recurrence/persistence of disease was found in 1.2% of RRA group and 2% in patients treated only with TT ($p = 0.59$). Conclusions: Our study shows that in low and intermediate-risk patients, RRA with 30 mCi seems to have no major advantage over patients who did not undergo RRA regarding response to initial therapy in each risk group and also in long term outcomes. Arch Endocrinol Metab. 2018;62(2):149-56

Keywords

Thyroid carcinoma; radioiodine ablation; low activity

[1] Serviço de Endocrinologia,
Instituto Nacional do Câncer
(Inca), Rio de Janeiro, RJ, Brasil
[2] Serviço de Endocrinologia,
Hospital das Clínicas,
Universidade Federal do Paraná
(UFPR), Curitiba, PR, Brasil
[3] Serviço de Medicina Nuclear,
Instituto Nacional do Câncer
(Inca), Rio de Janeiro, RJ, Brasil

Correspondence to:
Fernanda Vaisman
Praça da Cruz Vermelha, 23
8º andar, Centro
20230-130 – Rio de Janeiro, RJ, Brasil
fevaisman@globo.com

INTRODUCTION

Over the last decades, the incidence of DTC has increased significantly, especially of tumors smaller than 2 cm (1-3). Despite this, most of these patients have an excellent prognosis and a long follow-up during their lifetime (4,5). Nevertheless, rarely small tumors can metastasize and have an increased recurrence risk (6-8).

Recently, it has been advocated an individualized approach of DTC based on risk stratification (8-11) and a more selective use of RRA (12-15). In this sense, treatment for low-risk tumors tends to be less aggressive than high-risk tumors (16,17). Indeed, the use of RRA in low risk patients remains controversial, because it has not been shown to be beneficial in their management after complete surgical resection in some recent studies (18). More recent guidelines recommend a more careful use of radioiodine (RRA) due to its adverse effects, particularly chronic sialoadenitis and the increased risk of development of a second primary neoplasm (19,20).

In this sense, several studies have already shown that RRA with low RRA dose (30 mCi) is as effective as higher activities with excellent correlated remission rates (21-23). Mujammami and cols. summarizes the results of six studies, in which patients responded equally well to low iodine activity for RRA, when compared to higher activities, and the risk category was not a significant predictor of remission (low, intermediate and some high-risk patients without metastases) (7). However, there are authors who advocate the selective use of iodine, showing that it is not necessary in certain circumstances. In the study by Molinaro and cols., 63.6% of non-ablated low and intermediate risk patients evolved with remission during the follow-up period, without additional therapy, and all of these patients remained in remission through the study (24). Also, Schvartz and cols. failed to prove any benefit of RRA in survival in patients with low-risk DTC after thyroidectomy, reinforcing the idea that they should not be over-treated (22). Durante and cols., showed almost identical clinical response rates for low and intermediate risk patients, between subgroups with and without RRA (4). Similarly, our group had also previously shown that low and intermediate risk patients not treated with RRA had a very low risk of recurrence (25,26).

The aim of this study is to retrospectively analyze the follow-up of patients with thyroid carcinoma who were treated with TT and who did not receive RRA and compare them to patients who received a low dose of iodine (30 mCi).

SUBJECTS AND METHODS

We retrospectively reviewed the medical records of 189 patients with DTC > 18 years old treated with TT without RRA or with low dose RRA (30 mCi) between 1975 and 2015. We included 61 patients treated in Hospital das Clínicas da Universidade Federal do Paraná (HC-UFPR), Curitiba, Brazil and 128 patients treated in National Cancer Institute (Inca), Rio de Janeiro, Brazil. A minimum of 18 months of follow-up after initial therapy was required for entry into the study, unless one of the clinical outcomes was reached before that time point.

The initial thyroid surgery was total thyroidectomy (TT) in all patients. Therapeutic neck dissections were only performed for clinically apparent abnormal cervical lymphadenopathy, since in both institutions, it is not routinely performed prophylactic neck dissections for DTC. RRA was performed within two to six months after surgery in 87 patients and 102 patients did not receive RRA. RRA therapy was administrated after thyroid hormone withdrawal (TWH) for 30 days or with recombinant human TSH (TSHrh) administration in selected patients, and under a low iodine diet. Pre-ablation serum TSH, thyroglobulin (Tg) level and thyroglobulin-antibodies (Tg-Ab) titer were obtained in all patients and whole-body scans (WBS) were performed five to ten days after RRA.

This study was approved by the local research Ethics Committees.

Follow-up

Patients were followed every 6-8 months during the first year and at 6-12 months intervals thereafter at the discretion of the attending physician based on the risk of recurrence of the individual patient and the clinical course of the disease. Routine evaluation included serum TSH, serum Tg, Tg-Ab and neck ultrasound (US). For those patients with suspected local or distant metastasis, other imaging modalities such as computed tomography (CT) scan, or magnetic resonance imaging (MRI) and/or biopsies were performed as needed. Patients were treated and followed by the same group of physicians in each center.

Laboratory studies

Serum Tg was measured postoperative and during follow-up in regular bases. We considered postoperative Tg, measurements performed at a minimum of 6-8 weeks after TT, since Tg usually reaches its nadir by 3 to 4 weeks postoperatively (9,15). Trend of non-stimulated Tg was evaluated at the same TSH levels and defined as: stable, decreasing, or increasing (> 20% over baseline).

At Inca, from 1977 to 1985, the functional sensitivity of the serum Tg assays was approximately 5 ng/mL. Between 1986 and 1997, a variety of Tg assays was used with functional sensitivities of approximately 1 ng/mL. From 1998 to 2001, a Tg assay with a functional sensitivity of 0.5 ng/L was employed. Starting in 2001 until 2010, serum Tg was quantified by a immunometric assay (Immulite) with a functional sensitivity of 0.2 ng/mL, and from 2010 until today, the functional sensitivity dropped to 0.1 ng/mL.

At HC-UFPR, from 1990 to 2004, serum Tg was quantified by a radioimmunoassay assay with a functional sensitivity of 0.9 ng/mL. From 2004 until today, serum Tg was quantified by a chemiluminescence assay with a functional sensitivity of 0.1 ng/mL.

Risk stratification

Patients were stratified using the modified ATA 2015 risk stratification system (low or intermediate risk) (15).

Dynamic risk stratification was performed using the response to therapy assessment during the first 2 years of follow-up previous published by Tuttle and cols. and in the latest ATA guidelines (15,23). In patients treated with RRA, response to therapy were defined as: excellent response to therapy (negative imaging and suppressed Tg < 0.2 ng/mL and stimulated Tg < 1.0 ng/mL); indeterminate response (nonspecific findings on imaging studies, non-stimulated Tg detectable but < 1 ng/mL, stimulated Tg detectable but < 10 ng/mL); biochemical incomplete response (negative imaging and non-stimulated Tg > 1 ng/mL or stimulated Tg > 10 ng/mL); or structural incomplete response to therapy (structural or functional evidence of disease, with any Tg level) (9,15). For patients treated with TT without RRA, response to therapy definitions were: excellent response to therapy (undetectable Tg-Ab, negative imaging and non-stimulated Tg < 0.2 ng/mL or stimulated Tg < 2.0 ng/mL); indeterminate response (stable or declining Tg-Ab and/or nonspecific imaging findings and non-stimulated Tg detectable but 0.2-5 ng/mL, stimulated Tg detectable but 2-10 ng/mL); biochemical incomplete response (negative imaging and/or increasing Tg with similar TSH levels and/or increasing Tg-Ab and non-stimulated Tg > 5 ng/mL or stimulated Tg > 10 ng/mL); or structural incomplete response to therapy (structural or functional evidence of disease, with any Tg level) (9,11). Tg analysis were considered as following: Post operative undetectable Tg when Tg was below functional sensitivity of the Tg assay used at the time of surgery and to determinate the trend overtime we considered increase if either suppressed or stimulated Tg were rising, decline if both were declining or if one was stable and the other was falling and stable if both were stable. In those patients who did not have stimulated Tg repeated overtime, only suppressed Tg was considered. All of the patients had post operative stimulated Tg measured.

Clinical outcomes

Clinical outcomes were defined as:
- No evidence of disease (NED): the absence of suspected images and Tg levels used to classify as excellent response to therapy.
- Recurrent/persistent SD, defined as: positive cytology/histology, highly suspicious lymph-nodes or thyroid bed nodules on the US (hyper-vascularity, cystic areas, heterogeneous

content, rounded shape and enlargement on follow-up), or cross-sectional imaging highly suspicious for metastatic disease.
- Disease specific mortality: death related to the tumor or its treatment.

Additional outcomes evaluated were: need for additional therapy during follow-up (additional surgery and/or RRA), clinical outcomes after additional therapy and the trend of non-stimulated Tg after initial therapy without RRA.

Statistical analysis

Continuous data is presented as mean and standard deviations with median values. For comparing medians nonparametric Mann-Whitney test was used and for categories we used Chi2 to compare 2 or multiple groups and Fisher's exact tests. Analysis was performed using SPSS software (Version 20.0 for MAC; SPSS, Inc., Chicago IL).

RESULTS

The demographics, clinical features, risk stratification, initial management and clinical outcomes of the 189 patients included in the cohort are presented in Table 1. Considering the entire cohort, TT was performed as initial therapy in all patients, papillary thyroid cancer (PTC) was the most common histology and the majority of patients were female. Fifty-four percent (n = 102) of patients did not receive RRA and 46% (n = 87) did undergo low dose RRA (30 mCi). Patients treated with RRA were younger (49, range 18-86 years in the group without RRA vs 43, range 19-80 years for the RRA group) and microscopic extra-thyroidal extension (ETE) was more frequently observed (29.9% for RRA vs 14.7% without RRA) ($p = 0.04$ and $p = 0.01$, respectively). The groups did not differ in tumor size, presence of vascular invasion, lymph-node metastases (N1), tumor multifocality or ATA risk stratification. There was no statistical difference in median postoperative non-stimulated Tg and presence of Tg-Ab between the groups. However, presence of undetectable Tg postoperative during follow-up was significantly different ($p < 0.001$), observed in 65,7% of the patients treated without RRA and 49,4% of patients treated with low dose RRA. The Tg trend overtime decline in 67,6% of patients treated without RRA and 56,3% patients treated with low dose RRA ($p = 0.13$).

Table 1. Description of the cohort (n = 189)

	Without RRA (n = 102)	Low dose RRA (30mCi) (n = 87)	p-value
Age	49 (18-86)	43 (19-80)	**0.04**
Gender-female	93.1% (n = 94)	86.2% (n = 75)	0.09
Histology			
Papillary thyroid cancer	93.1% (n = 94)	95.4% (n = 83)	0.36
ETE	14.7% (n = 15)	29.9% (n = 26)	**0.01**
Multifocality	34.3% (n = 35)	39.1% (n = 34)	0.54
Size (cm)	1 (0.9-9)	1 (0.3-4.0)	0.21
Vascular invasion	8.8% (n = 9)	13.8% (n = 12)	0.35
N1	15.7% (n = 16)	23% (n = 20)	0.26
Post-operative non-stimulated Tg	1.25 (< 0.1-34)	0.77 (< 0.1-15)	0.59
Undetectable post-operative Suppressed Tg	65.7% (n = 67)	49.4% (n = 43)	**< 0.001**
Positive Anti-Tg	6.9% (n = 7)	8.0% (n = 7)	0.78
ATA 2016 risk stratification			
Low	78.4% (n = 80)	57.5% (n = 50)	**0.04**
Intermediate	20.5% (n = 21)	42.5% (n = 37)	
High	1% (n = 1)	0	
Median follow-up (months)	40.5 (1-488)	49.6 (4-321)	0.63
Recurrence/persistence structural disease	1% (n = 1)	1.1% (n = 1)	0.55
Additional therapy	1% (n = 1)	2.3% (n = 2)	0.59
Response to therapy – first 2 years of follow-up			
Excellent	68.6% (n = 70)	81.6% (n = 71)	0.08
Indeterminate	26.5% (n = 27)	13.8% (n = 12)	
Biochemical incomplete	2.9% (n = 3)	2.3% (n = 2)	
Structural incomplete	2% (n = 2)	2.3% (n = 2)	
Tg trend over time (suppressed and/or stimulated)			
Decline	67.6% (n = 69)	56.3% (n = 49)	0.13
Clinical status at final follow-up			
NED without additional therapy	98% (n = 100)	98,8% (n = 86)	0.59
NED after additional therapy	1% (n = 1)	1.2% (n = 1)	
Recurrent/persistent of disease after additional therapy	0%	0%	
Recurrent/persistent of disease without additional therapy	1% (n = 1)	0%	
Death from disease	0%	0%	

Data are presented percentage (number) or median (range). ETE: microscopic extra thyroid extension; N1: lymph node metastases; Tg: thyroglobulin; Anti-Tg: anti-Tg antibody; ATA: American Thyroid Association; NED: no evidence of disease.

During follow-up, recurrence/persistence of disease was similar between groups, with recurrence/persistence in 1% of patients not treated with RRA and 1.1% in patients treated with low dose RRA (30mCi) ($p = 0.55$). The median follow-up was 40.5 and 49.6 months respectively ($p = 0.63$) (Table 1). In both groups, the majority of patients had an excellent response to initial therapy followed by indeterminate and only few patients had incomplete response, either biochemical or structural. At final follow-up the majority of patients had no evidence of biochemical or structural disease without additional therapy. There were no cases of disease-related deaths.

Regarding response to therapy in patients classified as low risk by the ATA risk stratification system ($n = 130$), excellent response was found in 94 patients and indeterminate response in 30 patients, as presented in the univariate analysis shown in Table 1. Papillary was the most common histology and the majority was female in both groups. Similarly, age and size of tumor were not statistically different among them. The median postoperative non-stimulated Tg was significantly statistically different (0.1 ng/mL in patients with excellent response, ranging from < 0.1 to 3.4 ng/mL vs 1.0 ng/mL in patients with indeterminate response, ranging from < 0.1 to 3.0 ng/mL,

$p < 0.001$). The presence of lymph node metastasis at diagnosis was significantly different (7.4% in excellent response vs 13.3% in indeterminate response vs 66.7% and structural incomplete response, $p = 0.04$). When patients were analyzed according to their initial risk of recurrence (Tables 2 and 3), RRA treatment did not differ among patients with excellent and indeterminate response to initial therapy. Postoperative non-stimulated Tg was the only predictor of response to therapy in low and intermediate risk groups (Tables 2 and 3). Extrathyroidal extension, present only in the intermediate risk group, did not have impact on response to initial therapy even being more frequent in the group that underwent RRA.

Only 3 patients with low risk tumors had a biochemical incomplete response and 3 had structural incomplete within the first 2 years of follow-up. They are shown in Table 4. Also, 3 patients from the intermediate risk group had incomplete responses.

Stands out that the only patient with persistent disease (incomplete structural response) still survives with structural disease because it is a heterogeneous lymph node in the left anterior cervical region, near the sternal, which is suspect because of its characteristics (irregular margins) and size (1.4 x 1.2 x 1.3 cm), remains unchanged for more than one year; as well as without elevation of Tg.

DISCUSSION

This study showed that in properly selected low and intermediate risk DTC patients, low activities of RRA did not have a significant impact on response to therapy and also final status of being disease free. Furthermore, in response to initial therapy this difference was also not seen when patients were analyzed according to their initial risk of recurrence separately. Previous studies, Hilo and ESTIMABL, have shown in randomized trials

Table 2. Response to therapy in low risk patients (n = 130) during the first 2 years of follow-up

LOW RISK Patients	Excellent (n = 94)	Indeterminate (n = 30)	Biochemical incomplete (n = 3)	Structural incomplete (n = 3)	p-value
Age (years)	44.5 (20-86)	45.5 (26-76)	42 (32-57)	53 (39-79)	0.61
Gender-female	89.4% (n = 84)	90% (n = 27)	100% (n = 3)	100% (n = 3)	0.72
Histology Papillary thyroid cancer	91.5% (n = 86)	94.3% (n = 33)	100% (n = 3)	100% (n = 3)	0.88
Post operative non stimulated Tg	0.1 (< 0.1-3.4)	1.0 (< 0.1-3.0)	N/A	N/A	**< 0.001**
Size (cm)	2.0 (0.1-9.0)	1.0 (0.2-6)	1.7 (x-2.0)	1.2 (1.1-1.4)	0.78
N1	7.4% (n = 7)	13.3% (n = 4)	0%	66.7% (n = 2)	**0.04**
RRA	43.6% (n = 41)	26.7%% (n = 8)	0%	33.3% (n = 1)	0.24

Data are presented as percentage (number) or median (range). Tg: thyroglobulin, N1: lymph node metastases, RRA: radioiodine, N/A: non available.

Table 3. Response to therapy in intermediate risk patients (n = 58) during the first 2 years of follow-up

Intermediate risk patients	Excellent (n = 46)	Indeterminate (n = 9)	Biochemical incomplete (n = 2)	Structural incomplete (n = 1)	p-value
Age (years)	42 (18-69)	36 (34-43)	34.5 (19-50)	59	0.16
Gender-female	91.9% (42)	66.6% (n = 6)	100% (n = 2)	100% (n = 1)	0.48
Histology Papillary thyroid cancer	97.8% (n = 45)	100% (n = 9)	100% (n = 2)	100% (n = 1)	0.96
Post operative non stimulated Tg	< 0.1 (< 0.1-0.5)	0.1 (< 0.1-0.2)	1.4	3	**< 0.01**
ETE	69.6% (n = 32)	55.5% (n = 5)	100% (n = 2)	100% (n = 1)	**0.89**
Size (cm)	2.1 (1.0-4.7)	2.3 (2.1-3.0)	1.5 (0.6-2.4)	1.4	0.92
N1	37% (n = 17)	22.2% (n = 2)	50% (n = 1)	0%	0.80
RRA	65.2% (n = 30)	44.4% (n = 4)	50% (n = 1)	100% (n = 1)	0.66

Data are presented as percentage (number) or median (range). Tg: thyroglobulin; N1: lymph node metastases; RRA: radioiodine.

Table 4. Clinical characteristics of differentiated thyroid cancer patients with incomplete response to therapy within the first 2 years of follow-up (biochemical or structural)

	Pt1	Pt2	Pt3	Pt4	Pt5	Pt6	Pt7	Pt8	Pt9
Age (years)	79	53	39	57	42	32	59	50	19
Gender	F	F	F	F	F	F	F	F	F
Histology	PTC	PTC	PTC	PTC	PTC	PTC	PTC	PTC	PTC
Size (cm)	1.1	1.2	1.4	1.7	2.0	x	1,4	2,4	0,6
pN1	Yes	Yes	No	No	No	No	No	No	Yes
ATA risk	Low	Low	Low	Low	Low	Low	Intermediate	Intermediate	Intermediate
Radioiodine	No	Yes	No	Yes	No	No	Yes	No	Yes
Response to therapy	SI	SI	SI	BI	BI	BI	SI	BI	BI
Additional Therapy	No	Yes	Yes	No	No	No	No	No	Yes
Time to additional Therapy	x	18	120	x	x	x	x	x	34
Tg trend overtime	Decline	Decline	Decline	Decline	Decline	Decline	Stable	Stable	Increase
Follow-up (months)	20	18	384	16	28	139	12	23	39
Status at final follow-up	PD	NED-AT	NED-AT	NED	NED	NED	NED	NED	NED - AT

F: female; SI: structural incomplete; BI: biochemical incomplete; PD: persistent of disease; NED-AT: no evidence of disease-additional therapy; NED: no evidence of disease.

that low activities such as 30mCi are equally effective for low and intermediate risk patients as RRA (12,14). Vaisman and cols., thus, showed that the recurrence rate of properly selected low and intermediate risk DTC patients are very similar in patients who underwent RRA and those followed with no additional therapy after surgery (26). Furthermore, the study by Schvartz and cols., with a 10.3 years follow-up, showed no benefit of RRA after surgery on survival in a large cohort of patients with low-risk DTC (22). In the study by Durante and cols., the rates of complete clinical response were almost identical in the subgroup that received ablation and in the subgroup that did not receive (92.2% and 98.3%, respectively), reinforcing the low impact of RRA in response to therapy (4).

In the present study, patients treated with RRA were younger, and microscopic ETE was observed more frequently ($p = 0.04$ and $p = 0.01$, respectively). It is known that there is a tendency for an increase in the use of RRA in younger patients; however, most studies fail to show that isolated extra-thyroidal microscopic invasion increases recurrence significantly as an independent factor. Furthermore, the most recent recommendation is to avoid RRA in most patients when this is the only reason to treat with RRA (6). Moreover, in this present study, ETE did not have impact in response to initial therapy in the intermediate risk group, probably being only a factor that have influenced the decision of performing RRA, specially in the past.

In recent years, postoperative evaluation is becoming more important in decision making of RRA (13). This present study showed that the presence of undetectable non-stimulated Tg during follow-up was significantly different and more frequent in the non RRA group ($p < 0.001$), suggesting that independently of initial risk stratification, when postoperative Tg was negative, physicians were confortable to only follow these patients without RRA. Corroborating such findings, Webb and cols. concluded that low pre-ablation Tg should be considered a favorable risk factor in patients with DTC, suggesting that it may perhaps be used to select patients not candidates for RRA (15,27). In the same sense, Momesso and cols. (11) demonstrated that the value of non-stimulated Tg was the greatest predictor of recurrence/persistence of structural disease, which supports previous findings of patients not treated with RRA (10), in whom the decline or stability of non-stimulated Tg presented a good prognosis (18,26,28), being the best response in the first two years of follow-up, comparable to that at any time in the total follow-up of these patients (11). In the same study, there was no disease-specific mortality and low rates of recurrence/persistence of structural disease (11), as also occurred in the on-screen study, in which the majority of patients, more than 97%, had no evidence of disease (NED) at the end of the follow-up without additional therapy and without cases of death by the disease.

Over time, the trend of Tg values decreased by more than 55% in both groups. At the final follow-up, most patients had no evidence of biochemical or structural disease without additional therapy. In the study by Mujammami and cols., levels of pre-dose ablative Tg and biochemical response to primary therapy predicted favorable outcomes (7), with the majority of patients with elevated Tg levels and incomplete or indeterminate responses progressing to undetectable levels of Tg without further treatment (7). This has already been observed by Vaisman and cols. (10), who concluded that patients with incomplete biochemical response may be reclassified as without evidence of disease, without additional therapy beyond suppression of TSH with LT4. Similarly, Momesso and cols. showed that even patients with indeterminate response to therapy had a good prognosis, with no evidence of structural disease during follow-up, and could be observed conservatively (4,9,11,29). Current second generation Tg assays (0.05-0.1 ng/mL) have shown that patients with low-risk DTC with undetectable baseline Tg rarely recur (5). In this sense, study published in 2016 by Janovsky (1) concluded that an excellent response to treatment can be confirmed by the trend of Tg and US, these being the best follow-up approaches, showing that the use of RRA only to achieve negative levels of Tg for surveillance is not necessary because it is not an isolated value, but the tendency of Tg during follow-up, the determining factor for both (1). Therefore, based on the above, it should be emphasized that the trend of Tg is highly suggestive of being a predictor of disease-free follow-up.

When analyzing the low-risk patients separately, patients with excellent response had lower values of postoperative Tg than patients with indeterminate response. Webb and cols. (27) examined the predictive value of a single dose of serum Tg immediately prior to RRA as a subsequent disease free state and concluded that this evaluation is an inexpensive tool with a high negative predictive value which could be used to select patients not RRA candidates (15,27).

The presence of lymph node metastasis at the time of diagnosis was more frequent in those patients with indeterminate response to initial therapy and less frequently in those with excellent response, demonstrating that such presence may negatively interfere in the response to treatment. However, based on current ATA recommendations (15) there is no indication for RRA in low risk patients with up to 5 micro-metastases to lymph nodes. Furthermore, Wang and cols. demonstrated that properly selected patients, even with affected lymph nodes, should not necessarily receive RRA (30,31).

It should be noted that the present work has some limitations. As it is a retrospective and non-randomized trial, selection bias based on the assistant physician to perform RRA could occur. However, the basic characteristics are similar in both groups. Furthermore, there were changes in ultrasound technology and Tg assays as mentioned before that could interfere in initial response to therapy classification, however, the most clinically relevant endpoints, which are recurrence, and structural incomplete response is less influenced by Tg values. Other important limitation is the follow – up period. As known, the majority of the recurrences occur with the first 2-5 years, however, some of those can occur later on. Further prospective studies and with longer follow-up periods are needed to validate our findings. In addition, most of the studies with 30mCi (12,14) evaluate the efficacy of ablation not correlating this with recurrence rates. In our study, we correlate low activities with response to therapy, which is a parameter with well establish correlation with long term prognosis (8,9,10,15).

In conclusion, the present study shows that in low and intermediate risk patients, the treatment with 30mCi of radioiodine for ablation might appear to make a difference in response to therapy, however, when longer follow-up is analyzed, RRA activities at ablation seems to have no advantage over patients who did not undergo RRA with long term outcomes. As a secondary endpoint, in these patients an excellent response to treatment may be assured by the postoperative non-stimulated Tg values analyzed as predictors of disease-free follow-up.

REFERENCES

1. Janovsky CC, Maciel RM, Camacho CP, Padovani RP, Nakabashi CC, Yang JH, et al. A Prospective Study Showing an Excellent Response of Patients with Low-Risk Differentiated Thyroid Cancer Who Did Not Undergo Radioiodine Remnant Ablation after Total Thyroidectomy. Eur Thyroid J. 2016;5(1):44-9.

2. Brito JP, Hay ID, Morris JC. Low risk papillary thyroid cancer. BMJ. 2014;348:g3045.

3. Welsh L, Powell C, Pratt B, Harrington K, Nutting C, Harmer C, et al. Long-term outcomes following low-dose radioiodide ablation

for differentiated thyroid cancer. J Clin Endocrinol Metab. 2013;98(5):1819-25.

4. Durante C, Montesano T, Torlontano M, Attard M, Monzani F, Tumino S, et al. Papillary thyroid cancer: time course of recurrences during postsurgery surveillance. J Clin Endocrinol Metab. 2013;98(2):636-42.

5. Nakabashi CC, Kasamatsu TS, Crispim F, Yamazaki CA, Camacho CP, Andreoni DM, et al. Basal serum thyroglobulin measured by a second-generation assay is equivalent to stimulated thyroglobulin in identifying metastases in patients with differentiated thyroid cancer with low or intermediate risk of recurrence. Eur Thyroid J. 2014;3(1):43-50.

6. Lamartina L, Durante C, Filetti S, Cooper DS. Low-risk differentiated thyroid cancer and radioiodine remnant ablation: a systematic review of the literature. J Clin Endocrinol Metab. 2015;100(5):1748-61.

7. Mujammami M, Hier MP, Payne RJ, Rochon L, Tamilia M. Long-Term Outcomes of Patients with Papillary Thyroid Cancer Undergoing Remnant Ablation with 30 milliCuries Radioiodine. Thyroid. 2016;26(7):951-8.

8. Vaisman F, Tala H, Grewal R, Tuttle RM. In differentiated thyroid cancer, an incomplete structural response to therapy is associated with significantly worse clinical outcomes than only an incomplete thyroglobulin response. Thyroid. 2011;21(12): 1317-22.

9. Momesso DP, Tuttle RM. Update on differentiated thyroid cancer staging. Endocrinol Metab Clin North Am. 2014;43(2):401-21.

10. Vaisman F, Momesso D, Bulzico DA, Pessoa CH, Dias F, Corbo R, et al. Spontaneous remission in thyroid cancer patients after biochemical incomplete response to initial therapy. Clin Endocrinol (Oxf). 2012;77(1):132-8.

11. Momesso DP, Vaisman F, Yang SP, Bulzico DA, Corbo R, Vaisman M, et al. Dynamic Risk Stratification in Patients with Differentiated Thyroid Cancer Treated Without Radioactive Iodine J Clin Endocrinol Metab. 2016;101(7):2692-700.

12. Schlumberger M, Catargi B, Borget I, Deandreis D, Zerdoud S, Bridji B, et al. Strategies of radioiodine ablation in patients with low-risk thyroid cancer. N Engl J Med. 2012;366(18):1663-73.

13. Tuttle RM, Sabra MM. Selective use of RRA for ablation and adjuvant therapy after total thyroidectomy for differentiated thyroid cancer: a practical approach to clinical decision making. Oral Oncol. 2013;49(7):676-83.

14. Mallick U, Harmer C, Yap B, Wadsley J, Clarke S, Moss L, et al. Ablation with low-dose radioiodine and thyrotropin alfa in thyroid cancer. N Engl J Med. 2012;366(18):1674-85.

15. Haugen BR, Alexander EK, Bible KC, Doherty GM, Mandel SJ, Nikiforov YE, et al. 2015 American Thyroid Association Management Guidelines for Adult Patients with Thyroid Nodules and Differentiated Thyroid Cancer: The American Thyroid Association Guidelines Task Force on Thyroid Nodules and Differentiated Thyroid Cancer. Thyroid. 2016;26(1):1-133.

16. Iyer NG, Morris LG, Tuttle RM, Shaha AR, Ganly I. Rising incidence of second cancers in patients with low-risk (T1N0) thyroid cancer who receive radioactive iodine therapy. Cancer. 2011;117(19):4439-46.

17. Cho YY, Lim J, Oh CM, Ryu J, Jung KW, Chung JH, et al. Elevated risks of subsequent primary malignancies in patients with thyroid cancer: a nationwide, population-based study in Korea. Cancer. 2015;121(2):259-68.

18. Durante C, Montesano T, Attard M, Torlontano M, Monzani F, Costante G, et al. Long-term surveillance of papillary thyroid cancer patients who do not undergo postoperative radioiodine

19. Rosario PW, Ward LS, Carvalho GA, Graf H, Maciel RM, Maciel LM, et al. Thyroid nodules and differentiated thyroid cancer: update on the Brazilian consensus. Arq Bras Endocrinol Metabol. 2013;57(4):240-64.

20. Brito JP, Morris JC, Montori VM. Thyroid cancer: zealous imaging has increased detection and treatment of low risk tumours. BMJ. 2013;347:f4706.

21. Castagna MG, Cevenini G, Theodoropoulou A, Maino F, Memmo S, Claudia C, et al. Post-surgical thyroid ablation with low or high radioiodine activities results in similar outcomes in intermediate risk differentiated thyroid cancer patients. Eur J Endocrinol. 2013;169(1):23-9.

22. Schvartz C, Bonnetain F, Dabakuyo S, Gauthier M, Cueff A, Fieffe S, et al. Impact on overall survival of radioactive iodine in low-risk differentiated thyroid cancer patients. J Clin Endocrinol Metab. 2012;97(5):1526-35.

23. Tuttle RM, Tala H, Shah J, Leboeuf R, Ghossein R, Gonen M, et al. Estimating risk of recurrence in differentiated thyroid cancer after total thyroidectomy and radioactive iodine remnant ablation: using response to therapy variables to modify the initial risk estimates predicted by the new American Thyroid Association staging system. Thyroid. 2010;20(12):1341-9.

24. Molinaro E, Giani C, Agate L, Biagini A, Pieruzzi L, Bianchi F, et al. Patients with differentiated thyroid cancer who underwent radioiodine thyroid remnant ablation with low-activity (1)(3)(1)I after either recombinant human TSH or thyroid hormone therapy withdrawal showed the same outcome after a 10-year follow-up. J Clin Endocrinol Metab. 2013;98(7):2693-700.

25. Momesso DP, Vaisman F, Caminha LS, Pessoa CH, Corbo R, Vaisman M. Surgical approach and radioactive iodine therapy for small well-differentiated thyroid cancer. J Endocrinol Invest. 2014;37(1):57-64.

26. Vaisman F, Shaha A, Fish S, Michael Tuttle R. Initial therapy with either thyroid lobectomy or total thyroidectomy without radioactive iodine remnant ablation is associated with very low rates of structural disease recurrence in properly selected patients with differentiated thyroid cancer. Clin Endocrinol (Oxf). 2011;75(1):112-9.

27. Webb RC, Howard RS, Stojadinovic A, Gaitonde DY, Wallace MK, Ahmed J, et al. The utility of serum thyroglobulin measurement at the time of remnant ablation for predicting disease-free status in patients with differentiated thyroid cancer: a meta-analysis involving 3947 patients. J Clin Endocrinol Metab. 2012;97(8): 2754-63.

28. Vaisman F, Momesso D, Bulzico DA, Pessoa CH, da Cruz MD, Dias F, et al. Thyroid Lobectomy Is Associated with Excellent Clinical Outcomes in Properly Selected Differentiated Thyroid Cancer Patients with Primary Tumors Greater Than 1 cm. J Thyroid Res. 2013;2013:398194.

29. Padovani RP, Robenshtok E, Brokhin M, Tuttle RM. Even without additional therapy, serum thyroglobulin concentrations often decline for years after total thyroidectomy and radioactive remnant ablation in patients with differentiated thyroid cancer. Thyroid. 2012;22(8):778-83.

30. Wang LY, Palmer FL, Migliacci JC, Nixon IJ, Shaha AR, Shah JP, et al. Role of RRA in the management of incidental N1a disease in papillary thyroid cancer. Clin Endocrinol (Oxf). 2015.

31. Wang LY, Ganly I. Nodal metastases in thyroid cancer: prognostic implications and management. Future Oncol. 2016;12(7):981-94.

6

Cardiovascular risk in rural workers and its relation with body mass index

Joana Carolina Bernhard[1], Kely Lisandra Dummel[1], Éboni Reuter[1],
Miriam Beatris Reckziegel[1], Hildegard Hedwig Pohl[1]

ABSTRACT

Objective: Evaluate the propensity of cardiovascular risk in rural workers and, through the Framingham Risk Score (FRS), relate this risk with the classification of Body Mass Index (BMI). Subjects and methods: This study is characterized as descriptive and exploratory, with the participation of 138 subjects, ranging between 25-73 years old. Clinical and laboratory analysis of the risk factors contained in the FRS were performed, in addition to the determination of BMI, blood pressure, smoking and physical inactivity. Results: The procedures indicated a low risk of a coronary event in 10 years with 70.3% of the population. In contrast, 88.4% of the subjects were overweight. It was evidenced a risk improvement as the BMI increased, since 96.4% of high-risk cases were overweight or obese. Conclusion: Results suggest larger prevalence of intermediary or high FRS for women with higher BMI, which was not observed in men. Arch Endocrinol Metab. 2018;62(1):65-71

Keywords
Agribusiness; mortality; cardiovascular diseases

[1] Departamento de Educação Física e Saúde, Universidade de Santa Cruz do Sul (Unisc), Santa Cruz do Sul, RS, Brasil

Correspondence to:
Hildegard Hedwig Pohl
Av. Independência, 2293
96815-900 – Santa Cruz do Sul, RS, Brasil
hpohl@unisc.br

INTRODUCTION

Cardiovascular diseases are responsible for the high number of deaths, and recorded worldwide data in 2011 of 17 million, since 2000 leading the ranking of the ten leading causes of mortality. Mortality and morbidity levels in adults from 2008 to 2011, reported by WHO, show a significant increase of deaths due to cardiovascular disease, with production losses, and expenses with medical care, treatment and rehabilitation. Predictions are that by 2025 the risk of coronary heart disease and stroke will have increased by 120% for women and 137% for men living in developed countries (1). These figures reinforce the importance of effective primary measures for the prevention of these diseases (2).

Hypertension, diabetes mellitus, dyslipidemia, obesity and some habits related to lifestyle (poor diet, smoking, alcohol consumption, physical inactivity) are factors that predispose to cardiovascular risk (3). The Brazilian Society of Cardiology data indicate that 80% of individuals of the Brazilian adult population is sedentary and 52% are overweight, 11% obese, which reinforces the propensity of increased morbidity and mortality, since obesity is an independent risk factor associated with cardiovascular diseases (4).

These aspects combined with regional characteristics of the population and the changes processed in the labor world, with numerous effects on health and epidemiological profile of the working population (5), broaden the spectrum of health problems. Because, in addition to unhealthy lifestyles, inadequate working conditions, such as long working hours and high occupational stress, may predispose workers to high risk of cardiovascular diseases (6).

Rural workers have presented health problems. There is evidence that, by underreporting, the prevalence of diseases is higher in rural than in urban areas. Many factors could be related to health worsening, including restricted access to health system and work economic dependence, which subjects workers to long working days, frequent physical efforts, low income, assiduity even at physical adversities, and long term labor (increasing age group for this population) (7). For the International Labour Organization (ILO) rural work is of great significance, and more dangerous than other activities. It is estimated that millions of farmers suffer from serious health problems (8). Therefore, prevention measures are an important issue in promoting the health of these workers.

Given the complexity of these interactions, it is performed, in 1960, the first cohort study focusing on cardiovascular disease by identifying risk factors and pathophysiology, the Framingham Heart Study (FHS), a time when mortality and the incidence of cardiovascular disease showed progressive increases (9). As a result of advances in the FHS, which occurred from 1998, it is possible to stratify the risk of coronary events in 10 years, through a specific score for each risk factor, using clinical variables of daily practice. This indicative stratification of cardiovascular disease risk propensity is classified as low, intermediate and high risk (10). According to the Ministry of Health, the Framingham Score identifies the potential for developing cardiovascular disease even before the onset of symptoms (11).

In this context, the objective of this study is to evaluate the cardiovascular risk in farmers and their relation to the classification of Body Mass Index.

SUBJECTS AND METHODS

This is a descriptive exploratory study, developed from the database project "Screening of risk factors related to overweight in agribusiness workers using new analytical and health information technologies" developed at the University of Santa Cruz do Sul, approved by the Ethics Committee in Research with Human Beings, under the Protocol 2509/10. We evaluated 138 subjects with a mean age of 51.32 years (SD 10.32), who met the following inclusion criteria: be 18 years old and not be carriers coronary artery disease, stroke, heart failure and acute myocardial infarction.

Labor activities of the sample individuals are those typical of family farming workers, such as planting, farming maintenance, harvesting, animal husbandry, manufacturing of homemade products and trading of the production. Sample was obtained among residents in the municipalities of Santa Cruz do Sul, Passo do Sobrado, Vale Verde, Rio Pardo, Candelária, Encruzilhada do Sul e General Câmara, in the State of Rio Grande do Sul, Brazil. According to Bertê and cols. (12), the region has its rural sector dedicated mainly to monoculture, but receives incentives aiming to diversification of production and development of family agroindustry.

The screening of the subjects was performed by external seminar with the institutions involved in the study. Opportunity in which voluntary participants were informed about the purpose of the study and the conditions of involvement, when the lifestyle questionnaire was applied. Sampling was non-probabilistic and by convenience.

A survey form proposed by the Brazilian Association of Survey Companies (ABEP – 2014) (13) was used for economic classification, which consists on collecting data of movable and immovable property, domiciliary goods, as well as the graduation level of the householder. There are eight classification levels for Brazilian Criterion: A1, A2, B1, B2, C1, C2, D and E. In this study, subjects were divided in two groups, one of them formed by the members of A1, A2, B1 and B2, and the other one formed by the remaining categories.

Anthropometric, biochemical and physiological assessments were subsequently applied at the University. The body mass index (BMI) was calculated from the body mass obtained on the scale (Welmy) and height measured in a stadiometer, and calculated from dividing weight (kg) by height (m) squared. Systolic blood pressure (SBP) was measured after five minutes rest, with the subject seated, and the data categorized as normal SBP (< 129 mmHg), borderline (between 130 and 139 mmHg) or hypertension (above 140 mmHg) according to the VI Brazilian Guidelines of Hypertension (2010) (14).

Blood tests were performed at the Laboratory of Clinical Biochemistry at the University of Santa Cruz do Sul, using reactive of Labtest brand in semiautomated system (LabMax Progress – LabTest), observing, to the glycemic index the recommendations of the American Diabetes Association (15). Total cholesterol (TC) and high-density lipoprotein cholesterol (HDL-c) reference values of the Brazilian Cardiology Society (16). Blood collection was performed in the brachial vein, preceded by fasting for 12 hours using two *vacutainer*, one of them containing fluoride\oxalate (to obtain plasma) and another without additive (to obtain serum). Blood samples deposited in *vacutainer* without anticoagulants were incubated at 37°C for 15 minutes and centrifuged at 2500 rpm for five minutes to collect serum. The plasma samples were subjected to the determination of glucose (GLU), and the serum samples submitted to the determination of the TC and HDL-c. Diagnosis of diabetes was determined after the results of the glucose test.

According to the criteria proposed by the Framingham Heart Study (FHS) the following risk factors were considered: age, sex, diabetes, TC, HDL-c, smoking and SBP. Through the Framingham score

(FRS), the risk of occurrence of coronary events in 10 years was calculated. For each risk factor was applied a specific score as suggested by the FHS, obtaining the final score by the sum of individual points. The results were classified as low risk (LR) score < 10%, intermediate risk (IR) score between 10 and 20% and high risk (HR) > 20%. It is important to highlight that all those identified as diabetics were considered automatically as HR (6).

Data were analyzed using the Statistical Software for Social Sciences (SPSS, version 20.0), using descriptive statistics with central tendency and dispersion measures, for numeric variables, and frequency and percentage, for categorical variables. Pearson's chi-square test was used to the analytical statistics of the frequencies distribution between FRS and BMI as well as between FRS and sociodemographic characteristics, considering p < 0.05. In order to evaluate the prevalence ratio of BMI over the FRS, a Poisson Regression Test was used.

RESULTS

Most of the subjects is aged 40-55 (44.2%), married (75.4%), from C1-C2-D economic classes (58%), up to 7 years educated (73.2%) and women (62.3%). Regarding BMI, it is noteworthy that 88.4% of employees have some level of overweight (overweight or obese). Obesity prevails among women (51.2%) and overweight among men (65.4%). Regarding the FRS, 81.4% of women and 51.9% of men have low risk (Table 1).

Regarding the biochemical characteristics and BP, it can be seen that 58.0% has increased level of TC, HDL values within the desired standard in 83.3% of cases. Yet the glucose levels of 43.5% of workers are in the range of pre-diabetic and 15.9% in the diabetes range (Table 1).

By analyzing the average values of the indicators that compose the estimate of FRS and the average of risk score, we observed that the factors that had higher scores on the FRS were the mean age 51.32 ± 10.32 years and the total cholesterol 211.81 ± 48.98 mg/dL. It is important to state that 93.5% of workers had no smoking habit. As regards the systolic pressure, the mean value obtained was 131.67 ± 17.00 mmHg. The average score of 11.09 ± 6.19 points represents low risk for myocardial infarction or coronary heart disease within 10 years (Table 2) which is confirmed by the percentage of individuals rated as LR (Table 1).

Table 1. Characterization of the sample

Variables	Gender		Total* 138 (100)
	Female* 86 (62.3)	Male* 52 (37.7)	
Age range			
< 40 years	14 (16.3)	11 (21.2)	25 (18.1)
40-55 years	41 (47.7)	20 (38.5)	61 (44.2)
> 55 years	31 (36.0)	21 (40.4)	52 (37.7)
Marital status			
Single	6 (7.0)	8 (15.4)	14 (10.1)
Married	65 (75.6)	39 (75.0)	104 (75.4)
Others	15 (17.4)	5 (9.6)	20 (14.4)
Economic level			
B1-B2	32 (37.2)	26 (50.0)	58 (42.0)
C1-C2-D	54 (62.8)	26 (50.0)	80 (58.0)
Schooling			
Up to 7 years	64 (74.4)	37 (71.2)	101 (73.2)
8 to 10 years	9 (10.5)	6 (11.5)	15 (10.9)
11 years or more	13 (15.1)	9 (17.3)	22 (15.9)
BMI			
Recommended range	8 (09.3)	8 (15.4)	16 (11.6)
Overweight	34 (39.5)	34 (65.4)	68 (49.3)
Obesity	44 (51.2)	10 (19.2)	54 (39.1)
Total cholesterol			
Desirable	36 (41.9)	22 (42.3)	58 (42.0)
Increased	50 (58.1)	30 (57.7)	80 (58.0)
HDL			
Desirable	75 (87.2)	40 (76.9)	115 (83.3)
Decreased	11 (12.8)	12 (23.1)	23 (16.7)
SBP			
Recommended range	34 (39.6)	26 (50.0)	60 (43.5)
Bordering	22 (25.6)	10 (19.2)	32 (23.2)
Hypertension	30 (35.0)	16 (30.8)	46 (33.3)
Glucose			
Desirable	36 (41.9)	20 (38.5)	56 (40.6)
Pre-diabetes	38 (44.2)	22 (42.3)	60 (43.5)
Diabetes	12 (14.0)	10 (19.2)	22 (15.9)
FRS			
Low risk	70 (81.4)	27 (51.9)	97 (70.3)
Intermediate risk	1 (1.2)	12 (23.1)	13 (9.4)
High risk	15 (17.4)	13 (25.0)	28 (20.3)

*: frequency (percentage); BMI: body mass index; HDL: high density lipoprotein; SBP: systolic blood pressure; FRS: Framingham Risk Score.

When stratifying the risk of coronary artery disease, according to the FRS, it was observed that 70.3% of workers has low risk, 8.6% has intermediate risk and

22.3% has high risk When analyzing the risk related to BMI classification, statistical significance was found (p = 0.035) indicating relationship between the variables, while obesity is a preponderant factor in the definition of risk, there are other intervening variables that were not evidenced in this study. Although most of the subjects were rated low risk, it is noteworthy that among subjects with intermediate risk 69.2% are overweight, since those with high risk in 96.4% of the patients present weight excess: overweight (39.3%) or obese (57.1%). Another fact to highlight is the occurrence of high risk in the subject with recommended weight range, which was due to the presence of diabetes mellitus (Table 3).

When analyzing the prevalence ratio between BMI and FRS, it can be observed that overweight women have 14.7% greater risk prevalence than those rated as normal BMI. Obese women showed risk prevalence 25% greater than the eutrophic. This fact was neither observed for the male population, nor in whole sample (Table 4). From Table 5 it comes that, among sociodemographic characteristics, gender and age group are related to FRS, an expected fact, since this factors are component variables of FRS.

Table 2. Average values in the indicators that composse the Framingham Risk Score

FRS variables	Mean value (SD)	Mean score (SD)
Age	51.32 (10.32)	4.75 (5.51)
Cholesterol level	211.81 (48.98)	3.70 (2.55)
Smoke* [yes/no]	9 (6.5)/129 (93.5)	0.35 (1.51)
HDL	49.96 (10.97)	0.48 (0.94)
SBP	131.67 (17.00)	1.03 (1.00)
FRS	11.09 (6.19)	-

*: frequency (percentage); FRS: Framingham Risk Score; HDL: high density lipoprotein; SBP: systolic blood pressure; SD: standard deviation.

Table 3. Relation between BMI and the Framingham Risk Score

BMI	FRS			p*
	Low risk** 97 (70.3)	Intermediate risk** 13 (9.4)	High risk** 28 (20.3)	
Recommended range	12 (12.4)	3 (23.1)	1 (3.6)	
Overweight	48 (49.5)	9 (69.2)	11 (39.3)	0.035
Obesity	37 (38.1)	1 (7.7)	16 (57.1)	

*: Pearson's chi-square; **: frequency (percentage); FRS: Framingham Risk Score; BMI: body mass index.

Table 5. Relation between sociodemographic characteristics and the Framingham Risk Score

	FRS			p*
	Low risk** 97 (70.3)	Intermediate risk** 13 (9.4)	High risk** 28 (20.3)	
Gender				
Male	27 (27.7)	12 (92.3)	13 (46.4)	<0.001
Female	70 (72.2)	1 (7.7)	15 (53.6)	
Age range				
< 40 years	20 (20.6)	-	5 (17.9)	
40-55 years	53 (54.6)	3 (23.1)	5 (17.9)	<0.001
> 55 years	24 (24.7)	10 (76.9)	18 (64.3)	
Marital status				
Single	10 (10.3)	-	4 (14.3)	
Married	74 (76.3)	12 (92.3)	18 (64.3)	0.382
Others	13 (13.4)	1 (7.7)	6 (21.4)	
Economic level				
B1-B2	43 (44.3)	4 (30.8)	11 (39.3)	0.615
C1-C2-D	54 (55.7)	9 (69.2)	17 (60.7)	
Schooling				
Up to 7 years	69 (71.1)	11 (84.6)	21 (75.0)	
8 to 10 years	12 (12.4)	1 (7.7)	2 (7.1)	0.806
11 years or more	16 (16.5)	1 (7.7)	5 (17.9)	

*: Pearson's chi-square; **: frequency (percentage); FRS: Framingham Risk Score.

Table 4. Prevalence ratio of FRS high risk in relation to BMI

BMI	General		Gender			
			Male		Female	
	PR (CI 95%)	p	PR (CI 95%)	p	PR (CI 95%)	p
Recommended range	1	-	1	-	1	-
Overweight	1.035 (0.86-1.25)	0.719	0.961 (0.74-1.24)	0.762	1.147 (1.03-1.27)	0.010
Obesity	1.052 (0.87-1.28)	0.610	1.067 (0.79-1.44)	0.672	1.25 (1.13-1.38)	< 0.001

FRS: Framingham Risk Score; BMI: body mass index; PR: prevalence ratio; CI: confidence interval.

DISCUSSION

The results of this cross-sectional study show the prevalence of overweight and obesity among workers classified with intermediate and high cardiovascular risk. Regardless of overweight or obesity present in most of sample, the subjects were often classified with low cardiovascular risk. From the factors considered in the FHS, the ones who obtained the highest scores in the formation of the risk score were age and TC. Variables that may be related because the increase in TC may be associated with increased age, as in this study the subjects had higher mean age (51.32 years) compared with those obtained by workers in other economic sectors, such as studies industrialists (36.27 ± 10.21) (17) and commercial workers (27.65 ± 9.38) (18).

This mean age is characteristic of the demographic profile of Brazilian rural workers marked by continuous aging (19). This phenomenon stems from the migration of youth to urban centers, as has also been identified in France (20). This happens due to the migratory flow, which is common in contemporary societies, according to Dasre and cols. (21).

However, in addition to issues related to the logic of the organization and dynamics of production centered on family labor, factors that contribute to male dominance is the aging of the rural population. However, external elements to the family play an important role in the movement of young people to the cities, such as the increasing difficulty of access to basic health and education services (22).

With respect to the average value of TC, it was observed that this was above the recommended as desirable in half the subjects in this study. This result shows resemblance to a survey of urban bus drivers in Teresina (Piauí), in which approximately half of subjects had TC at levels above 200 mg/dL (10), as well as 39.4% of 678 drivers, working in alternating shifts in a mining company in Minas Gerais, had increased TC (23). A bi-racial study with women and African-American and white men, found above the recommended cholesterol (> 200 mg/dL) among white women (24).

Regarding HDL-c most of the subjects were classified at levels considered adequate (50.03 ± 10.96). Similar average results were found in a study applied with 2037 subjects (24). It is important to highlight that the small number of smokers (6.5%) led to the disregard of this variable in this study.

Although the highest percentage of subjects has presented systolic blood pressure in the proper range, a third of them (33.1%) was classified with hypertension. This finding may be associated with the age of the workers, since study in two rural communities identified 42.9% of hypertensive in 18-94-year-old subjects (25). These findings confirm the scientific evidence that high blood pressure increases progressively with age, being a common condition in people with older age, especially in people over 60 years old (26). The Framingham Heart Study states that the prevalence of hypertension increases from 27.3%, in patients younger than 60 years, to 74.0% in those aged over 80 years old (27).

In addition to the primary prevention, it is necessary more control and treatment of hypertension, especially in critically ill patients, as shown in a study of medical records of patients from the Cardiology Clinic of Anapolis/GO. The same authors stress the urgency of greater control over risk factors, such as physical inactivity and obesity, in order to avoid the emergence of CVD associated with SAH (28).

This recommendation is based on the influence of overweight in the prevalence of hypertension due to the risk that these changes represent a condition found in 87.8% of workers. This finding overcomes the data from a study that observed overweight and obesity in 65.5% of subjects in the hospital area (29) and 40.7% of farmers in Minnesota, United States (30). It is possible to observe that one of the factors prevalent among hypertensive individuals is the obesity (31).

Regarding BMI, studies show that the prevalence of most chronic diseases are associated with the increase of this anthropometrical measure. In addition, the cardiometabolic risk factors have been affecting both men and women with overweight and obesity (32), with this measure related to increased risk of premature death in subjects with severe obesity or above 35 kg/m² (33).

It is worth noting the risk posed by visceral fat and body fat for the development of coronary atherosclerosis, before the presence of comorbidities resulting from cardiovascular diseases (34). Thus, the Framingham score, for its ability to anticipate the identification of individuals at risk of developing cardiovascular events, is an important method for the primary prevention. Preventive interventions should be proposed and are indispensable in order to prevent the occurrence of any event.

Regarding the groups, no significant differences were observed between the clinical variables. According to the Framingham risk score, the average value found was 10.93 points, featuring intermediate risk of coronary events in 10 years. The results found in this study show that 22.3% of the subjects are at high risk of developing coronary event. Unlike the study of 309,955 workers in different economic sectors in Spain, with an average age of 36.5 years, in which 5.9% of the subjects were classified with high risk and 0.9% with moderate risk, those classified with high cardiovascular risk 7.6% were men and 1.7% were women, with a higher occurrence in agricultural (11.3%) and construction workers (8.2%), when compared to the industrial and services sector (35).

Finally, it is worth noting the presence of abnormal glucose (59.0%) with diabetic (15.8%) and pre-diabetic patients (43.2%) in the group assessed, highlighting the importance of primary actions that may reverse health complications through the assessment of cardiovascular risk in rural workers, using the Framingham risk Score, and stratify its distribution according to the classification of body mass index.

We considered the high number of diabetics in the sample was due to several factors, such as the advanced age of the individuals, the great number of overweight subjects and the fact that they referred not having regular attendance for this marker. Another point to be highlighted is the fact that men does not present risk increase as BMI increase. This fact points to weakness of BMI for part of this group, which could have been influenced by factors as lean mass increasing, what is not discriminated by BMI. Thus, we are sendend towards further investigations related to body composition and cardiovascular risk addressing the specifties of this population, especially regarding to the high average age.

The subjects of the study have a labor fairly active, mainly the men, which are more involved in heavy farm activities. Thus, men BMI might be biased, which could be explained by the overweight caused by lean body mass instead of fat body mass, since BMI does not tell which kind of body mass. This hypothesis could be investigated in future researches, using different anthropometric variables.

This study showed the presence of low risk for coronary events in the study population, estimated by the Framingham Risk Score. The influence of BMI on increasing cardiovascular risk was observed in the women workers. However, this fact was not identified in men. Nevertheless, these results show the importance of this variable when implementing actions that can stimulate healthier lifestyles, especially when addressed to a population with limited access to health care networks, as in the case of rural workers.

Acknowledgements: workers and organizers related to research subjects who have committed and provided their time to participate.

Financial support: this work was supported by *Secretaria de Desenvolvimento Econômico, Ciência e Tecnologia do Estado do Rio Grande do Sul*, by *Universidade de Santa Cruz do Sul*, by *Fundação de Amparo à Pesquisa do Estado do Rio Grande do Sul* (Fapergs) and the *Conselho Nacional de Desenvolvimento Científico e Tecnológico* (CNPq).

REFERENCES

1. Organização Mundial de Saúde. Estadísticas sanitarias mundiales. OMS; 2011.

2. Cesarino EJ, Vituzzo ALG, Sampaio JMC, Ferreira DAS, Pires HAF, Souza L. Assessment of cardiovascular risk of patients with arterial hypertension of a public health unit. Einstein. 2012;10(1):33-8.

3. Cesarino CB, Borges PP, Ribeiro RCHM, Ribeiro DF, Kusumota L. Avaliação do risco cardiovascular de pacientes renais crônicos segundo critérios de Framingham. Acta Paul Enferm. 2013;26(1):101-7.

4. Sociedade Brasileira de Cardiologia/Sociedade Brasileira de Hipertensão/Sociedade Brasileira de Nefrologia. VI Diretrizes Brasileiras de Hipertensão. Arq Bras Cardiol. 2010;95(supl. 1):1-51.

5. Wunsch VF. Perfil epidemiológico dos trabalhadores. Rev Bras Medicina Trab. 2004;2(2):103-17.

6. Huang JH, Huang SL, Li RH, Wang LH, Chen YL, Tang FC. Effects of nutrition and exercise health behaviors on predicted risk of cardiovascular disease among workers with different body mass index levels. Int J Environt Res Public Health. 2014;11(5):4664-75.

7. Moreira JPL, Oliveira BLCA, Muzi CD, Cunha CLF, Brito AS, Luiz RR. A saúde dos trabalhadores da atividade rural no Brasil. Cad Saúde Pública. 2015;31(8):1698-708.

8. Dias EC. Condições de vida, trabalho, saúde e doença dos trabalhadores rurais no Brasil. Saúde do Trabalhador Rural – RENAST. 2006.

9. Oliveira DS, Tannus LRM, Matheus ASM, Corrêa FH, Cobas R, Cunha EF, et al. Avaliação do risco cardiovascular segundo os critérios de Framingham em pacientes com diabetes tipo II. Arq Bras Endocrinol Metab. 2007;51(2):268-74.

10. Landim MBP, Victor EG. Escore de Framingham em Motoristas de Transporte Coletivo Urbano de Teresina, Piauí. Arq Bras Cardiol. 2006;87(3):315-20.

11. Ministério da Saúde. Protocolo clínico e diretrizes terapêuticas: dislipidemias em pacientes de alto risco de desenvolver eventos cardiovasculares; 2002.

12. 12. Bertê AMA, Lemos BO, Testa G, Zanella MAR, Oliveira SB. Perfil socioeconômico – COREDE Vale do Rio Pardo. Boletim Geográfico do Rio Grande do Sul. 2016;26:984-1024.

13. ABEP. Associação Brasileira de Empresas de Pesquisas. Critério de Classificação Econômica Brasil. 2014. Available from: http://www.abep.org/criterio-brasil. Accessed on: 25 Oct. 2016.

14. VI Diretriz Brasileira de Hipertensão. Rev Bras Hipertens. 2010;17(1):7-10.

15. American Diabetes Association. Standards of Medical Care in Diabetes. ADA. 2013.

16. Sociedade Brasileira de Cardiologia. III Diretrizes Brasileiras sobre Dislipidemias e Diretriz de Prevenção da Aterosclerose. Arq Bras Cardiol. 2001;77(supl. III):48.

17. Swarowsky I. A obesidade e os riscos à saúde de trabalhadores de uma indústria de Santa Cruz do Sul [dissertação]. Rio Grande do Sul. Universidade de Santa Cruz do Sul; 2012.

18. Pohl HH, Reckziegel MB, Reuter EM, Galliano LM, Corbellini VA, Stein MJ. Perfil de saúde dos trabalhadores do comércio: um estudo relacionado à aptidão física. Rev Bras Pesq Saúde. 2013;15(1):17-24.

19. Abramovay R (coord.). Os impasses da sucessão hereditária na agricultura familiar. Florianópolis. EPAGRI; NEAD/Ministério do Desenvolvimento Agrário; 2001.

20. Champagne P. Élargissement de l'espace social et crise de l'identité paysanne, Cahier d'Éco Soc Rur. 1986; déc.(3):73-89.

21. Dasre A, Kersuzan C, Caillot M, Bergouignan C. Sélectivité migratoire des populations selon leur âge et concentrations socio-spatiales. Espace Pop Soc. 2009;1:67-84.

22. Anderson JSN, Schneider S. Brazilian Demographic Transition and the Strategic Role of Youth. Espace Populations Societies. 2014;2-3.

23. Alves ME. Fatores de risco nutricionais, comportamentais, clínicos e bioquímicos para doenças cardiovasculares em trabalhadores de turnos alternantes da região dos inconfidentes, Minas Gerais, Brasil. 2012. 116f. Dissertação (Programa de Pós-Graduação em Ciências Biológicas) – Universidade Federal de Ouro Preto, Ouro Preto, 2012.

24. Barreira TV, Staiano AE, Harrington DM, Heymsfield SB, Smith SR, Bouchard C, et al. Anthropometric correlates of total body fat, abdominal adiposity, and cardiovascular disease risk factors in a biracial sample of men and women. Mayo Clin Proc. 2012;87(5):452-60.

25. Matozinhos FP, Mendes LL, Oliveira AGC, Velasquez-Melendez G. Fatores associados à hipertensão arterial em populações rurais. Rev Min Enferm. 2011;15(3):333-47.

26. Pimenta E, Oparil S. Management of hypertension in the elderly. Nat Rev Cardiol. 2012;9(5):286-96.

27. Lloyd-Jones DM, Evans JC, Levy D. Hypertension in adults across the age spectrum: current outcomes and control in the community. JAMA. 2005;294:466-72.

28. Tacon KC, Pereira AS, Santos HCO, Castro EC, Amaral WN. Perfil epidemiológico da hipertensão arterial sistêmica em pacientes atendidos em uma instituição de ensino superior. Rev Bras Clin Med. 2012;10(3):189-93.

29. Cavagioni L, Pierin AMG. Risco cardiovascular em profissionais de saúde de serviços de atendimento hospitalar. Esc Enferm. 2012;46(2):395-403.

30. Prokosch AJ, Dalleck LC, Pettitt RW. Cardiac Risk Factors between Farmers and Non-Farmers. JEPonline. 2011;14(3):91-100.

31. Radovanovic CAT, Santos LA, Carvalho MDB, Marcon SS. Hipertensão arterial e outros fatores de risco associados às doenças cardiovasculares em adultos. Rev Latino-Am Enfermagem. 2014;22(4):547-53.

32. Schienkiewitz A, Gert BMM, Scheidt-Nave C. Comorbidity of overweight and obesity in a nationally representative sample of German adults aged 18-79 years. BMC Public Health. 2012;12(1):658.

33. Schneider HJ, Friedrich N, Klotsche J, Pieper L, Nauck M, John U, et al. The predictive value of different measures of obesity for incident cardiovascular events and mortality. J Clin Endocrinol Metab. 2010;95(4):1777-85.

34. Lee SY, Chang HJ, Sung J, Kim KJ, Shin S, Cho IJ, et al. The impact of obesity on subclinical coronary atherosclerosis according to the risk of cardiovascular disease. Obesity. 2014;22(7):1762-68.

35. Chaparro MAS, Bonacho EC, Quintela AG, Cabrera M, Sáinz JC, Labander CF, et al. High cardiovascular risk in Spanish workers. Nut Met Card Dis. 2011;21(4):231-36.

7

Waist circumference is an effect modifier of the association between bone mineral density and glucose metabolism

Lygia N. Barroso[1], Dayana R. Farias[1], Marcia Soares-Mota[2],
Heloisa Bettiol[3], Marco Antônio Barbieri[3], Milton Cesar Foss[3],
Antônio Augusto M. da Silva[4], Gilberto Kac[1]

[1] Observatório de Epidemiologia Nutricional, Departamento de Nutrição Social e Aplicada, Instituto de Nutrição Josué de Castro, Universidade Federal do Rio de Janeiro (UFRJ), Cidade Universitária, Ilha do Fundão, Rio de Janeiro, RJ, Brasil
[2] Instituto de Nutrição Josué de Castro, Universidade Federal do Rio de Janeiro (UFRJ), Cidade Universitária, Ilha do Fundão, Rio de Janeiro, RJ, Brasil
[3] Departamento de Puericultura e Pediatria, Faculdade de Medicina de Ribeirão Preto, Universidade de São Paulo, Ribeirão Preto, SP, Brasil
[4] Departamento de Saúde Pública, Centro de Ciências da Saúde, Universidade Federal do Maranhão (UFMA), São Luís, MA, Brasil

Correspondence to:
Gilberto Kac
Departamento de Nutrição Social e Aplicada, Instituto de Nutrição Josué de Castro, Universidade Federal do Rio de Janeiro
Av. Carlos Chagas Filho, 367, CCS, Bloco J2, sala 29, Cidade Universitária, Ilha do Fundão, 21941-590 – Rio de Janeiro, RJ, Brasil
gilberto.kac@gmail.com

ABSTRACT

Objective: The role of bone markers on insulin resistance (IR) remains controversial. The objective of this study is to evaluate the association between bone mineral density (BMD) and glucose metabolism and investigate if visceral hyperadiposity, evaluated by waist circumference (WC), is an effect modifier of this association. Subjects and methods: Cross-sectional analysis with 468 young adults from the fourth follow-up of the 1978/79 Ribeirão Preto prospective birth cohort, Brazil. BMD, total osteocalcin (OC), fasting plasma glucose and insulin concentrations were assessed. IR, sensitivity (S) and secretion (β) were estimated by homeostasis model assessment (HOMA) indexes. Multiple linear regression models were constructed to estimate the association between BMD and glucose metabolism. Beta coefficient, R^2 and p-values were provided. WC was tested as an effect modifier and OC as a confounder. The covariates were selected based on Direct Acyclic Graph. Results: Significant interaction between BMD (femoral neck and proximal femur areas) and WC on glucose metabolism was observed in the adjusted models. Subjects with increased WC presented a positive association between BMD and log HOMA1-IR while an inverse association was found in those with normal WC (femoral neck $R^2 = 0.17$, p = 0.036; proximal femur $R^2 = 0.16$, p = 0.086). BMD was negatively associated with log HOMA2-S in individuals with increased WC and positively in those with normal WC (femoral neck $R^2 = 0.16$, p = 0.042; proximal femur $R^2 = 0.15$, p = 0.097). No significant associations between BMD, log HOMA2-β and OC and glucose metabolism markers were observed. Conclusions: BMD was associated with glucose metabolism, independently of OC, and WC modifies this association. Arch Endocrinol Metab. 2018;62(3):285-95

Keywords
Insulin resistance; glucose metabolism; bone mineral density; bone turnover markers; osteocalcin; bone formation markers

INTRODUCTION

Insulin resistance (IR) is characterized by a reduction of the action of the hormone in targets sites, such as muscle, adipose tissue and the liver, resulting in hyperglycemia. To maintain glucose homeostasis, the pancreas adapts through changes in the pancreatic β-cells, resulting in increased insulin secretion. However, exceeding the functional and adaptive capacity can result in the development of type 2 diabetes mellitus (DM2) (1).

Several factors, such as being overweight, age, sex, skin color and lifestyle (physical activity, smoking and alcohol intake) (2-8), may be involved in the etiology of IR. Visceral obesity, is associated with a chronic inflammatory response associated with the development

of IR (1). In addition to these classic factors, a possible role of bone markers in IR was found in experimental models (9).

Bone mineral density (BMD) results of the remodeling process, i.e., complex process of bone reabsorption and formation, which include the participation of calcitropic hormones that act directly on osteoblasts, osteoclasts and osteocytes. Osteocalcin (OC) is a protein synthesized by osteoblasts during bone formation and therefore affected by the concentration of calcitropic hormones, such as calcitonin and the parathyroid hormone (10). The visceral adipose tissue is associated with the genesis of osteoclasts and therefore with increased bone reabsorption (11). Thus, this tissue can affect bone turnover and the concentration of bone turnover markers, such as OC, which seems to be inversely associated with body fat in Chinese men (12). Recent investigations have studied the effects of bone turnover markers in glucose metabolism, adding evidence of the existence of a possible bone-pancreas endocrine axis (9,13). OC seems to be positively associated with proliferation of pancreatic β-cells, insulin secretion and sensitivity and inversely associated with IR in experimental models. In humans, these associations remains controversial in the literature (9,14,15).

The association between bone and glucose metabolism is not well defined and few studies have sought to study BMD in this context. We expect an inverse association between BMD and IR in young adults without visceral hyperadiposity, which also appear to have a higher concentration of OC (12), and tested if this is dependent of OC. In individuals with increased waist circumference (WC), we suspect that this association can be modified due to changes in bone metabolism. So we considered WC as a modifying effect on the association between bone and glucose metabolism.

The objective of this study was to evaluate if BMD predicts alterations in glucose metabolism, and assess the potential role of OC in this association. In addition, the relationship between OC and WC was tested in our sample.

SUBJECTS AND METHODS

Study design and participants

This cross-sectional study was developed with data collected in the fourth phase of the prospective cohort study of individuals born in Ribeirão Preto from the 1st of June 1978 to the 31st of May, 1979. At baseline, information was obtained from 9,067 live newborns delivered in the maternity hospitals of Ribeirão Preto. Infants born to mothers who did not reside in the municipality (n = 2,094) and twins (n = 146) were excluded from the original study. The initial sample comprised 6,827 infants born to mothers residing in Ribeirão Preto.

In 2002, when the fourth cohort follow-up was conducted, 5,665 young adults between 23 and 25 years of age were identified as living in the city. Ribeirão Preto consists of 4 geo-economic regions. A sub sample was created from the original study, of which one of

three individuals who lived in the same geo-economic area were invited to participate in this phase of the study, resulting in a total of 2,063 young adults.

Of the 2,063 individuals included in the fourth phase of the cohort, 513 agreed to undergo the BMD evaluation. Seventeen subjects were excluded due to the presence of a condition that would interfere with the clinical assessment or measures of bone metabolism (i.e., type 1 diabetes, asthmatics using corticosteroids, amaurosis, anorexia nervosa, scoliosis, urolithiasis and stroke). Additionally, 28 subjects were lost due to missing data or because their total OC and markers of glucose metabolism (fasting glucose and insulin) were not measured. The final sample of the present study comprised 468 individuals (females = 235) who underwent BMD, OC and HOMA [(homeostasis model assessment (HOMA), IR, insulin sensitivity (S), and β-cell function (β)] evaluations. More detailed information about this cohort can be obtained from previous publication (16).

Measurements

A 40-mL blood sample was collected after 12-hour fasting period. All laboratory tests (fasting insulin and glucose and OC) were analyzed at the time of data collection. Fasting glucose and insulin were determined using commercial kits by GOD/PAP human diagnostic colorimetric enzymatic method (Chronolab AG, Zug, Switzerland) and radioimmunoassay (Insulin kit, DPC, Los Angeles, CA, USA), respectively. OC was determined using an immunoradiometric method (DSL-7600, IRMA, Webster, TX, USA).

IR was estimated using the original HOMA1-IR, calculated according to the formula: fasting plasma glucose (mmol/L) x fasting plasma insulin (µU/mL)/22.5. To estimate insulin sensitivity (HOMA2-S) and secretion (HOMA2-β), we used the HOMA computer model (HOMA2 model), available from https://www.dtu.ox.ac.uk/homacalculator/.

BMD (g/cm^2) were obtained by dual-energy X-ray absorptiometry (DXA) using Hologic QDR-4500 (Waltham, MA, USA) equipment. Measurements of absolute precision error (and the percentage coefficient of variation) for BMD were 0.007 g/cm^2 (0.66%), 0.015 g/cm^2 (1.77%) and 0.007 g/cm^2 (0.70%) for the three evaluated anatomic areas: the lumbar spine, femoral neck and total proximal femur, respectively. The phantom coefficient of variation throughout the study was 0.38%. A standardized technician performed the quality control and all measurements. The analysis was performed in the nuclear medicine laboratory of the Clinics Hospital, Faculty of Medicine of Ribeirão Preto, University of São Paulo, Brazil.

The following socio-demographic and lifestyle variables were obtained through structured questionnaires: sex (male; female), age (23-25), self-classified skin color (white; mulatto/black/yellow), schooling (≤ 8; 9-11 and ≥ 12 years of study) and smoking (smokers; non-smokers).

Physical activity was measured using the short version of the International Physical Activity Questionnaire (IPAQ), validated for the Brazilian population, and categorized as low, moderate, or high activity (17).

Caloric intake (kcal/day) was estimated based on an adaptation of a validated food frequency questionnaire (FFQ) (18). The software Dietsys version 4.0 was used (National Cancer Institute, Bethesda, MD, USA). Alcohol consumption was estimated based on the FFQ, expressed as a percentage of total dietary energy per day.

Adult weight and height were obtained using standardized techniques. A mechanical scale (Filizola, São Paulo, Brazil) with an accuracy of 100 g and a freestanding wood stadiometer (University of São Paulo, Ribeirão Preto, Brazil) with an accuracy of 0.1 cm were used. Body mass index (BMI) was categorized as < 25 (underweight or normal weight), 25 to 29.9 (overweight) and ≥ 30 kg/m^2 (obesity) (19).

Waist circumference (WC) was measured by a D-loop non-stretch fiberglass tape as the smallest circumference between the ribs and the iliac crest while the subject stood with the abdomen relaxed at the end of a normal expiration. The individuals were classified as normal/increased WC (women: < 80 cm; ≥ 80 cm; men: < 94 cm; ≥ 94 cm) according to cutoff points of WC proposed by the World Health Organization (WHO) (20).

Ethics

This study was approved by the Research Ethics Committee of the Clinics Hospital, Faculty of Medicine of Ribeirão Preto, University of São Paulo, Brazil, in February 2000 (protocol no. 7606/99).

Statistical analyses

The subject characteristics were described using means (standard deviation) and p-value refers to the Student's

t-test or median (interquartile range) and Mann-Whitney U test. Categorical variables are expressed as absolute and relative frequency and compared by qui-squared test.

The study outcomes were described using medians and interquartile ranges stratified by categories of potentially associated factors. Continuous variables were categorized into tertiles, and comparisons between categories were performed using Mann-Whitney U and Kruskal-Wallis tests.

To evaluate the association between BMD and IR (HOMA1-IR), sensitivity (HOMA2-S) and secretion (HOMA2-β), multiple linear regression models were fitted for each outcome. For this analysis, HOMA1-IR, HOMA2-S and HOMA2-β were log-transformed.

WC was tested as an effect modifier in multiple linear regression models considering that inflammation associated with visceral adipose tissue can affect bone metabolism markers, which may explain the association between BMD and IR. We constructed linear prediction plots of the associations between each anatomic bone area (spinal, femoral neck and proximal femur) and the outcomes, stratified by WC cutoff points (normal/increased), in order to interpret the interactions.

The covariates were selected for inclusion in the final model based on a directed acyclic graph [(DAG, www.dagitty.net), Figure S1]. A DAG is a graphic model in which potential confounding factors that can distort the causal inference process can be identified and included as covariates in adjusted models (21). DAGs can make more explicit the relationship between exposure and outcome and help avoid inappropriate adjustments.

OC concentration was included in the models as a confounder because of its association with both the exposure and the outcome. We tested whether the association between BMD and glucose metabolism is dependent of OC or if there is an independent pathway linking BMD and IR. The relationship between OC and WC was tested by Pearson correlation test, stratified by sex.

In the analysis, associations with p-value < 0.05 were considered significant, except in the evaluation of interactions, in which a p-value < 0.1 was considered significant (22). The regression analysis provided a beta coefficient, the co-variable for the p-value, the R^2 (variation explained by the models) for each model, and the p-value of all the multiple models. All analyses were performed using Stata Data Analysis and Statistical Software (STATA) version 12.0, 2011, College Station, TX (StataCorp LP).

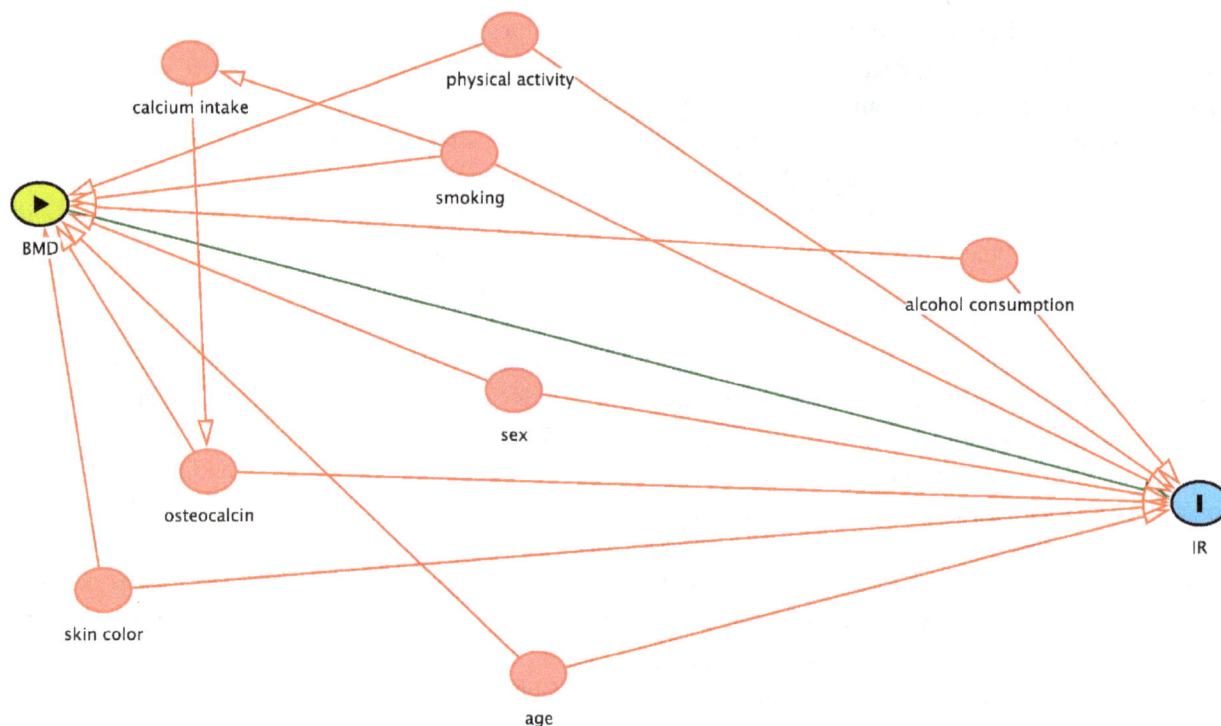

Figure S1. Causal diagram of the association between BMD and IR. Minimal sufficient adjustment sets for estimating the total effect of BMD and IR, suggested by DAG – age, alcohol consumption, osteocalcin, physical activity, sex, skin color and smoking. Colors of variables: green – exposure; blue – outcome; red – co variables.

RESULTS

We evaluated 468 (233 men and 235 women) adults. The study participants had a mean age of 23.5 (0.5) years and a mean BMI of 23.7 (4.2) kg/m². The majority of the sample was white (65%), presented normal WC (78%), had more than 8 years of schooling (88%), reported moderate or high physical activity (74%) and were non-smokers (85%). The mean calorie intake and alcohol consumption were 2,188.9 (713.4) kcal/day and 1.8% (2.3) of EI/day, respectively. The median (interquartile range) of IR, insulin sensitivity and β-cell function were 1.1 (0.7:1.7), 136.6 (92.7:217.9) and 98.1 (73.7:132.4), respectively. Men presented higher IR and lower insulin secretion compared to women (p < 0.05). The mean OC concentration was 12.6 (5.1) ng/mL, and the BMD was 1.0 (0.1) g/cm² for the spinal anatomic area, 0.9 (0.2) g/cm² for the femoral neck and 1.0 (0.2) g/cm² for the proximal femur.

Higher mean of OC and BMD (spinal, femoral neck and proximal femur) were detected among men (p < 0.001) (Table 1).

A positive association between nutritional status markers (BMI and WC) and HOMA1-IR and HOMA2-β and an inverse association with HOMA2-S was found (p < 0.001 for all). Individuals who reported low physical activity had higher median HOMA1-IR (p = 0.007) and HOMA2-β values (p < 0.001) and lower HOMA2-S values (p = 0.002) than those reporting moderate or high levels of physical activity. The median HOMA1-IR and HOMA2-β levels differed between the sexes, i.e., men presented higher mean IR values (p = 0.016) and lower hormone secretion (p = 0.024) than women. Subjects classified in the 1st tertile of OC presented significantly higher median levels of HOMA2-β than those in the 2nd and 3rd tertiles (p = 0.018). The femoral neck and proximal femur BMD were inversely associated with insulin sensitivity

Table 1. Descriptive characteristics of a young adults sample, 2002-2004 Ribeirão Preto cohort, Brazil, fourth follow-up

Characteristics	Total (n = 468)	Men (n = 233)	Women (n = 235)	p-value[1]
Age (years)	23.5 (0.5)	23.5 (0.03)	23.5 (0.03)	0.312
BMI (kg/m²)	23.7 (4.2)	24.7 (0.27)	22.7 (0.26)	**< 0.001**
WC (cm)[2]				**0.025**
Normal	363 (78.0)	180 (49.6)	183 (50.4)	
Increased	105 (22.0)	53 (50.5)	52 (49.5)	
Skin color				0.070
White	304 (65.0)	142 (46.7)	162 (53.3)	
Black/mullato/yellow	164 (35.0)	91 (55.5)	73 (44.5)	
Schooling (years)				0.277
≤ 8	58 (12.0)	27 (46.5)	31 (53.5)	
9-11	262 (56.0)	139 (53.0)	123 (47.0)	
≥ 12	148 (32.0)	67 (45.3)	81 (54.7)	
Energy intake (kcal/day)	2188.9 (713.4)	2415.9 (45.8)	1963.8 (42.6)	**< 0.001**
Alcohol consumption (% of EI/day)	1.8 (2.3)	2.44 (0.16)	1.13 (0.12)	**< 0.001**
Physical activity				**0.002**
Low	121 (26)	46 (38.0)	75 (62.0)	
Moderate	200 (43)	99 (49.5)	101 (50.5)	
High	147 (31)	88 (59.9)	59 (40.1)	
Smoking				**0.016**
Yes	68 (85.0)	43 (63.2)	25 (36.8)	
No	400 (15.0)	190 (47.5)	210 (52.5)	
HOMA1-IR	1.1 (0.7;1.7)	1.26 (0.78;1.92)	1.1 (0.7;1.5)	**0.016**
HOMA2-S	136.6 (92.7;217.9)	131.5 (83.1;204.8)	140.2 (100;223.6)	0.104
HOMA2-β	98.1 (73.7;132.4)	92.4 (69.9;131)	104.3 (76.5;134.2)	**0.024**
Osteocalcin (ng/mL)	12.6 (5.1)	14.01 (0.33)	11.22 (0.31)	**< 0.001**
BMD Spinal (g/cm²)	1.0 (0.1)	1.06 (0.00)	0.99 (0.00)	**< 0.001**
BMD Femoral neck (g/cm²)	0.9 (0.2)	1.00 (0.01)	0.84 (0.00)	**< 0.001**
BMD Proximal femur (g/cm²)	1.0 (0.2)	1.09 (0.01)	0.90 (0.00)	**< 0.001**

Continuous variables are expressed as mean (standard deviation) and [1] p-value refers to the Student's t-test or median (interquartile range) and Mann-Whitney U test. Categorical variables are expressed as absolute and relative frequency and compared by qui-squared test. [2] Categorized using World Health Organization cutoff points, normal WC: < 80 cm for women and < 94 cm for men; increased WC: ≥ 80 cm for women and ≥ 94 cm for men.
For EI variable, we had 1 exclusion due to high calorie value (> 6000 kcal/day).
BMI: body mass index; WC: waist circumference; EI: energy intake; HOMA: homeostatic model assessment; HOMA1-IR: insulin resistance; HOMA2-S: insulin sensitivity; HOMA2-β: β-cell function (insulin secretion); BMD: bone mineral density.

(p = 0.036 and p = 0.002) and were positively associated with IR (p = 0.013 and p < 0.001) (Table 2).

A significant inverse correlation between OC and WC was observed in men (r = -0.23, p = 0.002) and women (r = -0.15, p = 0.020) (data not shown).

We found a significant interaction between BMD (femoral neck and proximal femur) and WC in the fully adjusted regression (p < 0.1). We observed a positive association between BMD and the log HOMA1-IR level in individuals with increased WC and an inverse association in those with normal WC (femoral neck R^2 = 0.17, p=0.036; proximal femur R^2 = 0.16, p = 0.086). BMD was negatively associated with the log HOMA2-S level in subjects with increased WC and positively associated in those with normal WC (femoral neck R^2 = 0.16, p = 0.042; proximal femur R^2 = 0.15, p = 0.097). We did not observe significant associations between BMD (spinal, femoral neck and proximal femur) and the log HOMA2-β level and OC and the log HOMA1-IR, HOMA2-S and HOMA2-β levels (Table 3 and Figures 1 and 2).

Table 2. Distribution of insulin resistance (HOMA1-IR[1]), insulin sensitivity (HOMA2-S[2]) and β cell function (HOMA2-β[2]) in 468 young adults according to categories of selected variables, 2002-2004 Ribeirão Preto cohort, Brazil, fourth follow-up

	n	HOMA1–IR	p1	HOMA2-S	p1	HOMA2-β	p1
BMI (kg/m²)							
< 25	312	1.0 (0.6;1.4)[a]		157.9 (110.6;247.2)[a]		92.0 (70.2;122.2)[a]	
≥ 25-29.9	116	1.4 (0.9;1.9)[b]		116.3 (84.9;170.1)[b]		108.9 (77.9;139.5)[b]	
≥ 30	40	2.5 (1.5;3.3)[c]	**< 0.001**	68.9 (50.3;100.0)[c]	**< 0.001**	144.4 (109.8;182.0)[c]	**< 0.001**
WC[2]							
Normal	363	1.0 (0.6;1.5)		154.5 (108.0;242.7)		92.3 (70.5;122.0)	
Increased	105	1.8 (1.1;3.2)	**< 0.001**	88.9 (55.4;135.4)	**< 0.001**	129.4 (95.0;165.5)	**< 0.001**
Sex							
Women	235	1.1 (0.7;1.5)		140.2 (100.0;224.8)		104.3 (76.5;134.2)	
Men	233	1.3 (0.8-1.9)	**0.016**	131.5 (83.1;204.8)	0.105	92.4 (69.9;131.0)	**0.024**
Physical activity							
Low	121	1.3 (0.9;2.0)[a]		118.5 (80.9;174.7)[a]		111.8 (88.5;147.5)[a]	
Moderate	200	1.1 (0.7;1.6)[b]		136.7 (101.4;228.0)[b]		94.6 (72.8;126.3)[b]	
High	147	1.0 (0.6;1.7)[b]	**0.007**	152.1 (93.9;262.4)[b]	**0.002**	87.5 (67.0;125.8)[b]	**< 0.001**
Smoking							
No	400	1.1 (0.7;1.7)		136.0 (95.0;217.9)		98.7 (73.7;131.3)	
Yes	68	1.1 (0.7;1.9)	0.907	146.5 (82.5;214.1)	0.890	94.5 (69.9;147.9)	0.955
Skin color							
White	304	1.1 (0.7;1.6)		141.1 (97.8;223.9)		95.1 (72.4;129.3)	
Black/mullato/yellow	164	1.2 (0.8;2.0)	0.055	128.8 (81.2;194.3)	0.055	100.4 (74.9;141.5)	0.154
Schooling (years)							
≤ 8	58	1.2 (0.7;2.0)		117.6 (77.2;208.6)		104.9 (76.4;135.8)	
9-11	262	1.2 (0.7;1.7)		133.6 (90.2;211.9)		97.5 (72.9;131.7)	
≥ 12	148	1.1 (0.7;1.6)	0.177	151.2 (100.7;221.6)	0.117	95.6 (73.8;132.5)	0.349
Alcohol consumption (% of EI/day)							
1st and 2nd tertiles (0.0-2.1)	315	1.1 (0.7;1.7)		136.1 (93.9;217.5)		98.3 (74.8;134.0)	
3rd tertile (2.2-12.1)	153	1.1 (0.7;1.7)	0.727	139.8 (89.6;218.4)	0.857	98.0 (69.1;130.2)	0.479
Energy intake (kcal/day)							
1st and 2nd tertiles (851.1-2377.6)	313	1.1 (0.7;1.6)		141.3 (96.6;211.9)		98.9 (73.8;134.2)	
3rd tertile (2394.1-4940.7)	154	1.3 (0.7;1.8)	0.221	125.7 (88.5;219.1)	0.363	96.5 (72.1;131.0)	0.602
Osteocalcin (ng/mL)							
1st tertile (2.9-9.6)	151	1.2 (0.8;1.9)		131.8 (83.5;197.6)		106.6 (78.5;144.6)[a]	
2nd tertile (9.8-14.3)	161	1.1 (0.7;1.6)		139.8 (99.7;219.1)		93.8 (72.9;130.2)[b]	
3rd tertile (14.4-32.9)	156	1.1 (0.6;1.7)	0.174	151.1 (95.0;238.6)	0.110	93.4 (68.6;120.7)[b]	**0.018**
BMD Spinal (g/cm²)							
1st and 2nd tertiles (0.7-1.1)	309	1.1 (0.7;1.6)		141.0 (97.2;224.3)		98.5 (73.1;130.2)	
3rd tertile (1.1-1.4)	159	1.2 (0.7;1.8)	0.062	123.0 (85.4;200.0)	0.089	97.0 (74.5;134.6)	0.415
BMD Femoral neck (g/cm²)							
1st and 2nd tertiles (0.5-1.0)	310	1.1 (0.7;1.6)		140.6 (99.4;229.5)		99.9 (73.7;130.9)	
3rd tertile (1.0-1.5)	158	1.3 (0.8;1.9)	**0.013**	125.7 (80.9;197.2)	**0.036**	95.3 (73.7;135.8)	0.864
BMD Proximal femur (g/cm²)							
1st and 2nd tertiles (0.6-1.0)	309	1.1 (0.7;1.5)		147.2 (100.0;229.5)		99.0 (73.7;129.3)	
3rd tertile (1.0-1.5)	159	1.4 (0.9;2.3)	**< 0.001**	115.7 (75.0;180.8)	**0.002**	96.3 (73.7;141.4)	0.447

[1] p-value refers to Kruskall Wallis test and Mann-Whitney U test. Values with differing superscript letters (a, b, c) denote statistically significant differences across the categories.

[2] Categorized using World Health Organization cutoff points, normal WC: < 80 cm for women and < 94 cm for men; increased WC: ≥ 80 cm for women and ≥ 94 cm for men.

Data are expressed as median (interquartile range). For EI variable, we had 1 exclusion due to high calorie value (> 6000 kcal/day).

HOMA: homeostatic model assessment; HOMA1-IR: insulin resistance; HOMA2-S: insulin sensitivity; HOMA2-β: β-cell function (insulin secretion); BMI: body mass index; WC: waist circumference; EI: energy intake; BMD: bone mineral density.

Table 3. Linear regression between bone mineral density (BMD; g/cm²) and insulin resistance (HOMA1-IR[1]), insulin sensitivity (HOMA2-S[2]) and β cell function (HOMA2-β[2]) in 468 young adults, 2002-2004 Ribeirão Preto cohort, Brazil, fourth follow-up

	HOMA1-IR				HOMA2-S				HOMA2-β			
	Model 1 β¹ (95% CI)	p²	Model 2 β¹ (95% CI)	p²	Model 1 β¹ (95% CI)	p²	Model 2 β¹ (95% CI)	p²	Model 1 β¹ (95% CI)	p²	Model 2 β¹ (95% CI)	p²
BMD - Spinal												
Spinal (g/cm²)	-0.2 (-0.8;0.4)	0.510	-0.5 (-1.1;0.1)	0.133	0.2 (-0.3;0.8)	0.432	0.4 (-0.2;1.0)	0.160	-0.2 (-0.6;0.1)	0.196	-0.2 (-0.5;0.2)	0.424
WC (normal/increased)³	-0.0 (-1.4;1.3)	0.936	-0.2 (-1.6;1.2)	0.763	0.1 (-1.2;1.4)	0.885	0.2 (-1.1;1.5)	0.760	-0.1 (-1.0;0.7)	0.735	-0.1 (-1.0;0.8)	0.836
Interaction term												
Spinal#WC	0.6 (-0.7;1.9)	0.344	0.8 (-0.5;2.0)	0.246	-0.6 (-1.8;0.6)	0.324	-0.7 (-1.9;0.5)	0.256	0.4 (-0.4;1.2)	0.322	0.3 (-0.5;1.2)	0.401
Osteocalcin (ng/mL)	-0.0 (-0.0;0.0)	0.230	-0.0 (-0.0;0.0)	0.114	0.0 (-0.0;0.0)	0.189	0.0 (-0.0;0.0)	0.139	-0.0 (-0.0;0.0)	0.079	-0.0 (-0.0;0.0)	0.364
R²⁴	0.13		0.16		0.12		0.15		0.08		0.11	
BMD - Femoral neck (FN)												
FN (g/cm²)	-0.1 (-0.6;0.3)	0.553	-0.5 (-1.0;0.0)	0.052	0.2 (-0.2;0.6)	0.385	0.5 (-0.0;1.0)	0.066	-0.2 (-0.5;0.1)	**0.038**	-0.2 (-0.5;0.1)	0.245
WC (normal/increased)³	-0.4 (-1.3;0.5)	0.395	-0.3 (-1.3;0.5)	0.440	0.4 (-0.5;1.3)	0.383	0.3 (-0.5;1.2)	0.457	-0.2 (-0.8;0.3)	0.392	-0.1 (-0.7;0.4)	0.606
Interaction term												
FN#WC	1.0 (0.1;1.9)	**0.032**	1.0 (0.1;1.9)	**0.036**	-1.0 (-1.9;-0.1)	**0.033**	-0.9 (-1.8;-0.0)	**0.042**	0.6 (-0.0;1.2)	**0.061**	0.4 (-0.1;1.0)	0.135
Osteocalcin (ng/mL)	-0.0 (-0.0;0.0)	0.269	-0.0 (-0.0;0.0)	0.119	0.0 (-0.0;0.0)	0.228	0.0 (-0.0;0.0)	0.144	-0.0 (-0.0;0.0)	0.110	-0.0 (-0.0;0.0)	0.378
R²⁴	0.13		0.17		0.13		0.16		0.09		0.11	
BMD - Proximal femur (PF)												
PF (g/cm²)	-0.1 (-0.5;0.4)	0.799	-0.5 (-1.0;0.0)	0.080	0.1 (-0.3;0.5)	0.571	0.4 (-0.1;0.9)	0.098	-0.2 (-0.5;0.2)	0.047	-0.2 (-0.5;0.2)	0.307
WC (normal/increased)³	-0.2 (-1.2;0.7)	0.617	-0.2 (-1.2;0.7)	0.638	0.2 (-0.7;1.1)	0.605	0.2 (-0.7;1.1)	0.647	-0.1 (-0.7;0.5)	0.591	-0.1 (-0.7;0.5)	0.726
Interaction term												
PF#WC	0.8 (-0.1;1.7)	**0.090**	0.8 (-0.1;1.7)	**0.086**	-0.8 (-1.6; 0.1)	**0.091**	-0.7 (-1.6;0.1)	**0.097**	0.4 (-0.1;1.0)	0.137	0.4 (-0.2;1.0)	0.205
Osteocalcin (ng/mL)	-0.0 (-0.0; 0.0)	0.248	-0.0 (-0.0;0.0)	0.113	0.0 (-0.0;0.0)	0.212	0.0 (-0.0;0.0)	0.138	-0.0 (-0.0;0.0)	0.106	-0.0 (-0.0;0.0)	0.373
R²⁴	0.13		0.16		0.12		0.15		0.08		0.11	

[1] Linear regression coefficient; [2] p-value refers to linear regression. [3] Categorized using World Health Organization cutoff points, normal WC: < 80 cm for women and < 94 cm for men; increased WC: ≥ 80 cm for women and ≥ 94 cm for men. [4] R² refers to the outcome variation explained by the models.

Model 1 was adjusted only for osteocalcin. Model 2 was further adjusted for physical activity, smoking, alcohol intake, sex, age and skin color. All the multiple models were statically significant (p-value < 0.001).

CI: confidence interval; HOMA: homeostatic model assessment; HOMA1-IR: insulin resistance; HOMA2-S: insulin sensitivity; HOMA2-β: β-cell function (insulin secretion); WC: waist circumference; BMD: bone mineral density.

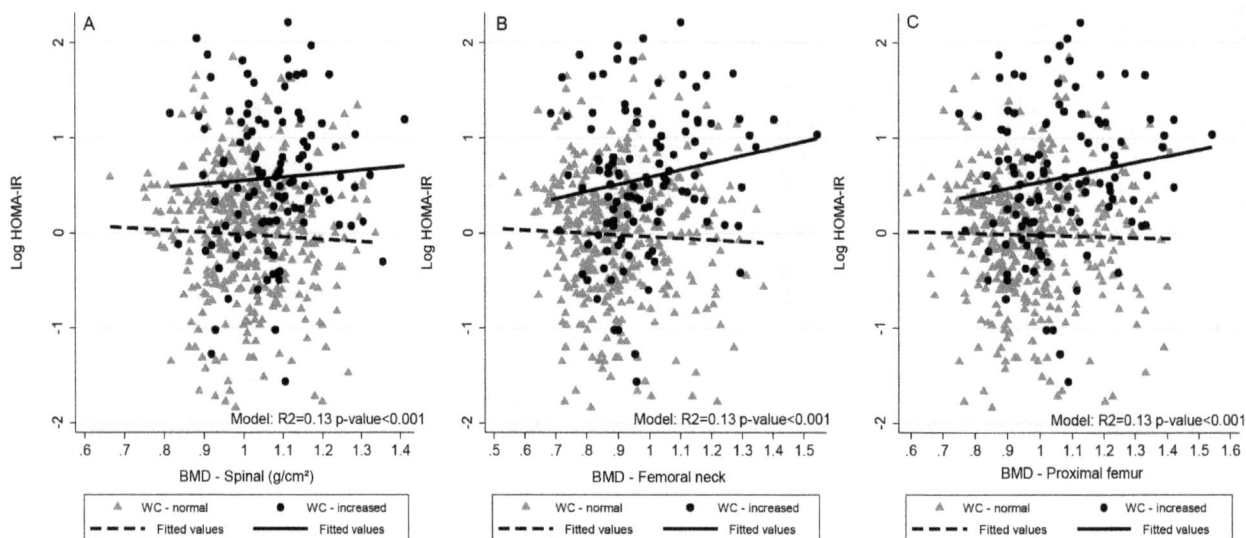

Figure 1. Scatter and linear prediction between BMD and Log HOMA1-IR according to WC in 468 young adults, 2002-2004 Ribeirão Preto, Brazil, fourth cross-sectional evaluation. **A)** Spinal BMD. **B)** Femoral neck BMD. **C)** Proximal femur BMD.
HOMA1-IR: homeostatic model assessment – insulin resistance; WC: waist circumference; BMD: bone mineral density.
Fitted values were predicted using linear regression models; WC was categorized using World Health Organization cutoff points, normal WC: < 80 cm for women and < 94 cm for men; increased WC: ≥ 80 cm for women and ≥ 94 cm for men.

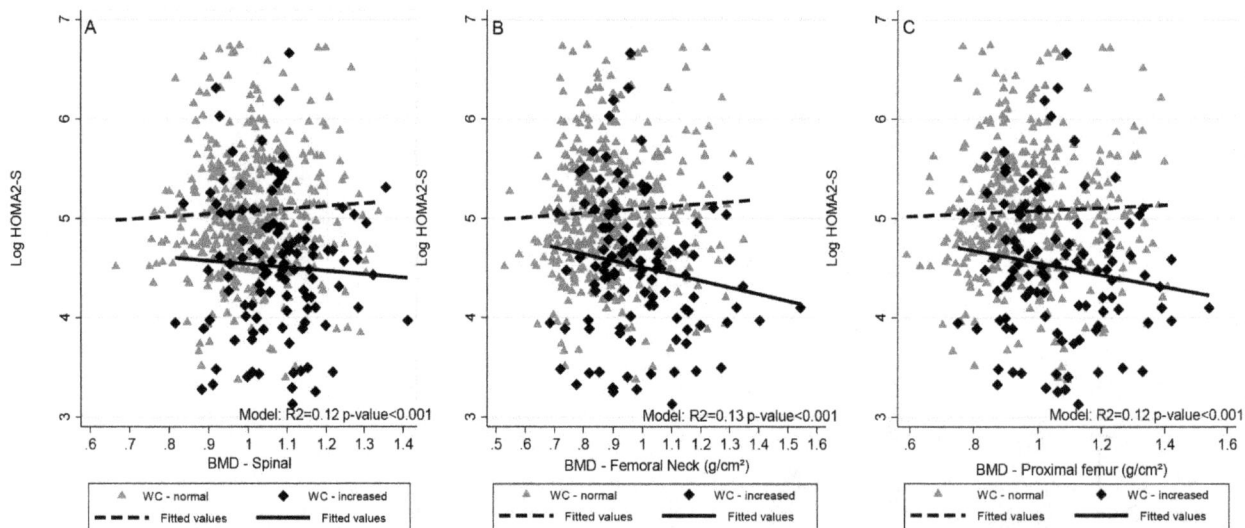

Figure 2. Scatter and linear prediction between BMD and Log HOMA2-S according to WC in 468 young adults, 2002-2004 Ribeirão Preto, Brazil, fourth cross-sectional evaluation. **A)** Spinal BMD. **B)** Femoral neck BMD. **C)** Proximal femur BMD.
HOMA2-S: homeostatic model assessment – insulin sensitivity; WC: waist circumference; BMD: bone mineral density.
Fitted values were predicted using linear regression models; WC was categorized using World Health Organization cutoff points, normal WC: < 80 cm for women and < 94 cm for men; increased WC: ≥ 80 cm for women and ≥ 94 cm for men.

DISCUSSION

The present study has three main results. First, we found that BMD predict alterations in glucose metabolism in young adults. Second, we observed that the direction of the association differed according to WC classification,

i.e., adults with increased WC had a positive association between BMD and IR, while those with normal WC had an inverse association between these two markers. The association between BMD and insulin sensitivity occurred in the opposite direction, i.e., we observed an inverse association in individuals with increased WC and a positive association in those with normal WC. Finally, we did not observe any significant association between OC and glucose metabolism in the adjusted models.

This study has some potential limitations. Although we used a large sample size from a birth cohort, only 24.9% (n = 513/2,063) of the individuals evaluated in the fourth phase of the birth cohort follow-up consented to undergo DXA assessments, and after exclusions, the final sample comprised 468 subjects who had valid BMD measurements. In addition, although WC is a very practical and internationally used tool to evaluate the deposition of intra-abdominal fat, recommended by WHO (20), its use has as a limitation the fact that it does not separate visceral adipose tissue of the subcutaneous tissue. Moreover, it was not possible to use the WHO protocol to measure waist circumference (WC) in our study, because data collection occurred from 2002 to 2004, while the WHO STEPS protocol was published in 2008 (23). Additionally, this study was based on a cross-sectional analysis, a study design that cannot determine whether the results are merely associations or if BMD exerts a causal effect on glucose metabolism in these young adults. Finally, although in experimental studies OC uncarboxilated has been reported to be the metabolically active form (9,13), we did not differentiate plasma OC by gamma-carboxylation status, and our assessment included all forms of OC. The strength of this study is the number of young adults evaluated by DXA, a very accurate procedure for measuring bone density. Moreover, in the multivariate analysis, we evaluated the inclusion of co-variables based on a DAG that allows for the minimization of bias in epidemiological studies. DAGs allows the identification of the minimum sufficient adjustment to estimate the total and direct effect of a certain exposure on the studied outcome (21). To the best of our knowledge, this is only the second study that has evaluated if BMD, assessed by a gold standard measure (DXA), predict alterations in glucose metabolism (IR, sensitivity and secretion) in young adults.

This study provides new information about the association between bone and glucose metabolism. We found a significant association between BMD and IR and insulin sensitivity and a significant interaction between BMD and WC. A non-significant association between BMD and glucose metabolism (plasma glucose and serum insulin) has been found in the unadjusted

model, which persisted after adjusting the analysis in 155 healthy young adults (24). In that study, although fat mass was considered a confounder, the adipose tissue was not tested as an effect modifier in the association between bone and glucose metabolism (24), as done in our study.

It is known that body fat, particularly visceral fat, may affect bone metabolism markers and BMD. Chronic low-grade inflammation associated with visceral fat is related to the genesis of osteoclasts, increased bone resorption and decreased OC concentration (11,12). Individuals with obesity present increased risk of fractures possibly associated with metabolic dysfunction that result in reduction of bone turnover and bone quality (25). Therefore, considering the effects of inflammation on bone turnover and mass, our conceptual framework considers that WC plays an important role in the association between BMD and IR. We have hypothesized that WC acts as an effect modifier and not as a confounder, and for this reason, this marker of visceral fat deposition was not included in the DAG that depicted the theoretical relationship between all involved variables.

OC is one of the most studied bone biomarkers in the association with glucose metabolism. In the current study, it was observed an inverse correlation between OC and WC in a sample of predominantly white young adults of both sexes (data not shown). These results corroborates with the inverse relationship between OC and visceral fat area found in Chinese men (12) and an inverse relationship between OC and trunk fat in men with obesity (26). These findings suggest a negative effect of adipose tissue, especially visceral fat, on OC.

Despite this, we did not find a significant association between OC concentrations and HOMA1-IR or HOMA2-S in either the crude or adjusted analysis. Animal studies, however, have demonstrated the positive effect of OC on insulin secretion and the sensitivity and proliferation of pancreatic β-cells (9,27). To exert these effects, OC binds to its receptor GPCR6a in pancreatic β-cells and can also increase the expression of anti-inflammatory adipokines and reduce the secretion of pro-inflammatory cytokines (13). In humans, the findings remain controversial. In line with our results, 137 young adults (18.6 years) were evaluated and no association was found between OC and HOMA1-IR (28). In addition, other studies found no association between OC and HOMA1-IR, HOMA2-β, QUICKI insulin sensitivity marker, blood glucose and insulin in pre- and post-menopausal women (14,29). On the other hand, some studies have found an inverse association between OC and IR and a positive association between OC and insulin sensitivity and secretion (12,26,30). The differences between these studies and ours may be explained by the fact that we studied healthy young adults while the others studies investigated older people (approximately 50 years of age) and/or individuals with obesity, which tend to have higher IR. Moreover, we also found methodological differences as most studies used only correlation statistical procedures (12,26), and only one study performed adjusted regression models like ours (30). Unlike our study, none of the published articles evaluated the selection of covariates with a DAG model. Finally, we expected that the addition of OC in the regression model could explain the association between BMD and IR, however, we observed that associations between bone and glucose metabolism is independent of this bone metabolism marker (because the inclusion of OC in the regression model did not affect the association between BMD and glucose metabolism).

Some studies have demonstrated that osteoprotegerin (OPG), that promotes bone formation, appears to be increased in metabolic disorders, such as obesity (31), and in individuals with obesity was found a positive association between OPG and HOMA1-IR (32). In experimental study, OPG increased inflammation in adipose tissue (33). This association of OPG with inflammation may explain its association with IR. In addition to OPG, the amino terminal propeptide of procollagen type 1 (P1NP), a marker of bone formation as OC, was also positively associated with HOMA1-IR in young women with overweight or obesity (15). In view of this, we suggest that further studies be performed to investigate the action of biomarkers other than OC, that may explain the positive association between BMD and HOMA1-IR observed in our study.

Individuals in the accrual phase present higher speed of bone mass gain, especially until reaching peak bone mass. Considering that in our study we found a positive effect of BMD on IR in young individuals with increased WC, it can be concluded that this is a critical phase of life, associated with increased metabolic risk. It is recognized that IR is involved in the pathophysiology of DM2, a global public health problem. The association between bone and IR suggests the existence of bone-pancreas axis. However, the exact mechanism that links bone mass and glucose metabolism is not fully understood, and this study sought to contribute evidence to clarify this relation. We believe that a better understanding of this association can contribute to improve IR. Corroborating this statement, other studies have been developed with the aim of modulating pharmacologically bone metabolism markers to improve glycemic control (34). Additionally, disorders associated with IR, such as obesity, seem related to reduced bone quality and formation and increased bone fracture risk (25). Thus, the investigation of the relationship between bone and glucose metabolism may not only contribute to the glycemic control but also to bone fragility prevention.

Moreover, as expected, we found that subjects with obesity and those with increased WC present higher IR and secretion and lower insulin sensitivity. Individuals with obesity were evaluated and it was identified that those with a higher percentage of lean mass also had higher insulin sensitivity and lower inflammatory status (35). Greater insulin secretion was found in individuals who have greater IR, which characterizes the pancreatic response in compensation of IR (1).

It is known that the increased secretion of adiponectin and the positive effect of estrogen on glucose homeostasis contributes to the lower IR observed in women compared to men (6), as found in our results. In addition, we found that men had a higher mean BMI compared to women, which may also explain the higher rate of IR in this group.

We conclude that BMD was associated with glucose metabolism and this association is independent of OC. We also found that the WC modifies the association between BMD and IR and sensitivity. These results indicate that bone may play a role in the metabolic profile of IR and obesity. However, further studies are needed to assess the direction of the association between BMD and IR and to test the possible mechanisms involved in this relationship.

Author contributions: all authors have made substantial contributions on analysis and interpretation of data; have drafted the article and revised it critically; have seen and approved the contents of the submitted manuscript.

Funding: this study was funded by the São Paulo Research Foundation – Fapesp, National Council for Scientific and Technological Development (CNPq), and Brazilian Coordination Body for the Training of University Level Personnel (Capes).

REFERENCES

1. Kahn SE, Hull RL, Utzschneider KM. Mechanisms linking obesity to insulin resistance and type 2 diabetes. Nature. 2006;444(7121):840-6.

2. Willi C, Bodenmann P, Ghali WA, Faris PD, Cornuz J. Active smoking and the risk of type 2 diabetes: a systematic review and meta-analysis. JAMA. 2007;298(22):2654-64.

3. Kim JY, Lee DY, Lee YJ, Park KJ, Kim KH, Kim JW, et al. Chronic alcohol consumption potentiates the development of diabetes through pancreatic β-cell dysfunction. World J Biol Chem. 2015;6(1):1-15.

4. Li L, Yin X, Yu D, Li H. Impact of physical activity on glycemic control and insulin resistance: a study of community-dwelling diabetic patients in Eastern China. Intern Med. 2016;55(9):1055-60.

5. Jung UJ, Choi MS. Obesity and its metabolic complications: the role of adipokines and the relationship between obesity, inflammation, insulin resistance, dyslipidemia and nonalcoholic fatty liver disease. Int J Mol Sci. 2014;15(4):6184-223.

6. Geer EB, Shen W. Gender differences in insulin resistance, body composition, and energy balance. Gend Med. 2009;6 Suppl 1:60-75.

7. Piccolo RS, Subramanian SV, Pearce N, Florez JC, McKinlay JB. Relative contributions of socioeconomic, local environmental, psychosocial, lifestyle/behavioral, biophysiological, and ancestral factors to racial/ethnic disparities in type 2 diabetes. Diabetes Care. 2016;39(7):1208-17.

8. Barzilai N, Ferrucci L. Insulin resistance and aging: a cause or a protective response? J Gerontol A Biol Sci Med Sci. 2012;67(12):1329-31.

9. Lee NK, Sowa H, Hinoi E, Ferron M, Ahn JD, Confavreux C, et al. Endocrine regulation of energy metabolism by the skeleton. Cell. 2007;130(3):456-69.

10. De Paula FJA, Rosen CJ. Back to the future: revisiting parathyroid hormone and calcitonin control of bone remodeling. Horm Metab Res. 2010;42(5):299-306.

11. Aguirre L, Napoli N, Waters D, Qualls C, Villareal DT, Armamento-Villareal R. Increasing adiposity is associated with higher adipokine levels and lower bone mineral density in obese older adults. J Clin Endocrinol Metab. 2014;99(9):3290-7.

12. Bao Y, Ma X, Yang R, Wang F, Hao Y, Dou J, et al. Inverse relationship between serum osteocalcin levels and visceral fat area in Chinese men. J Clin Endocrinol Metab. 2013;98(1):345-51.

13. Ferron M, Lacombe J. Regulation of energy metabolism by the skeleton: osteocalcin and beyond. Arch Biochem Biophys. 2014;561:137-46.

14. Lu C, Ivaska KK, Alen M, Wang Q, Törmäkangas T, Xu L, et al. Serum osteocalcin is not associated with glucose but is inversely associated with leptin across generations of nondiabetic women. J Clin Endocrinol Metab. 2012;97(11):4106-14.

15. Lucey AJ, Paschos GK, Thorsdottir I, Martínez JA, Cashman KD, Kiely M. Young overweight and obese women with lower circulating osteocalcin concentrations exhibit higher insulin resistance and concentrations of C-reactive protein. Nutr Res. 2013;33(1):67-75.

16. Barbieri MA, Bettiol H, Silva AA, Cardoso VC, Simões VM, Gutierrez MR, et al. Health in early adulthood: the contribution of the 1978/79 Ribeirão Preto birth cohort. Braz J Med Biol Res. 2006;39(8):1041-55.

17. Craig CL, Marshall AL, Sjöström M, Bauman AE, Booth ML, Ainsworth BE, et al. International physical activity questionnaire: 12-country reliability and validity. Med Sci Sports Exerc. 2003;35(8):1381-95.

18. Ribeiro AB, Cardoso MA. Construção de um questionário de frequência alimentar como subsídio para programas de prevenção de doenças crônicas não transmissíveis. Rev Nutr. 2002;15(2):239-45.

19. World Health Organization (WHO). Physical status: the use and interpretation of anthropometry. Geneva: WHO; 1995. [Technical Report Series 854]

20. World Health Organization (WHO). Obesity: prevention and managing the global epidemic. Geneva: WHO; 1998. [Report of the WHO Consultation on Obesity]

21. Textor J, Hardt J, Knüppel S. DAGitty: a graphical tool for analyzing causal diagrams. Epidemiology. 2011;22(5):745.

22. Twisk J. Applied multilevel analysis: a practical guide. United Kingdom: Cambridge University Press; 2006.

23. World Health Organization (WHO). Waist circumference and waist-hip ratio. Geneva: WHO; 2008. [Report of a WHO expert consultation, 8-11]

24. Pirilä S, Taskinen M, Turanlahti M, Kajosaari M, Mäkitie O, Saarinen-Pihkala UM, et al. Bone health and risk factors of cardiovascular disease – a cross-sectional study in healthy young adults. PLoS One. 2014;9(10):e108040.

25. Nielson CM, Marshall LM, Adams AL, LeBlanc ES, Cawthon PM, Ensrud K, et al.; Osteoporotic Fractures in Men Study Research Group. BMI and fracture risk in older men: the osteoporotic fractures in men study (MrOS). J Bone Miner Res. 2011;26(3):496-502.

26. Migliaccio S, Francomano D, Bruzziches R, Greco EA, Fornari R, Donini LM, et al. Trunk fat negatively influences skeletal and testicular functions in obese men: clinical implications for the aging male. Int J Endocrinol. 2013;2013:182753.

27. Ferron M, Hinoi E, Karsenty G, Ducy P. Osteocalcin differentially regulates beta cell and adipocyte gene expression and affects the development of metabolic diseases in wild-type mice. Proc Natl Acad Sci U S A. 2008;105(13):5266-70.

28. Polgreen LE, Jacobs DR Jr, Nathan BM, Steinberger J, Moran A, Sinaiko AR. Association of osteocalcin with obesity, insulin resistance, and cardiovascular risk factors in young adults. Obesity (Silver Spring). 2012;20(11):2194-201.

29. Caglar GS, Ozdemir ED, Kiseli M, Demirtas S, Cengiz SD. The association of osteocalcin and adiponectin with glucose metabolism in nondiabetic postmenopausal women. Gynecol Obstet Invest. 2014;77(4):255-60.

30. Gravenstein KS, Napora JK, Short RG, Ramachandran R, Carlson OD, Metter EJ, et al. Cross-sectional evidence of a signaling pathway from bone homeostasis to glucose metabolism. J Clin Endocrinol Metab. 2011;96(6):E884-90.

31. Suliburska J, Bogdanski P, Gajewska E, Kalmus G, Sobieska M, Samborski W. The association of insulin resistance with serum osteoprotegerin in obese adolescents. J Physiol Biochem. 2013;69(4):847-53.

32. Gannagé-Yared MH, Yaghi C, Habre B, Khalife S, Noun R, Germanos-Haddad M, et al. Osteoprotegerin in relation to body weight, lipid parameters insulin sensitivity, adipocytokines, and C-reactive protein in obese and non-obese young individuals: results from both cross-sectional and interventional study. Eur J Endocrinol. 2008;158(3):353-9.

33. Bernardi S, Fabris B, Thomas M, Toffoli B, Tikellis C, Candido R, et al. Osteoprotegerin increases in metabolic syndrome and promotes adipose tissue proinflammatory changes. Mol Cell Endocrinol. 2014;394(1-2):13-20.

34. D'Amelio P, Sassi F, Buondonno I, Spertino E, Tamone C, Piano S, et al. Effect of intermittent PTH treatment on plasma glucose in osteoporosis: A randomized trial. Bone. 2015;76:177-84.

35. Fornari R, Francomano D, Greco EA, Marocco C, Lubrano C, Wannenes F, et al. Lean mass in obese adult subjects correlates with higher levels of vitamin D, insulin sensitivity and lower inflammation. J Endocrinol Invest. 2015;38(3):367-72.

8

Effect of one time high dose "stoss therapy" of vitamin D on glucose homeostasis in high risk obese adolescents

Preneet Cheema Brar[1], Maria Contreras[2], Xiaozhou Fan[3], Nipapat Visavachaipan[4]

ABSTRACT

Objective: To study the effect of using a one time high dose "stoss therapy" of vitamin D2 (ergocalciferol: VD2) on indices of insulin sensitivity {whole body sensitivity index: WBISI} and secretion {insulinogenic index: IGI} measured during an oral glucose tolerance test (OGTT) in obese adolescents with VDD (25 OHD; serum metabolite of vit D: < 30 ng/dL). Subjects and methods: In a randomized placebo controlled cross over design 20 obese adolescents with vitamin D deficiency (VDD) had baseline OGTT. Arm A received one time high dose 300,000 IU of ergocalciferol and Arm B received placebo. After 6 weeks the adolescents were reassigned to Arm A if they were in Arm B and vice versa. 25OHD, calcium, parathyroid hormone, comprehensive metabolic panel, urine calcium creatinine ratio were measured at each study visit. OGTTs to assess indices of sensitivity and secretion were done at baseline, 6 weeks and 12 weeks respectively. Results: Adolescents were obese and insulin resistant (mean ± SD: mean age = 15.1 ± 1.9 years; BMI: 32.7 ± 9.8; homeostatic model of insulin resistance: HOMA-IR: 4.2 ± 2.8). Stoss therapy with VD2 increased 25OHD from baseline (16.7 ± 2.9 to 19.5 ± 4.5; p = 0.0029) when compared to the placebo. WBISI (2.8 ± 1.9) showed a trend towards improvement in Rx group (p = 0.0577) after adjustment for covariates. IGI (3 ± 2.2) showed an improvement in both Rx and placebo groups. Conclusions: Our study demonstrated that using a high dose of VD2 (300,000 IU) did not have any beneficial effect on insulin sensitivity (whole body sensitivity index {WBISI}) and secretory indices (insulinogenic index {IGI}) in obese adolescents. High dose "stoss therapy" of VD2 did not appear to have any beneficial effect on glucose homeostasis on obese adolescents. Arch Endocrinol Metab. 2018;62(2):193-200

Keywords
Vitamin D; insulin resistance; prediabetes; obesity

[1] Department of Pediatrics, Division of Pediatric Endocrinology, New York University School of Medicine, New York, USA
[2] Texas Tech University Health Science Center, Department of Pediatrics, Amarillo, Texas, USA
[3] Department of Population Health, New York University School of Medicine, New York, USA
[4] Bumrungrad International Hospital, Bangkok, Thailand

Correspondence to:
Preneet Cheema Brar
160 East 3nd street, L3,
New York 100016, New York,
United States of America
Preneet.Brar@nyumc.org

INTRODUCTION

Low vitamin D levels are consistently seen in 32-50% of obese adolescents (1-3). It is also thought that these low levels could be due to differences in vitamin D metabolizing enzymes in adipose tissue (4,5) and higher volumetric dilution of serum vitamin D, rather than just sequestration in adipose tissue, which could explain these lower levels of vitamin D in obese adolescents when compared to their lean peers.

Vitamin D has been shown in both in vivo and in vitro studies to have effects on beta cell function and insulin sensitivity (6,7). The role of vitamin D in glucose homeostasis is well established and prospective studies have shown that vitamin D deficiency has an inverse and significant association with prediabetes and/or Type 2 diabetes (8,9).

There have been inconsistent results in randomized controlled trials done to study the effect of vitamin D supplementation on parameters of glucose homeostasis in insulin resistance states, in both adults and children, with some showing beneficial effects on insulin sensitivity (10-13) while others did not (14). In adults, the effect of vitamin D on prediabetes and/or T2DM showed beneficial effect in a study by Neyestani and cols. (15) and no effect in another (16). More recently studies using high dosing vitamin D (150,000-300,000 units) over a short duration (4-8 weeks) have also shown conflicting results on insulin sensitivity and secretion in adults with prediabetes (17,18).

There has been no RCT which has been done in obese adolescents with vitamin D deficiency, defined as a 25(OH) D level of < 30 ng/dL (75 nmol/L) (19) and insulin resistance to assess the efficacy of using one time high dose of VD2 on indices of insulin sensitivity and secretion over a short period of time. To summarize we tested whether one time high dose of ergocalciferol (300,000 units) corrected the vitamin D deficiency and improved glucose homeostasis in obese adolescents with insulin resistance.

SUBJECTS AND METHODS

This was a randomized placebo controlled cross over design trial with inclusion criteria that were: a) obese adolescents (BMI: ≥ 95th percentile for age) who were 12-18 years; b) > Tanner 2 for puberty and had vitamin D deficiency defined as a 25(OH)D of ≤ 20 ng/mL (50 nmol/L). Exclusion criteria were: a) treatment with medication known to effect vitamin D, calcium and glucose metabolism, such as glucocorticoids, thiazolidinediones, metformin, anticonvulsants metabolized through cytochrome P-450 (phenytoin, carbamazepine, phenobarbital, sodium valproate); b) vitamin D supplementation greater than 400 IU daily in the preceding 3 months; c) history of nephrolithiasis or hypercalcemia; pregnancy; d) attendance at a tanning salon. The study was approved by the Ethics committee at New York University School of Medicine and consent was obtained from parents and patients.

We chose to use "stoss" therapy {German word stossen means "to push"} based on a recent global consensus for management of vitamin D deficiency (20). The Endocrine society consensus statement recommended 50,000 for 6 weeks for children and adolescents with vitamin D deficiency. Much higher dosing was recommended for obese adults at least 6,000-10,000 per day for 8 weeks (19). We decided to give 300,000 IU as a "stoss dose", a practical choice to improve compliance. Subjects selected for the study were randomized, half to the treatment group (A) and half to the placebo group (B). At week 7, subjects were switched over and reassigned to receive vitamin D if they are in Group B and placebo if they were in Group A and the study lasted 12 weeks from start to completion.

Ergocalciferol (50,000 IU) capsules and placebo capsules were provided at the study visit based on the randomization scheme. Each subject got 6 capsules of study drug or placebo at the study visit totaling 300,000 IU of ergocalciferol or no ergocalciferol at all in the placebo capsules. Each arm of trial lasted 6

weeks with no washout period. Patients were blinded to treatment assignment during the entire study. Study design and recruitment are shown in the study consort diagram (Figure 1).

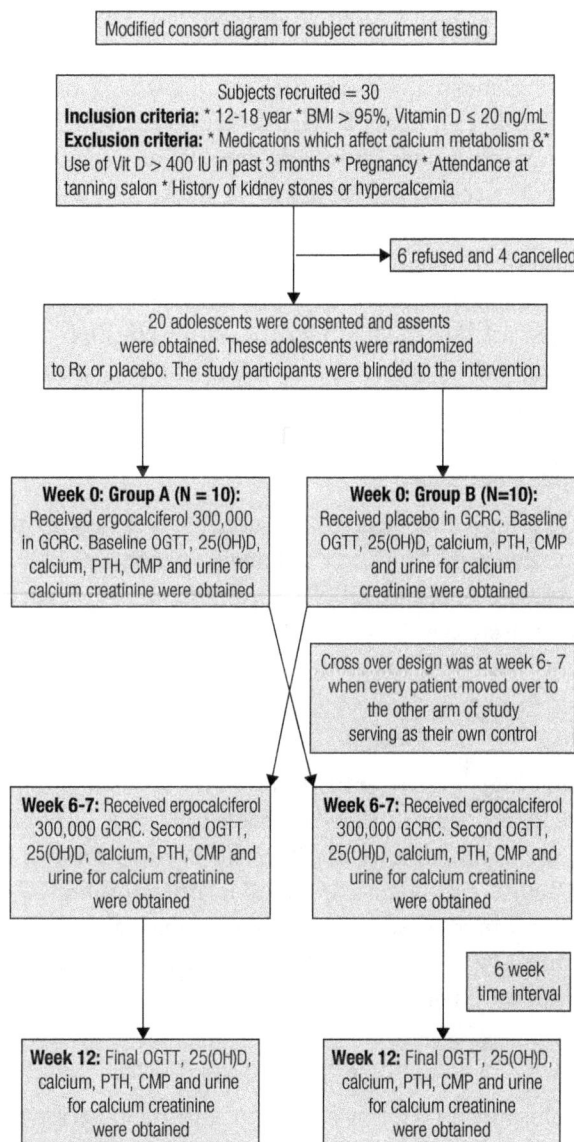

GCRC: General Clinical Research Center.

Figure 1. Consort diagram to show recruitment and study design.

The study subjects had an oral glucose tolerance test with 75 g of glucose solution (OGTT) and screening labs were drawn at baseline, at week 7 and then again week 12 at the completion of the study. Plasma glucose and insulin will were measured using Luminex technology. Serum 25-OH vitamin D were measured using liquid chromatography, tandem mass spectrometry (LC/MS/MS), which consists of extraction via protein precipitation, separation via high-performance liquid chromatography (HPLC), detection and quantitation via tandem mass spectrometry. $25OHD_2$ and $25OHD_3$ concentrations were used to calculate total 25OHD levels. Glycosylated hemoglobin (HbA1C) were measured in red blood cells using HPLC method. Serum calcium (mg/dL), albumin (g/dL) and intact parathyroid hormone (PTH) (pg/mL were measured. Calcium was corrected for the serum albumin {([4-albumin (g/dL)] x 0.8) + calcium (mg/dL)} (21). Intact PTH, 25(OH) D and spot urine calcium/creatinine ratio were checked at completion of the 6 week treatment phase (in week 7) to exclude vitamin D toxicity including hypercalciuria (urine calcium/creatinine ratio ≥ 0.2), hyperphosphatemia (serum phosphate > 5.7 mg/mL), hypercalcemia (serum calcium > 10.5 mg/dL), serum 25(OH) D > 150 ng/mL. Baseline labs were drawn at the same time as 0 minute OGTT.

Primary outcome

OGTT was done glucose solution (1.75 g/kg up to a maximum of 75 g) over a 2-minute period and blood samples were obtained at 0, 10, 30, 60, 90 and 120 minutes. Indices were calculated from OGTTs done at three time points: baseline; 7 week and 12 week time points.

Calculated insulin sensitivity parameter from OGTT

Whole body insulin sensitivity (WBISI) (22) is an insulin sensitivity measure that has been validated in obese children and adolescents (23) calculated as follows = $10,000/\sqrt{(\text{fasting glucose mg/dl} \times \text{fasting insulin}\mu IU/ml) \times (\text{mean glucose} \times \text{mean insulin})}$ during OGTT 1 during OGTT. Higher WBISI levels indicate greater insulin sensitivity.

Calculated insulin secretory parameters from OGTT

Insulin index (IGI): is a measure of insulin secretion that has been validated in children against the hyperglycemic clamp [7], calculated as followed: IGI = [30-minute insulin − fasting plasma insulin (uIU/mL)/[30-minute glucose − fasting plasma glucose (mg/dL)]. Adolescents with Type 2 diabetes have a significant reduction in IGI (24).

Secondary outcome

a. Pre- and post treatment 25 OHD; b. change in serum PTH; c. Biochemical evidence of vitamin D toxicity such hypercalciuria (urine calcium/creatinine ratio ≥ 0.2), serum phosphate > 5.7 mg/mL, serum calcium > 10.5 mg/dL, serum 25(OH) D > 150 ng/mL.

Statistical analysis

To estimate the effect of vitamin D treatment on the clinical features in this crossover study, we first examined the within patient comparison by using paired t-test. We next examined the treatment given one period (treatment/placebo) adjusted for the baseline values by using mixed regression models controlling for baseline measurements, age, gender, race, BMI, and seasons [winter: Dec-Feb; spring: Mar-May; summer: Jun-Aug; fall: Sep-Nov]. Koch's test was used to examine the crossover effect on the association of treatment and clinical features. We further conducted stratified analyses according to baseline diabetes and pre-diabetes status, using the criteria plasma glucose at 0 minute ≥ 100 mg/dL or at 120 minutes ≥ 140 in oral glucose tolerance test (OGTT), HbA1C ≥ 5.7% and HOMA -IR ≥ 3.4, and intact PTH ≥ 44 pg/mL. At last, plasma glucose concentration and insulin level at times 0, minutes, 30 minutes, 60 minutes, 90 minutes, and 120 minutes in insulin sensitivity test were compared between treatment and placebo groups by using the mixed regression models described above, as well as the mean levels at the first-phase (at and before 30 minutes), second phase (after 30 minutes), and whole period (0-120 minutes). All statistical tests were two-sided, and all statistical analyses were carried out using SAS 9.3.

RESULTS

Of the twenty participants, 80% (n = 16) were females, and 75% (n = 15) were Hispanic, with mean age 15 year-old. The study participants were predominantly overweight, with mean BMI 32.7 (Table 1). The baseline clinical features of all participants were shown in Table 1 as well: Serum 25-OH vitamin D levels were 16.7 ± 2.9 ng/mL (reference range 12-20 ng/mL) (25); and WBISI were 2.8 ± 1.9 (reference range 1.84 ± 0.17); and IGI were 3.0 ± 2.2; and PTH were 50.9 ± 15.8 (reference range 15 – 75 pg/mL).

We first examined the effect of vitamin D treatment on the serum 25-OH vitamin D levels (Table 2). Treatment group had significant increased serum 25-OH vitamin D levels (19.5 ± 4.5 ng/mL; p from paired t-test = 0.0029) compared to baseline levels. This increase in serum 25-OH vitamin D levels after treatment was significantly different relative to placebo group, after further adjusted for covariates (adjusted p from mixed model = 0.0059), and did not due to crossover effect (p from Koch's analysis = 0.4506).

Table 1. Baseline characteristics and clinical features of the study population

Characteristics and clinical features	Study participants (n = 20)	
	Mean/N	SD/%
Age (year)	15.1	1.9
Gender*		
Male	4	20
Female	16	80
Ethnicity*		
African American	3	15
Bangladesh	1	5
Caucasian	1	5
Hispanic	15	75
Height (cm)	162.5	7.8
Weight (kg)	90.7	19.2
BMI	32.7	9.8
25 OH vitamin D (ng/mL)	16.7	2.9
WBISI	2.8	1.9
IGI	3.0	2.2
Intact, PTH (pg/mL)	50.9	15.8
HbA1C	5.7	0.3
HOMA-B%	452.2	343.3
HOMA-IR	4.2	2.8
Serum calcium (mg/dL)	9.4	0.4
Albumin (g/dL)	4.2	0.3
Albumin-adjusted serum calcium (mg/dL)	9.2	0.4
Alkaline phosphatase (U/L)	110.0	46.8
AST (U/L)	29.2	14.1
ALT (U/L)	42.3	39.8
Serum phosphorus (mg/dL)	4.5	0.6
Random urine calcium (mg/dL)	6.5	4.6
Random urine creatinine (mg/dL)	217.9	107.2

* Numbers of participants and percentage were calculated.

We next examined that if the vitamin D treatment were associated with insulin sensitivity and secretory parameters (Table 2). The means of whole body insulin sensitivity (WBISI) tend to be increased (Δ_{mean} = 0.1, $p_{t\text{-test}}$ = 0.5377) in treatment group and decreased (Δ_{mean} = 0.3, $p_{t\text{-test}}$ = 0.3855) in placebo group compared to baseline levels, however, without statistical significance. Whereas, the difference in WBISI between treatment and placebo group was marginally significant after adjusted for covariates (adjusted p from mixed model = 0.0577). The means of insulin index (IGI) increased with 0.1 in both treatment and placebo group compared to baseline, and these differences were not statistically

significant. Intact PTH decreased in treatment group (Δ_{mean} = -6.0, $p_{t\text{-test}}$ = 0.0538); however, this decrease was not significant compared to the changes in placebo group (adjusted p from mixed model = 0.1290). Additionally, alkaline phosphatase levels decreased in both treatment group (Δ_{mean} = -6.5, $p_{t\text{-test}}$ = 0.0334) and placebo group (Δ_{mean} = -7.5, $p_{t\text{-test}}$ = 0.0034), and AST and ALT only decreased in treatment group (Δ_{mean} = -2.0, $p_{t\text{-test}}$ = 0.0209 for AST, and Δ_{mean} = -4.0, $p_{t\text{-test}}$ = 0.0106 for ALT). However, the decrease were not significant compared to the changes in placebo group.

Since childhood diabetes and pre-diabetes status may have effects of vitamin D treatment on insulin sensitivity, we stratified the associations of VD2 treatment with WBISI and IGI by clinical diabetes measurements (Table 3). In contrast to the overall analysis, the means of IGI decreased in treatment (Δ_{mean} = -0.70, $p_{t\text{-test}}$ = 0.5606) in children with fasting serum glucose level ≥ 100 or ≥ 140 at time 0 and 120 minutes during the OGTT, although these differences were not significant. Children with HOMA-IR ≥ 3.4 and HbA1C ≥ 5.7% had similar trend of in both treatment and placebo group with the overall changes. When stratified by PTH, the treatment group with PTH ≤ 44 pg/mL had increased mean of WBISI (Δ_{mean} = 0.10, $p_{t\text{-test}}$ = 0.5040), and decreased mean of IGI (Δ_{mean} = -0.30, $p_{t\text{-test}}$ = 0.5722).

In the comparisons of the mean differences between treatment and placebo group at each time point of OGTT (Table 4: 0 min, 10 min, 30 min, 60 min, 90 min, 120 min), serum glucose level decreased slower in treatment group (Δ_{mean} = -5.5, $p_{t\text{-test}}$ = 0.2162) than placebo (Δ_{mean} = -18.5, $p_{t\text{-test}}$ = 0.0007) at 30 minutes, with p value from mixed model equals to 0.0236. While, insulin level increased in treatment group (Δ_{mean} = 9.0, $p_{t\text{-test}}$ = 0. 7864), and decreased in placebo (Δ_{mean} = -6.0, $p_{t\text{-test}}$ = 0.1270) at 30 minutes (p from mixed model = 0.0197). No significant differences between treatment and placebo at other time point of OGTT was found, as well as the mean values of all time points in both glucose and insulin levels.

DISCUSSION

Our study demonstrated that using high dose of VD2 (300,000 IU) in a cross over design trial did not have any beneficial effect on insulin sensitivity and secretory indices in obese adolescents when measured using an oral glucose tolerance test.

Table 2. Baseline values and changes after treatment in clinical features and the placebo group

| | Baseline | | Treatment group (N = 20) | | | | | Placebo group (N = 20) | | | | | | |
| | | | Δ after treatment | | | | | Δ after treatment | | | | | | |
	Mean	SD	Mean	SD	Median*	IQR*	p†	Mean	SD	Median*	IQR*	p†	p‡	p§
25 OH vitamin D (ng/mL)	16.7	2.9	19.5	4.5	2.4	4.7	0.0029	17.2	4.7	0.0	2.2	0.5262	0.0059	0.4506
WBISI	2.8	1.9	2.7	1.4	-0.1	1.1	0.5377	3.1	1.5	0.3	1.9	0.3855	0.0577	0.4205
IGI	3.0	2.2	3.5	2.7	0.1	1.8	0.2878	4.3	6.3	0.1	1.2	0.3069	0.5971	0.0030
Intact, PTH (pg/mL)	50.9	15.8	45.6	11.8	-6.0	19.0	0.0538	50.3	14.3	0.5	16.0	0.8327	0.1290	0.1075
HbA1C	5.7	0.3	5.7	0.4	0.1	0.2	0.2674	5.7	0.4	0.1	0.3	0.3264	0.9052	0.2918
HOMA-B%	452.2	343.3	483.5	258.2	19.8	173.8	0.3889	543.9	532.2	34.2	288.5	0.2769	0.5740	0.0004
HOMA-IR	4.2	2.8	5.2	3.6	0.9	2.3	0.1079	4.9	4.5	0.2	1.3	0.2829	0.3403	0.3396
Serum calcium (mg/dL)	9.4	0.4	9.3	0.4	0.0	0.4	0.4936	9.2	0.3	-0.1	0.5	0.0909	0.1287	0.2258
Albumin (g/dL)	4.2	0.3	4.2	0.9	-0.3	0.4	0.8346	4.1	0.3	-0.2	0.3	0.1670	0.8932	0.0200
Albumin-adjusted serum calcium	9.2	0.4	9.1	0.7	0.1	0.4	0.8927	14.7	25.6	0.0	0.6	0.3750	0.3975	< 0.0001
Alkaline phosphatase (U/L)	110.0	46.8	103.6	43.5	-6.5	13.0	0.0344	99.6	37.6	-7.5	15.0	0.0034	0.3105	0.4072
AST (U/L)	29.2	14.1	25.2	11.9	-2.0	5.5	0.0209	29.1	15.8	-0.5	6.0	0.9374	0.0870	< 0.0001
ALT (U/L)	42.3	39.8	36.2	32.4	-4.0	9.5	0.0106	40.6	36.7	-1.0	9.0	0.6514	0.2704	< 0.0001
Serum phosphorus (mg/dL)	4.5	0.6	4.5	0.6	-0.1	0.5	0.7354	4.5	0.5	0.0	0.4	0.5965	0.6586	0.9649
Random urine calcium (mg/dL)	6.5	4.6	8.6	7.8	2.7	6.2	0.1733	14.0	21.4	1.0	7.0	0.1411	0.3369	0.0007
Random urine creatinine (mg/dL)	217.9	107.2	274.6	441.8	-12.7	106.5	0.5034	199.2	108.3	-9.9	89.7	0.4150	0.3292	< 0.0001

* Medians and IQR of the difference between treatment/placebo group and baseline were calculated.
† p values were calculated from exact comparison (paired t-test) of measurements to baseline.
‡ p values were calculated from mixed regression models, adjusted for baseline measurements, age, gender, race, BMI, and season [winter: Dec-Feb; spring: Mar-May; summer: Jun-Aug; fall: Sep-Nov].
§ p values were calculated from Koch's analysis testing for crossover effects.

Table 3. Changes after treatment in WBISI and IGI and the placebo group stratified according to diabetes status

| | Treatment group | | | | | | Placebo group | | | | | | | |
| | | | Δ after treatment | | | | | | Δ after treatment | | | | | |
	N	Mean	SD	Median*	IQR*	p†	N	Mean	SD	Median*	IQR*	p†	p‡	p§
G_0 ≥ 100 mg/dL and/or G_120 ≥ 140 mg/dL	5						5							
WBISI		1.38	0.80	-0.20	0.30	0.1293		1.56	1.04	-0.10	0.50	0.6213	0.4718	0.5477
IGI		5.18	4.51	-0.70	1.20	0.5606		2.94	2.43	-0.60	1.60	0.1376	0.1236	0.1126
HOMA-IR ≥ 3.4 & HbA1C ≥ 5.7%	6						6							
WBISI		2.27	1.44	-0.25	0.30	0.8226		2.32	1.06	0.25	0.90	0.4391	0.2516	0.1764
IGI		5.70	3.52	2.30	5.60	0.2714		8.40	10.69	0.95	5.60	0.2636	0.1735	0.8965
Intact, PTH ≤ 44 pg/mL	9						9							
WBISI		2.15	1.18	0.10	0.35	0.5040		2.86	1.69	0.30	2.00	0.0765	0.3445	< 0.0001
IGI		3.26	2.20	-0.30	1.10	0.5722		2.64	1.88	-0.55	1.40	0.0389	0.3450	< 0.0001
Intact, PTH > 44 pg/mL	11						11							
WBISI		3.05	1.43	-0.30	1.90	0.4458		3.34	1.46	0.20	1.60	0.7871	0.2312	0.4084
IGI		3.74	3.20	0.65	3.20	0.2286		5.61	8.24	0.50	1.50	0.1978	0.7405	0.1898

N: number; SD: standard deviation; IQR: inter quartile range; p: *p* value.

Table 4. Baseline values and changes after treatment in plasma glucose and insulin levels and the placebo group at each time point

| | Baseline | | Treatment group (N = 20) | | | | | Placebo (N = 20) | | | | | | |
| | | | | | Δ after treatment | | | | | Δ after treatment | | | | |
	Mean	SD	Mean	SD	Mean*	SD*	p†	Mean	SD	Mean*	SD*	p†	p‡	p§
Plasma glucose														
At fasting	82.0	7.2	82.0	5.6	0.0	8.5	0.9698	81.2	5.5	-0.5	7.0	0.4466	0.3645	0.2856
At 10 min	102.4	16.1	100.6	13.3	1.5	9.5	0.5910	96.7	13.5	-2.5	12.0	0.0589	0.2423	0.1161
At 30 min	139.8	25.4	133.4	22.6	-5.5	33.0	0.2162	122.5	22.1	-18.5	25.0	0.0007	0.0236	0.4265
At 60 min	139.8	28.5	128.7	38.9	-3.5	55.5	0.1202	119.8	34.0	-21.0	37.0	0.0067	0.2243	0.0452
At 90 min	127.5	29.4	123.4	34.9	-10.5	53.0	0.5524	117.7	39.9	-10.5	29.0	0.2737	0.4540	0.1342
At 120 min	123.3	31.2	110.5	31.0	-13.5	28.5	0.0568	111.8	35.1	-11.0	19.0	0.0419	0.9691	0.0700
Mean	119.1	18.4	113.1	20.1	-6.9	27.0	0.0684	108.3	22.0	-10.7	19.4	0.0037	0.1754	0.1741
Insulin														
At fasting	20.9	13.3	25.2	16.7	4.0	10.0	0.0749	24.1	21.7	0.5	6.5	0.2686	0.4555	0.7516
At 10 min	77.7	63.4	74.2	49.5	5.0	27.0	0.7478	71.9	61.7	3.5	52.0	0.6103	0.8206	0.6579
At 30 min	183.5	147.6	176.9	110.1	9.0	117.0	0.7864	151.4	116.7	-6.0	108.5	0.1270	0.0197	0.3541
At 60 min	213.9	183.6	187.0	181.3	-8.0	95.0	0.2746	145.8	136.3	-41.5	105.5	0.0178	0.1340	0.3023
At 90 min	207.6	253.6	204.7	253.6	-17.5	133.0	0.3248	148.0	185.0	-58.0	117.0	0.0245	0.0604	0.0242
At 120 min	231.3	352.4	138.7	116.3	-37.0	109.5	0.1919	165.7	250.4	-31.0	80.5	0.0487	0.6277	0.0135
Mean	156.0	158.9	136.0	115.7	-5.5	54.4	0.2027	117.8	121.6	-2970.0	59.8	0.0215	0.2580	0.1541
First-phase (≤ 30 m)	49.3	35.3	52.1	34.9	5.5	17.8	0.6396	48.0	40.3	0.8	33.0	0.8336	0.5587	0.5024
Second-phase (> 30 m)	211.8	225.3	175.4	153.8	-20.3	83.3	0.1284	152.7	164.2	-36.8	87.0	0.0167	0.2367	0.3730

* Medians and IQR of the difference between treatment/placebo group and baseline were calculated.

† p values were calculated from exact comparison (paired t-test) of measurements to baseline.

‡ p values were calculated from mixed regression models, adjusted for baseline measurements, age, gender, race, BMI, and season [winter: Dec-Feb; spring: Mar-May; summer: Jun-Aug; fall: Sep-Nov].

§ p values were calculated from Koch's analysis testing for crossover effects.

Prediabetes was found in 10-39% of obese adolescents (24,26), which parallels the rise of obesity (27). Vitamin D has shown to have effects on insulin secretion and action and in both pediatric and adult studies an inverse association between vitamin D levels and development of prediabetes and/or T2DM have been demonstrated (10,21).

Long term randomized control trials (3 months-7 years) have studied whether giving vitamin D prevents the progression of insulin resistance to prediabetes to Type 2 diabetes due to its effects on augmenting insulin action and secretion. Von Hurst and cols. studied 42 South Asian women with insulin resistance using 4000 IU of D3 for 6 months. Fasting insulin and HOMA-IR improved in the cases versus controls (p values = 0.02). Davidson and cols. used a weight and vitamin D based formula to calculate vitamin D dosing (average of 88000 IU/week) for 12 months and showed improvement in Hba1c (decrease by 0.2%) but the intervention affected no other parameters of any OGTT derived secretory and sensitivity indices in this cohort of pre diabetic adults. These studies (more than 6 months

of vitamin D treatment) have been equivocal to truly establish any real benefit of using vitamin D on indices of beta cell function and insulin sensitivity, the caveat being the variations in the dosing of vitamin D used, compliance concerns and whether the vitamin D truly reached an optimal level (i.e. > 30 ng/mL) to effect the aspects of function of beta cell. It is clear that in this obese cohort of female adolescents (average BMI = 32.1) we found that treatment did increase the vitamin D level when compared to the placebo arm (19.5 vs. 17.2 ng/dL; p = 0.0029) and this significance stayed after adjustments for covariates: BMI, age sex, gender, race and season. However our intervention of 300,000 IU was not able to optimize the vitamin D levels to levels of sufficiency i.e. ≥ 30 ng/mL in all except one subjects. Levels reached ≥ 20 ng/mL in six subjects by the end of the three month intervention. This dosing was based on the Endocrine society guidelines of using 50,000 IU for 6 weeks for deficient states (19).

We wanted to test the effect of using high dose of vitamin D effect on insulin sensitivity and secretory indices. WBISI did show an increase in the Rx group (delta mean increase 0.1) though this difference was not significant when compared to the placebo. IGI increased in both groups while PTH decreased to a greater extent when compared to the placebo though in the mixed model analysis the difference was not significant. In a similar study designed by Ashraf and cols. obese adolescents (average age 14.9 ± 1.8 years) were given 50,000 IU of vitamin D per week for 8 weeks to observe effects on glucose parameters. While HOMA-IR and WBISI did not improve on the follow up OGTT fasting glucose showed statistical improvement (p = 0.05) in cases when compared to controls. In a dose titration study (400 IU to 4000 IU) of 323 early pubertal children (age = 11.3 years; BMI% 70% and 25 (OH) levels 28 ng/mL) fasting insulin and HOMA-IR correlated with baseline levels of 25(OH) D (r = 0.14 and 0.15 respectively). Rx with vitamin D had no significant positive impact on glucose and insulin parameters over a 12 week period. In this study by Ferira and cols. among these children only 15% were vitamin D deficient and obese respectively and therefore making comparisons with our study results would not be reasonable (28).

In a noteworthy study by Wagner and cols. investigated the effect of high-dose vitamin D3 treatment on beta-cell function, insulin sensitivity, and glucose tolerance in subjects with prediabetes or diet-treated type 2 diabetes adults (n = 43, BMI 28.6) randomized to 30,000 IU of cholecalciferol or placebo drops weekly for 8 weeks. They studied first and second phase insulin response (I Sec_{0-12}, I Sec_{12-12}), disposition index {DI} (measured with hyperglycemic clamp) and WBISI using pre and post Rx OGTT. The investigators did not find any improvement I Sec_{0-12}, I Sec_{12-120} results which are in line with our results which showed no improvements in the indices derived either from the clamp or OGTT. The difference between this study in adults and ours in adolescents is that their vitamin D levels rose from 17.2 ng/mL (43 mmol/L) at baseline to 34 ng/mL at the end of the 8 week study (29). The fact that they normalized the vitamin D levels supports their findings that vitamin D given in high doses over a short period does not improve metabolic profile of prediabetes and T2DM adults.

To further analyze the data we stratified and looked at the associations between vitamin D levels and metabolic parameters which reflect emerging decompensation such as: Glucose ≥ 100 mg/dL or ≥ 140 mg/dL at 0 and 120 minutes of the OGTT,

HbA1c ≥ 5.7%-6.4% (defined as prediabetes by American Diabetes Association). No differences were found in the Rx group using this stratification analysis. No significant differences between treatment and placebo at other time point of OGTTs were found, as well as the mean values of all time points (10, 30, 60, and 90 min) in both glucose and insulin levels. These results further reiterate that the intervention had no effects in the variables of interest.

The cross-over of our RCT was designed to balance the exposure to vitamin D and placebo in sequence based on the arm that the adolescents were assigned to. Each patient served as their own control which allowed for a smaller sample size. The limitations were the "order" and "carry over" effect of a cross over study and we recognize that we did not have a wash out period which could have affected our results. A strength of the study was that we did adjust for seasonal variation in our analysis of the data. We were not able to normalize 25 OHD level and that is a major limitation of our study. 25 OHD has a threshold effect on the beta cell function and we speculate that this is reason why we could find any improvements in insulin secretory and sensitivity parameters. Also, given emerging information on pharmacokinetics studies on available formulations found that ergocalciferol was not as good a choice as cholecalciferol which is more effective in increasing the serum 25(OH) D pools (30).

Our results are aligned to the negative results found in the recent studies showing no beneficial effect of vitamin D on glucose and insulin indices derived from OGTT. We suggest considering much higher dosing for obese adolescents based on adult studies (31) accepting the fact that these are adult sized adolescents. Based on our study there is no evidence to support the use of high dose vitamin D over a short term period to improve glucose homeostasis.

Acknowledgments: supported in part by the NYU CTSA grant UL1 TR000038 from the National Center for Advancing Translational Sciences, National Institutes of Health.

REFERENCES

1. Olson ML, Maalouf NM, Oden JD, White PC, Hutchison MR. Vitamin D deficiency in obese children and its relationship to glucose homeostasis. J Clin Endocrinol Metab. 2012;97(1):279-85.

2. Reis JP, von Muhlen D, Miller ER 3rd, Michos ED, Appel LJ. Vitamin D status and cardiometabolic risk factors in the United States adolescent population. Pediatrics. 2009;124(3):e371-9.

3. Alemzadeh R, Kichler J, Babar G, Calhoun M. Hypovitaminosis D in obese children and adolescents: relationship with adiposity, insulin sensitivity, ethnicity, and season. Metabolism. 2008;57(2):183-91.

4. Wamberg L, Christiansen T, Paulsen SK, Fisker S, Rask P, Rejnmark L, et al. Expression of vitamin D-metabolizing enzymes in human adipose tissue -- the effect of obesity and diet-induced weight loss. Int J Obes (Lond). 2013;37(5):651-7.

5. Drincic AT, Armas LA, Van Diest EE, Heaney RP. Volumetric dilution, rather than sequestration best explains the low vitamin D status of obesity. Obesity (Silver Spring). 2012;20(7):1444-8.

6. Norman AW, Frankel JB, Heldt AM, Grodsky GM. Vitamin D deficiency inhibits pancreatic secretion of insulin. Science (New York, NY). 1980;209:823-5.

7. Chiu KC, Chu A, Go VL, Saad MF. Hypovitaminosis D is associated with insulin resistance and beta cell dysfunction. Am J Clin Nutr. 2004;79(5):820-5.

8. Deleskog A, Hilding A, Brismar K, Hamsten A, Efendic S, Ostenson CG. Low serum 25-hydroxyvitamin D level predicts progression to type 2 diabetes in individuals with prediabetes but not with normal glucose tolerance. Diabetologia. 2012;55(6):1668-78.

9. Song Y, Wang L, Pittas AG, Del Gobbo LC, Zhang C, Manson JE, et al. Blood 25-hydroxy vitamin D levels and incident type 2 diabetes: a meta-analysis of prospective studies. Diabetes Care. 2013;36(5):1422-8.

10. Pittas AG, Lau J, Hu FB, Dawson-Hughes B. The role of vitamin D and calcium in type 2 diabetes. A systematic review and meta-analysis. J Clin Endocrinol Metab. 2007;92(6):2017-29.

11. von Hurst PR, Stonehouse W, Coad J. Vitamin D supplementation reduces insulin resistance in South Asian women living in New Zealand who are insulin resistant and vitamin D deficient - a randomised, placebo-controlled trial. Br J Nutr. 2010;103(4):549-55.

12. Belenchia AM, Tosh AK, Hillman LS, Peterson CA. Correcting vitamin D insufficiency improves insulin sensitivity in obese adolescents: a randomized controlled trial. Am J Clin Nutr. 2013;97(4):774-81.

13. Nader NS, Aguirre Castaneda R, Wallace J, Singh R, Weaver A, Kumar S. Effect of vitamin D3 supplementation on serum 25(OH) D, lipids and markers of insulin resistance in obese adolescents: a prospective, randomized, placebo-controlled pilot trial. Horm Res Paediatr. 2014;82:107-12.

14. Wamberg L, Kampmann U, Stodkilde-Jorgensen H, Rejnmark L, Pedersen SB, Richelsen B. Effects of vitamin D supplementation on body fat accumulation, inflammation, and metabolic risk factors in obese adults with low vitamin D levels - results from a randomized trial. Eur J Intern Med. 2013;24(7):644-9.

15. Neyestani TR, Nikooyeh B, Alavi-Majd H, Shariatzadeh N, Kalayi A, Tayebinejad N, et al. Improvement of vitamin D status via daily intake of fortified yogurt drink either with or without extra calcium ameliorates systemic inflammatory biomarkers, including adipokines, in the subjects with type 2 diabetes. J Clin Endocrinol Metab. 2012;97(6):2005-11.

16. Kampmann U, Mosekilde L, Juhl C, Moller N, Christensen B, Rejnmark L, et al. Effects of 12 weeks high dose vitamin D3 treatment on insulin sensitivity, beta cell function, and metabolic markers in patients with type 2 diabetes and vitamin D insufficiency - a double-blind, randomized, placebo-controlled trial. Metabolism. 2014;63(9):1115-24.

17. Nazarian S, St Peter JV, Boston RC, Jones SA, Mariash CN. Vitamin D3 supplementation improves insulin sensitivity in subjects with impaired fasting glucose. Transl Res. 2011;158(5):276-81.

18. Wagner H, Alvarsson M, Mannheimer B, Degerblad M, Ostenson CG. No Effect of High-Dose Vitamin D Treatment on β-Cell Function, Insulin Sensitivity, or Glucose Homeostasis in Subjects With Abnormal Glucose Tolerance: A Randomized Clinical Trial. Diabetes Care. 2016;39(3):345-52.

19. Holick MF, Binkley NC, Bischoff-Ferrari HA, Gordon CM, Hanley DA, Heaney RP, et al. Evaluation, treatment, and prevention of vitamin D deficiency: an Endocrine Society clinical practice guideline. J Clin Endocrinol Metab. 2011;96(7):1911-30.

20. Munns CF, Shaw N, Kiely M, Specker BL, Thacher TD, Ozono K, et al. Global Consensus Recommendations on Prevention and Management of Nutritional Rickets. J Clin Endocrinol Metab. 2016;101(2):394-415.

21. Pittas AG, Dawson-Hughes B. Vitamin D and diabetes. J Steroid Biochem Mol Biol. 2010;121(1-2):425-9.

22. Matsuda M, DeFronzo RA. Insulin sensitivity indices obtained from oral glucose tolerance testing: comparison with the euglycemic insulin clamp. Diabetes Care. 1999;22(9):1462-70.

23. Yeckel C, Weiss R, Dziura J, Taksali S, Dufour S, Burgert T, et al. Validation of insulin sensitivity indices from oral glucose tolerance test parameters in obese children and adolescents. J Clin Endocrinol Metab. 2004;89(3):1096-101.

24. Sinha R, Fisch G, Teague B, Tamborlane WV, Banyas B, Allen K, et al. Prevalence of impaired glucose tolerance among children and adolescents with marked obesity. N Engl J Med. 2002;346(11): 802-10.

25. Ross AC, Manson JE, Abrams SA, Aloia JF, Brannon PM, Clinton SK, et al. The 2011 report on dietary reference intakes for calcium and vitamin D from the Institute of Medicine: what clinicians need to know. J Clin Endocrinol Metab. 2011;96(1):53-8.

26. Nowicka P, Santoro N, Liu H, Lartaud D, Shaw M, Goldberg R, et al. Utility of hemoglobin a1c for diagnosing prediabetes and diabetes in obese children and adolescents. Diabetes Care. 2011;34(6):1306-11.

27. Ogden CL, Carroll MD, Flegal KM. High body mass index for age among US children and adolescents, 2003-2006. JAMA. 2008;299(20):2401-5.

28. Ferira AJ, Laing EM, Hausman DB, Hall DB, McCabe GP, Martin BR, et al. Vitamin D Supplementation Does Not Impact Insulin Resistance in Black and White Children. J Clin Endocrinol Metab. 2016;101(4):1710-8.

29. Herpertz S, Albus C, Wagener R, Kocnar M, Wagner R, Henning A, et al. Comorbidity of diabetes and eating disorders. Does diabetes control reflect disturbed eating behavior? Diabetes Care. 1998;21(7):1110-6.

30. Itkonen ST, Skaffari E, Saaristo P, Saarnio EM, Erkkola M, Jakobsen J, et al. Effects of vitamin D2-fortified bread v. supplementation with vitamin D2 or D3 on serum 25-hydroxyvitamin D metabolites: an 8-week randomised-controlled trial in young adult Finnish women. Br J Nutr. 2016;115(7):1232-9.

31. Barger-Lux MJ, Heaney RP, Dowell S, Chen TC, Holick MF. Vitamin D and its major metabolites: serum levels after graded oral dosing in healthy men. Osteoporos Int. 1998;8(3):222-30.

9

Effectiveness and safety of carbohydrate counting in the management of adult patients with type 1 diabetes mellitus

Eliege Carolina Vaz[1], Gustavo José Martiniano Porfírio[2],
Hélio Rubens de Carvalho Nunes[3], Vania dos Santos Nunes-Nogueira[1]

[1] Departamento de Clínica Médica, Faculdade de Medicina de Botucatu, Universidade Estadual de São Paulo (Unesp), Botucatu, SP, Brasil
[2] Centro Cochrane do Brasil, Disciplina de Medicina de Urgência e Medicina Baseada em Evidências, Universidade Federal de São Paulo (Unifesp), São Paulo, SP, Brasil
[3] Departamento de Saúde Pública, Faculdade de Medicina de Botucatu, Universidade Estadual de São Paulo (Unesp), Botucatu, SP, Brasil

Correspondence to:
Vania dos Santos Nunes Nogueira
Departamento de Clínica Médica, Faculdade de Medicina de Botucatu, Universidade Estadual de São Paulo
Av. Prof. Mário Rubens Guimarães Montenegro, s/nº
Unesp, Campus de Botucatu
18618-687 – Botucatu, SP, Brasil
vsnunes@fmb.unesp.br

ABSTRACT

Objective: This study aimed to evaluate the effectiveness and safety of carbohydrate counting (CHOC) in the treatment of adult patients with type 1 diabetes mellitus (DM1). Materials and methods: We performed a systematic review of randomized studies that compared CHOC with general dietary advice in adult patients with DM1. The primary outcomes were changes in glycated hemoglobin (HbA1c), quality of life, and episodes of severe hypoglycemia. We searched the following electronic databases: Embase, PubMed, Lilacs, and the Cochrane Central Register of Controlled Trials. The quality of evidence was analyzed using the Grading of Recommendations Assessment, Development and Evaluation (GRADE). Results: A total of 3,190 articles were identified, and two reviewers independently screened the titles and abstracts. From the 15 potentially eligible studies, five were included, and 10 were excluded because of the lack of randomization or different control/intervention groups. Meta-analysis showed that the final HbA1c was significantly lower in the CHOC group than in the control group (mean difference, random, 95% CI: -0.49 (-0.85, -0.13), p = 0.006). The meta-analysis of severe hypoglycemia and quality of life did not show any significant differences between the groups. According to the GRADE, the quality of evidence for severe hypoglycemia, quality of life, and change in HbA1c was low, very low, and moderate, respectively. Conclusion: The meta-analysis showed evidence favoring the use of CHOC in the management of DM1. However, this benefit was limited to final HbA1c, which was significantly lower in the CHOC than in the control group. Arch Endocrinol Metab. 2018;62(3):337-45

Keywords
Type 1 diabetes mellitus; carbohydrate counting; quality of life; systematic review; meta-analysis

INTRODUCTION

Diabetes mellitus (DM) comprises a heterogeneous group of metabolic disorders that commonly feature hyperglycemia, which results from disturbances in insulin secretion, insulin action, or both (1). In most cases, type 1 DM (DM1) is an autoimmune disease characterized by the destruction of insulin-producing beta cells, accounting for 5% to 10% of all DM cases (1). In Brazil, eight of every 100,000 people under the age of 20 have DM1 (2).

The therapeutic treatment and control of DM1 includes the use of insulin for glycemic control, balanced diet, and regular physical activity. Daily insulin requirements vary based on age, diet, patient self-monitoring of blood glucose and daily routines.

Glycemic control of patients with DM is important because it impacts the development of diabetic complications (3). Diabetes control is evaluated mainly according to the levels of HbA1c, fasting blood glucose, and postprandial blood glucose (blood glucose measured two hours after meal consumption). Borderline normal values without the risk of hypoglycemia, impaired mental status, and patient welfare indicate good glycemic control (4).

The American Diabetes Association recommends the following levels for nonpregnant adults: HbA1c < 7%, preprandial capillary plasma glucose between 80 mg/dL and 130 mg/dL, and peak postprandial capillary plasma glucose < 180 mg/dL (4). The Diabetes Control and Complications Trial (DCCT) showed that adequate glycemic control in patients with DM1 (e.g., fasting blood glucose levels up to 110 mg/dL, postprandial glucose levels lower than 180 mg/dL, and HbA1c < 6.5%) delays the onset and progression of microvascular complications, such as retinopathy, nephropathy, and neuropathy, and reduces the risk of any cardiovascular event by 42% and that of nonfatal infarction, stroke, and death by 57% (3).

The treatment of patients with DM1 facilitates proper development in children and adolescents and improves the quality of life (QOL) of patients in general (5).

DM1 control cannot be achieved solely via regular insulin use. Combining insulin use with diet and physical activity is important. In particular, adjusting insulin therapy to an individualized food plan is key to proper metabolic control (3). Conventional nutritional advice for patients with DM1 is the same as for the general population. Specifically, a balanced nutrition with appropriate concentrations of macro- and micronutrients should be based on the goals of treatment (i.e., total carbohydrate (CHO), 45%-60% of total energy intake (VET); protein, 15%-20% of VET; total fat (GT), up to 30% of VET; and minimum dietary fiber, 20 g/day or 14 g/1000 kcal) (6).

In addition to conventional nutritional DM1 treatments, carbohydrate counting (CHOC) is a meal planning tool that allows for great variation in food choices among individuals with DM (7), with the main objective of providing flexibility in food intake (8). Few dietary restrictions and the option to decide the number of meals (traditional treatment plans recommend eating six meals per day) may improve acceptance of the disease and overall QOL (9).

CHOC consists of measuring the amount of carbohydrates to be eaten during every meal in grams. Based on that count and preprandial blood glucose levels, the patient calculates the dose of fast or regular insulin they need before each meal (10,11). This method can be used for any patient with diabetes in combination with the use of varying doses of rapid-acting insulin or continuous subcutaneous insulin infusion (12). Two CHOC methods are widely used: listing carbohydrate equivalents (A) and measuring the carbohydrate in grams (B). In method A, foods are grouped so that each food portion chosen by the patient corresponds to 15 g of carbohydrate, classifying them as equivalents. Method B consists of the sum of carbohydrate grams in each food per meal based on information in food labels and tables (13).

To improve glycemic control and decrease the frequency of acute and chronic complications, CHOC is now recommended as another nutritional tool (3,14).

Regarding the efficacy of the CHOC method in metabolic DM1 control in the DCCT study, individuals who adjusted their pre-meal insulin doses based on carbohydrate counts had a 0.5% decrease in HbA1c compared to the group that used a fixed dose (15). Dias and cols. (16) showed that HbA1c levels were reduced in a group of 55 adult patients, and although the total daily dose of insulin increased, no weight gain was observed. Waller and cols. (17) also evaluated CHOC in children and adolescents with DM1 and reported no changes in HbA1c, body mass index (BMI), or frequency of hypoglycemic episodes. However, the children and their parents showed an improvement in QOL.

We hypothesized that the CHOC method in adult individuals with DM1 may be more effective and efficient for glycemic control and better improve QOL compared to conventional nutritional guidance.

This study aimed to evaluate the effectiveness and safety of CHOC in the treatment of adult patients with DMI using a systematic literature review.

MATERIALS AND METHODS

This review was performed according to Cochrane Methodology (18) and reported according to the PRISMA Statement (19).

Eligibility criteria

We included randomized controlled trials with at least three months of follow-up, and evaluation of outcomes in which patients were randomly divided into two groups, intervention or comparison. Data were interpreted based on patient-characteristics, intervention, comparison, and outcomes (PICO) as described below.

Patients

Patients consisted of men and women aged over 18 years old who had been diagnosed with DM1 for at least six months and were not in the "honeymoon period", in which the pancreas can produce small amounts of insulin that can be enough to achieve adequate glycemic control at a daily dose of less than 0.5 IU insulin/kg in 24 hours. Patients had standard nutritional counseling with a professional nutritionist and took slow-acting or intermediate and multiple fast or regular insulin doses before meals (breakfast, lunch, and dinner) or continuous subcutaneous insulin infusion (CSII). Studies that included pregnant women, individuals with a BMI > 40 kg/m², kidney failure, or HbA1c >14% were excluded from analysis.

Intervention

Individuals in the intervention group had nutritional counseling for CHOC to determine the amount of fast or regular insulin that they would need before each main meal.

Comparison

The comparison group included individuals who had conventional nutritional advice and used fixed doses of fast or regular insulin before meals.

Outcomes

Assessed outcomes were reduction in HbA1c, frequency of severe hypoglycemia, improved QOL, body weight or BMI gain, lipid profile, and total daily dose of insulin. Validated questionnaires were used to evaluate QOL: Audit of Diabetes-Dependent Quality of Life (ADDQoL), Diabetes Treatment Satisfaction Questionnaire (DTSQ), and Diabetes Quality of Life Measure (DQoL).

Search strategy and selection

No language restriction was imposed. We searched the following electronic databases through November 30, 2016 to identify randomized clinical trials involving CHOC versus conventional nutritional advice in the treatment of DM1 patients: Embase (1980-2016), PubMed (1966-2016), Lilacs (1982-2016), and the Cochrane Central Register of Controlled Trials (CENTRAL, the Cochrane Library, issue 2016). We also searched for ongoing clinical trials on the clinicaltrials. gov website. Medical Subject Heading terms used included "Type 1 Diabetes Mellitus", "Carbohydrates", "Nutrition Therapy", and "Randomized Controlled Trial".

Two reviewers (ECV and VSNN) independently screened the titles and abstracts identified in the literature search. Studies potentially eligible for inclusion in the review were selected for complete reading.

Data extraction and risk of bias

Both reviewers assessed the study quality and extracted data using an extraction template. For each trial, we assigned the risk of bias considering the quality scores for random sequence generation, allocation concealment, blinding of outcome assessment, and incomplete outcome data. We used the criteria described in the Cochrane Reviewer's Handbook (18) to classify these scores as adequate (low risk of bias), unclear, and inadequate (high risk of bias).

Data synthesis and analysis

We performed the meta-analysis by using a random-effects model in Review Manager 5.3 software. For dichotomous outcomes, the relative risk was calculated with a 95% confidence interval and continuous variables were expressed as a weighted mean difference with 95% confidence intervals. Potential causes of heterogeneity among studies were also analyzed. The I^2 statistic was used to measure the impact of heterogeneity for each outcome (where an $I^2 \geq 50$ indicates a considerable level of heterogeneity) (18). When we found heterogeneity, we attempted to determine possible reasons for it via subgroup analysis or by examining individual studies.

Quality assessment

The quality of evidence per outcome measurement was graded according to the Grading of Recommendations Assessment, Development and Evaluation (GRADE) Working Group. The confidence of the GRADE system decreases if randomized studies have major limitations that may interfere with treatment effect estimates (20). These limitations include risk of bias for each study, inconsistency, indirectness, imprecision, and publication bias of each evaluated outcome per GRADE considerations.

RESULTS

From the database searches, 3190 articles were identified (Figure 1). Fifteen articles were potentially eligible for inclusion in the analysis and were selected for full review. Five of the 15 studies were included for analysis (7,10,15,21,22). Of the 10 excluded studies, three were not randomized (23-25), three compared two different methods for mealtime insulin dosing; no group had conventional nutritional advice using a fixed dose of fast or regular insulin before meals (8,26,27). In three studies, patients were children or adolescents (28-30), and one study compared three different possibilities of insulin self-adjustments, without a group using a fixed dose of fast or regular insulin before meals (31).

The baseline characteristics of study participants and eligibility criteria of the included studies are presented in Tables 1 and 2, respectively. P values < 0.05 were considered statistically significant.

Dafne and cols. (7) performed a single-center study in England. A total of 169 patients with DM1 who had been diagnosed more than two years prior without chronic complications and intensive insulin therapy were randomized to CHOC or conventional nutritional treatment. The main outcome measures after a

six-month follow-up were: HbA1c, severe hypoglycemia, and the impact of diabetes on QOL as assessed using the ADDQoL questionnaire.

Laurenzi and cols. (10) recruited patients from a clinic in Milan, Italy. A total of 61 adult patients with DM1 who had been treated with CSII were randomly assigned to learn CHOC in the intervention group or to estimate pre-meal insulin doses empirically for six months. The main outcome measures were: HbA1c, fasting glucose, BMI, waist circumference, daily insulin dose, hypoglycemic events, and analysis of QOL through the Diabetes-Specific Quality-of-life Scale, which evaluates individual treatment goals in patients with DM1.

In the study of Scavone and cols. (Italy) (21), 256 patients with DM1 who had been diagnosed for more than five years were randomized to a CHOC group or a control group. Weight, BMI, HbA1c, lipid profile, uric acid, creatinine, microalbuminuria, daily insulin requirements, and number of episodes of hypoglycemia (blood glucose < 70 mg/dL) were the main outcomes evaluated.

Schmidt and cols. (15) recruited patients from two centers in Denmark. The authors randomized 63 adults with DM1 and poor metabolic control (HbA1c: 8.0% to 10.5%) to the CHOC or control groups for more than 12 months using analogues of basal and fast insulin. The main outcome measures were: change in HbA1c, weight, satisfaction with the treatment of diabetes, and perceived frequency of hyper- and hypoglycemia. The parameters were measured according to the Diabetes Treatment Satisfaction status version and version change questionnaires (DTSQs and DTSQc, respectively). QOL was analyzed using the ADDQoL questionnaire.

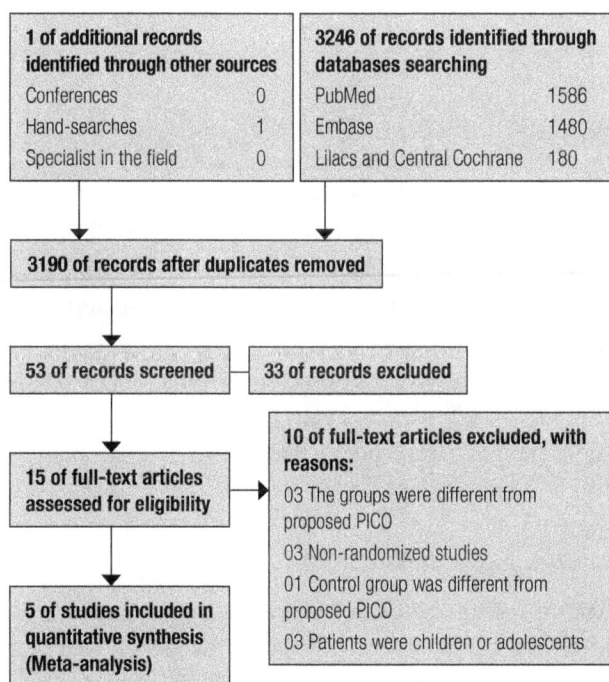

Figure 1. Flowchart for identifying eligible studies

Table 1. Baseline characteristics of patients in each included study

Study	Number of randomized patients	Male/Female	Age (SD)	HbA1C (SD)	Fasting Glucose nmol/L (SD)	BMI or weight (kg) (SD)	Insulin dose (SD)
Dafne, 2002	G1 = 84 G2 = 85	-	-	G1- 9.4 (1.2) G2 = 9.3 (1.1)	-	G1 = 80.5 (1.7) G2 = 77.4 (13.4)	-
Laurenzi, 2011	G1 = 28 G2 = 28	G1 = 15/13 G2 = 09/19	G1 = 41.2 (10.0) G2 = 39.8 (9.8)	G1 = 7.9 (0.9) G2 = 8.1 (1.5)	-	G1 = 23.7 (21-25.2) G2 = 23.8 (20.8-26.8)	**G1 = 36 (24.5-49) **G2 = 33 (28.5-39.5)
Scavone, 2010	G1 = 100 G 2 = 156	G1 = 49/51 G2 = 74/82	G1 = 39 (11) G2 = 39 (11)	G1 = 7.8 (1.3) G2 = 7.5 (0.8)	-	-	-
Schmidt, 2012	G1 = 26 G2 = 09	G1 = 10/11 G2 = 06/02	G1= 41 (10) G2 = 46 (09)	G1 = 9.2 (0.6) G2 = 9.1 (0.7)	-	-	*G1 = 0.6 (0.2) *G2 = 0.7 (0.17)
Trento, 2009	G1 = 27 G2 = 29	G1= 18/9 G2 = 12/17	G1 = 37.33 (12.6) G2 = 36.76 (7.9)	G1 = 7.6 (1.3) G2 = 7.7 (1.24)	G1 = 9.64 (5.17) G2 = 9.05 (5.08)	G1 = 24.4 (2.6) G2 = 23.5 (3.3)	**G1 = 47.9 (10.6) **G2 = 45.7 (12.6)

G1: intervention group; G2: control group. * Daily insulin dose per kg; ** Total insulin dose (basal and bolus). - No information provided.

Table 2. Length of follow-up, inclusion criteria, and outcomes of included studies

Study	Follow-up	Inclusion criteria	Outcomes
DAFNE, 2002	6 months	> 18 years of HbA1c from 7.5% to 12% and diagnosis greater than 2 years without advanced complications	Change in HbA1C (HPLC), severe hypoglycemia and hyperglycemia, quality of life (ADDQoL, DTSQ, and W-BQ12), weight, blood pressure, lipid profile, injections, glucose monitoring, and daily total dose of insulin
Laurenzi, 2011	3 and 6 months	Age between 18 and 65 years and treatment with continuous insulin infusion pump for more than 3 months	Change in HbA1C (HPLC), hypoglycemia, quality of life (DSQOLS), BMI, waist, fasting glucose, and daily insulin dose
Scavone, 2010	9 months	Diagnosis of type 1 diabetes mellitus over 5 years	Changes in HbA1c, hypoglycemia, daily insulin dose, weight, lipid profile, creatinine, and microalbuminuria
Schmidt, 2012	4 months	Age between 18 and 65 years, poor metabolic control, diabetes duration over 12 months, and use of basal and fast analogue insulin.	Changes in HbA1C, severe hypoglycemia, treatment satisfaction and perceived frequency of hypo- and hyperglycemia (DTSQs and DTSQc), quality of life (ADDQoL), change in the perception of problem areas (PAID), and change in fear of hypoglycemia (HFS)
Trento, 2009	30 months	Age <70 years, onset of diabetes before 30 years of age, and onset of insulin use within the first year of the diagnosis	Changes in HbA1C (HPLC), severe hypoglycemia and hyperglycemia, quality of life (DQOL, GISED, CSI), BMI, and lipid profile and fasting glucose

Trento and cols. (22) included 56 patients with DM1 who had all been diagnosed before age 30 years. Twenty-seven subjects were randomized to a CHOC program and the remaining patients were assigned to the control group. Body weight, fasting glucose, HbA1c, total cholesterol, high-density lipoprotein cholesterol, triglycerides and creatinine, frequency of hypoglycemia, and QOL were the main outcome measures.

Risk of bias

Dafne and cols. (7) and Laurenzi and cols. (10) randomized patients using a computer-generated random number. Schmidt and cols. (15) performed the random distribution with a 1: 3: 3 ratio in blocks of 14 with sealed, opaque envelopes containing group assignments. Scavone and cols. (21) and Trento and cols. (22) did not describe how the randomization sequence was generated.

Only Dafne, Laurenzi, and Schmidt described allocation concealment and as such were classified as low risk of bias. The other two studies did not provide any information regarding the allocation process.

Most of the studies included did not report blinding for outcome evaluation. However, except for severe hypoglycemia, most were laboratory assessments, which were not susceptible to bias. QOL questionnaires were self-applied and could not be blinded.

Only Laurenzi and cols. reported that patients who did not complete the treatment regimen were included in the final analysis (low risk) (10). Trento and cols. (22) reported that all participants completed the

treatment (low risk). In the study of Dafne and cols. (7), 28 patients were lost to follow-up and were not included in the final analysis, although the number of patients who were lost was not significantly different between the groups (15 in the intervention group and 13 in the control group) (low risk). Scavone and cols. (21) had a 27% loss of patients in the intervention group, and they were not included in the final analysis (high risk). Schmidt and cols. (15) had a 19% loss, and these patients were not included in the final analysis (high risk).

Meta-analysis of outcomes

The five studies included analyzed changes in HbA1c levels at the end of the study. Meta-analysis showed that the final HbA1c was significantly lower in the CHOC group than in the control group (mean difference, random, 95% CI: -0.49 (-0.85, -0.13), p = 0.006, I^2 = 72%) (Figure 2).

In the four trials, the number of patients who experienced at least one episode of severe hypoglycemia can be assessed (7,15,21,22). The meta-analysis of this outcome was not significantly different between groups (risk ratio, random, 95% CI: 0.94 (0.55, 1.6), p = 0.82, I^2 0%) (Figure 3).

Regarding QOL, two studies (7,15) used the ADDQoL instrument, but no difference was noted between groups (mean difference, random, 95% CI: -0.23 (-1.4, 0.94), p = 0.7, I^2 = 84%). The same studies also used the DTSQs questionnaire and found no difference between groups (mean difference, random, 95% CI: 3.53 (-7.11, 14.16), p = 0.52, I^2 = 95%).

Study or Subgroup	Carbohydrate Counting			General Dietary Advice			Weight	Mean Difference IV, Random, 95% CI	Mean Difference IV, Random, 95% CI
	Mean	SD	Total	Mean	SD	Total			
Dafne 2002	8.4	1.2	67	9.4	1.3	72	21.7%	-1.00 [-1.42, -0.58]	
Laurenzi 2011	7.6	0.6	28	7.9	0.6	28	24.8%	-0.30 [-0.61, 0.01]	
Scavone 2009	7.4	0.9	73	7.5	1.1	156	26.1%	-0.10 [-0.37, 0.17]	
Schmidt 2012	8.4	0.9	21	8.9	1.1	8	11.2%	-0.50 [-1.35, 0.35]	
Trento 2010	7.2	0.9	27	7.9	1.4	29	16.2%	-0.70 [-1.31, -0.09]	
Total (95% CI)			216			293	100.0%	-0.49 [-0.85, -0.13]	

Heterogeneity: Tau² = 0.11; Chi² = 14.08, df = 4 (P = 0.007); I² = 72%
Test for overall effect: Z = 2.65 (P = 0.008)

Favours [experimental]   Favours [control]

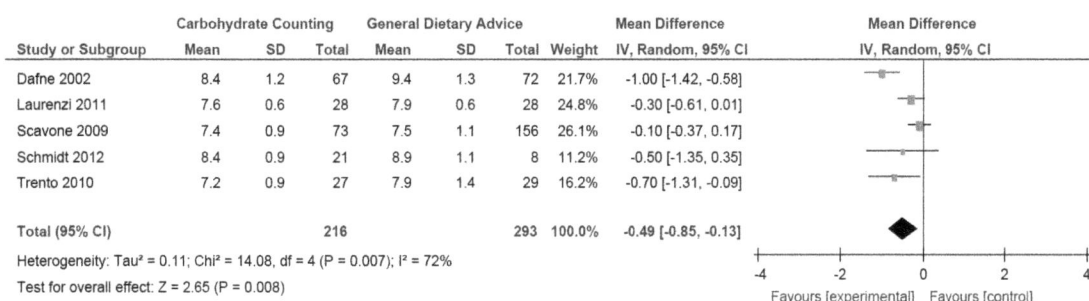

Figure 2. Meta-analysis of change in HbA1c.

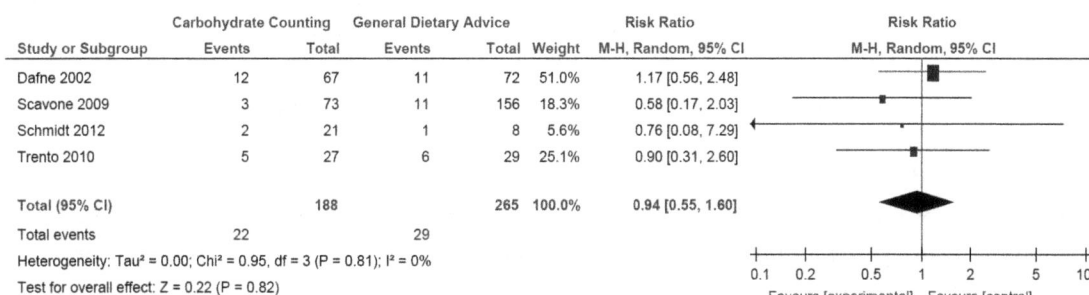

Study or Subgroup	Carbohydrate Counting		General Dietary Advice		Weight	Risk Ratio M-H, Random, 95% CI	Risk Ratio M-H, Random, 95% CI
	Events	Total	Events	Total			
Dafne 2002	12	67	11	72	51.0%	1.17 [0.56, 2.48]	
Scavone 2009	3	73	11	156	18.3%	0.58 [0.17, 2.03]	
Schmidt 2012	2	21	1	8	5.6%	0.76 [0.08, 7.29]	
Trento 2010	5	27	6	29	25.1%	0.90 [0.31, 2.60]	
Total (95% CI)		188		265	100.0%	0.94 [0.55, 1.60]	
Total events	22		29				

Heterogeneity: Tau² = 0.00; Chi² = 0.95, df = 3 (P = 0.81); I² = 0%
Test for overall effect: Z = 0.22 (P = 0.82)

Favours [experimental]   Favours [control]

Figure 3. Meta-analysis of episodes of severe hypoglycemia.

We plotted the QOL outcomes using different questionnaires (DQOL and DTSQs) cited in three studies (7,15,22,23) and found no significant differences between groups (std. mean difference, random, 95% CI: 0.64 (-0.7, 1.98), p = 0.35, I² = 94%).

Meta-analysis of total cholesterol, HDL-C, and triglycerides could only be performed based on the results reported in the study of Dafne and cols. (7) and Trento and cols. (22); no significant differences were noted among groups.

According to the GRADE, the quality of evidence of the primary outcomes was moderate for changes in HbA1c, low for episodes of severe hypoglycemia, and very low for QOL (Table 3).

DISCUSSION

Most individuals with DM1 have a hard time managing fasting and postprandial blood glucose levels. In addition, many patients with this disease have poor compliance to dietary advice.

Poor disease control can increase the risk of complications, such as retinopathy and other microvascular conditions (3). Ahola and cols. (32) reported that only one-third of patients maintained controlled blood glucose levels after a meal and that approximately 40% experienced frequent hyperglycemia despite having seemingly normal metabolic control. As such, the search for tools to improve these health issues

Table 3. Quality of evidence of primary outcomes according to GRADE approach

Outcomes	Risk of bias	Inconsistency	Indirectness	Imprecision	Publication bias	Intervention vs comparator 95% CI	Participants (studies)	Quality of evidence
Severe hypoglycemia	Serious* (-1)	No	No	Serious (-1)***	Unlikely	RR 0.92 (0.54 a 1.56)	453 (4)	+Low
Quality of Life (ADDQoL)	Serious* (-1)	Serious (-1)**	No	Serious (-1)****	Unlikely	MD 3.53 (-7,11 a 14.16)	168 (2)	+++Very low
Change in HbA1c	Serious* (-1)	No	No	No	Unlikely	MD -0.45 (-0.77, -0.13)	535 (5)	+ Moderate

* Most of the included studies did not report about allocation concealment, and they did not perform an intention-to-treat analysis. ** Presence of statistical heterogeneity (I² > 75%). *** 95% CI overlaps no effect but includes important benefit or important harm. **** Optimal information size criterion was not meet. ADDQOL: Audit of Diabetes – Dependent Quality of Life. RR: Relative risk. MD: Mean difference. ++ **Low evidence**: The authors are not confident in the effect estimate, and the true value may be substantially different from it. ++ **Very low evidence**: The authors do not have any confidence in the estimate, and it is likely that the true value is substantially different from it. + **Moderate evidence**: Further research is likely to have an important impact on our confidence in the estimate of effect and may change the estimate.

has increased, and CHOC may be the only effective option for adherence to dietary requirement in patients with variable dietary habits.

To reduce postprandial blood glucose, protocols from the DAPHNE program and the Diabetes Teaching and Treatment have used the CHOC method for nutritional counseling (33). Some studies reported that CHOC can provide better glycemic control and lead to an improved QOL for patients (3,17). Patients using this method have greater flexibility in food choices without the concern of postprandial hyperglycemia given that the amount of carbohydrates ingested is considered when computing the amount of insulin to be administered before meals.

In daily clinical practice, the goal is to maintain good long-term disease control, prevent chronic complications from DM, and reduce the frequency of hypoglycemia to improve overall QOL. We performed a systematic review focusing on the efficacy and safety of the CHOC method in the management of patients with DM1. We included randomized trials that compared the CHOC method with conventional nutritional guidance in the treatment of patients with DM1.

Five studies met the established inclusion criteria and were included in qualitative and quantitative analyses. Most of the studies assessed changes in HbA1c, frequency of hypoglycemia, and QOL as primary endpoints. Meta-analysis showed a significant difference in final HbA1c favoring the intervention group.

A criticism of HbA1c is that even though levels are associated with the frequency of chronic complications and rate of morbidity and mortality, the value of this laboratory outcome is often discussed without considering glycemic variability. Although it is important for HbA1c levels to be lower than the cutoff values that indicate disease control, blood glucose levels can range from high to low. An association between glycemic variability and development of micro diabetes-related complications has been shown in type 2 DM and has also been studied as a possibility in DM1 (34). If confirmed, HbA1c values in DM1 would be inadequate to determine the superiority of one treatment to another. However, in this present review, the frequency of hypoglycemia was the same between the groups, which means that the relevance of lowering HbA1c would not be reduced.

Regarding QOL outcomes, several different instruments were used in the studies included, which negatively affected the single meta-analysis of this parameter. However, independent of the instrument used, an improvement in QOL from baseline compared with the final visit in most of the studies was noted, although no difference was observed between the intervention and control groups. Improvement in QOL can be more associated with follow-up programs and nutritional guidance than the initial methods evaluated.

Applying the GRADE approach for the outcomes "change in HbA1c" and "severe hypoglycemia," it was necessary to rate down for the risk of bias because five out of the six studies lost patients to follow-up without an intention to treat analysis. In addition, concealment allocation and randomization processes were unclear in two of the studies. Similarly, imprecision was rated down for both, because optimal information size criterion was not met and 95% CI overlaps no effect but includes important benefit or important harm, respectively. Rating down for indirectness and publication bias was unnecessary. The quality of evidence for "change in HbA1c" and "severe hypoglycemia" was moderate and low, respectively, indicating that further research is likely to have an important impact on our confidence and authors are not confident in the effect estimate. The quality of the evidence regarding QOL outcomes was very low, and any estimate of its effect is uncertain.

Bell and cols. (35) recently published a similar systematic review. They included a study that was not included in our analysis because the comparison groups were different from the proposed PICO (31) They also included another study that we excluded because patients in the control group were predominantly children, and they were provided nutritional guidance of low glycemic index (36). Finally, Bell and cols. did not use the GRADE. The results of the previous study favored the intervention group, and the authors interpreted the results in support of recommending CHOC instead of general dietary advice in patients with DM1.

Considering the studies included in the present systematic review, the meta-analysis showed evidence favoring the use of CHOC in the management of adult patients with DM1. However, this benefit was limited to final HbA1c, which was significantly lower in the CHOC group than in the control group. Therefore, new randomized trials with greater internal and external validation and long-term outcomes are needed to analyze whether or not a significant difference exists between these two nutritional guidance tools in terms of other important diabetes-related outcomes, such as mortality, QOL, and diabetes complications.

REFERENCES

1. American Diabetes Association. Diagnosis and classification of diabetes mellitus. Diabetes Care. 2014;37 Suppl 1:S81-90.

2. DIAMOND Project Group. Incidence and trends of childhood type 1 diabetes worldwide 1990-1999. Diabet Med. 2006;23(8):857-66.

3. Diabetes Control and Complications Trial Research Group, Nathan DM, Genuth S, Lachin J, Cleary P, Crofford O, Davis M, et al. The effect of intensive treatment of diabetes on the development and progression of long-term complications in insulin-dependent diabetes mellitus. N Engl J Med. 1993;329(14):977-86.

4. American Diabetes Association. 6. Glycemic Targets. Diabetes Care. 2017;40(Suppl 1):S48-S56.

5. Diet, nutrition and the prevention of chronic diseases. World Health Organ Tech Rep Ser. 2003;916:i-viii, 1-149, backcover.

6. Evert AB, Boucher JL, Cypress M, Dunbar SA, Franz MJ, Mayer-Davis EJ, et al. Nutrition therapy recommendations for the management of adults with diabetes. Diabetes Care. 2014;37 Suppl 1:S120-43.

7. DAFNE Study Group. Training in flexible, intensive insulin management to enable dietary freedom in people with type 1 diabetes: dose adjustment for normal eating (DAFNE) randomised controlled trial. BMJ. 2002;325(7367):746.

8. Rabasa-Lhoret R, Garon J, Langelier H, Poisson D, Chiasson JL. Effects of meal carbohydrate content on insulin requirements in type 1 diabetic patients treated intensively with the basal-bolus (ultralente-regular) insulin regimen. Diabetes Care. 1999;22(5):667-73.

9. Rossi MC, Nicolucci A, Di Bartolo P, Bruttomesso D, Girelli A, Ampudia FJ, et al. Diabetes Interactive Diary: a new telemedicine system enabling flexible diet and insulin therapy while improving quality of life: an open-label, international, multicenter, randomized study. Diabetes Care. 2010;33(1):109-15.

10. Laurenzi A, Bolla AM, Panigoni G, Doria V, Uccellatore A, Peretti E, et al. Effects of carbohydrate counting on glucose control and quality of life over 24 weeks in adult patients with type 1 diabetes on continuous subcutaneous insulin infusion: a randomized, prospective clinical trial (GIOCAR). Diabetes Care. 2011;34(4):823-7.

11. Hegar K, Heiber S, Brandle M, Christ E, Keller U. Carbohydrate counting of food. Swiss Med Wkly. 2011;141:w13224.

12. Bell KJ, King BR, Shafat A, Smart CE. The relationship between carbohydrate and the mealtime insulin dose in type 1 diabetes. J Diabetes Complications. 2015;29(8):1323-9.

13. Nutricionistas Membros do Departamento de Nutrição da SBD. Manual de contagem de carboidratos para pessoas com diabetes. Sociedade Brasileira de Diabetes, 2016.

14. Diretrizes da Sociedade Brasileira de Diabetes (2015-2016). Rio de Janeiro: AC Farmacêutica Ltda.; 2016. Princípios para Orientação Nutricional no Diabetes Mellitus; p. 91-110.

15. Schmidt S, Meldgaard M, Serifovski N, Storm C, Christensen TM, Gade-Rasmussen B, et al. Use of an automated bolus calculator in MDI-treated type 1 diabetes: the BolusCal Study, a randomized controlled pilot study. Diabetes Care. 2012;35(5):984-90.

16. Dias VM, Pandini JA, Nunes RR, Sperandei SL, Portella ES, Cobas RA, et al. Effect of the carbohydrate counting method on glycemic control in patients with type 1 diabetes. Diabetol Metab Syndr. 2010;2:54.

17. Waller H, Eiser C, Knowles J, Rogers N, Wharmby S, Heller S, et al. Pilot study of a novel educational programme for 11-16 year olds with type 1 diabetes mellitus: the KICk-OFF course. Arch Dis Child. 2008;93(11):927-31.

18. Cochrane Handbook for Systematic Reviews of Interventions Version 5.1.0 [updated March 2011] [Internet]. 2011.

19. Liberati A, Altman DG, Tetzlaff J, Mulrow C, Gotzsche PC, Ioannidis JP, et al. The PRISMA statement for reporting systematic reviews and meta-analyses of studies that evaluate health care interventions: explanation and elaboration. Ann Intern Med. 2009;151(4):W65-94.

20. Guyatt GH, Oxman AD, Kunz R, Vist GE, Falck-Ytter Y, Schünemann HJ; GRADE Working Group. What is "quality of evidence" and why is it important to clinicians? BMJ. 2008;336(7651):995-8.

21. Scavone G, Manto A, Pitocco D, Gagliardi L, Caputo S, Mancini L, et al. Effect of carbohydrate counting and medical nutritional therapy on glycaemic control in Type 1 diabetic subjects: a pilot study. Diabet Med. 2010;27(4):477-9.

22. Trento M, Trinetta A, Kucich C, Grassi G, Passera P, Gennari S, et al. Carbohydrate counting improves coping ability and metabolic control in patients with Type 1 diabetes managed by Group Care. J Endocrinol Invest. 2011;34(2):101-5.

23. Bao J, Gilbertson HR, Gray R, Munns D, Howard G, Petocz P, et al. Improving the estimation of mealtime insulin dose in adults with type 1 diabetes: the Normal Insulin Demand for Dose Adjustment (NIDDA) study. Diabetes Care. 2011;34(10):2146-51.

24. Chiesa G, Piscopo MA, Rigamonti A, Azzinari A, Bettini S, Bonfanti R, et al. Insulin therapy and carbohydrate counting. Acta Biomed. 2005;76 Suppl 3:44-8.

25. Dubé MC, Lavoie C, Galibois I, Weisnagel SJ. Nutritional strategies to prevent hypoglycemia at exercise in diabetic adolescents. Med Sci Sports Exerc. 2012;44(8):1427-32.

26. Rossetti P, Ampudia-Blasco FJ, Laguna A, Revert A, Vehì J, Ascaso JF, et al. Evaluation of a novel continuous glucose monitoring-based method for mealtime insulin dosing – the iBolus – in subjects with type 1 diabetes using continuous subcutaneous insulin infusion therapy: a randomized controlled trial. Diabetes Technol Ther. 2012;14(11):1043-52.

27. Gilbertson HR, Brand-Miller JC, Thorburn AW, Evans S, Chondros P, Werther GA. The effect of flexible low glycemic index dietary advice versus measured carbohydrate exchange diets on glycemic control in children with type 1 diabetes. Diabetes Care. 2001;24(7):1137-43.

28. Gökşen D, Atik Altınok Y, Ozen S, Demir G, Darcan S. Effects of carbohydrate counting method on metabolic control in children with type 1 diabetes mellitus. J Clin Res Pediatr Endocrinol. 2014;6(2):74-8.

29. Albuquerque IZ, Stringhini SMF, Marques RMB, Mundim CA, Rodrigues MLD, Campos MRH. Carbohydrate counting, nutritional status and metabolic profile of adolescents with type 1 diabetes mellitus. Sci Med. 2014;24(4).

30. Enander R, Gundevall C, Strömgren A, Chaplin J, Hanas R. Carbohydrate counting with a bolus calculator improves post-prandial blood glucose levels in children and adolescents with type 1 diabetes using insulin pumps. Pediatr Diabetes. 2012;13(7):545-51.

31. Kalergis M, Pacaud D, Strychar I, Meltzer S, Jones PJ, Yale JF. Optimizing insulin delivery: assessment of three strategies in intensive diabetes management. Diabetes Obes Metab. 2000;2(5):299-305.

32. Ahola AJ, Mäkimattila S, Saraheimo M, Mikkilä V, Forsblom C, Freese R, Groop PH; FinnDIANE Study Group. Many patients with type 1 diabetes estimate their prandial insulin need inappropriately. J Diabetes. 2010;2(3):194-202.

33. Speight J, Amiel SA, Bradley C, Heller S, Oliver L, Roberts S, et al. Long-term biomedical and psychosocial outcomes following DAFNE (Dose Adjustment For Normal Eating) structured education to promote intensive insulin therapy in adults with sub-optimally controlled type 1 diabetes. Diabetes Res Clin Pract. 2010;89(1):22-9.

34. American Diabetes Association. Executive summary: standards of medical care in diabetes – 2011. Diabetes Care. 2011;34 Suppl 1:S4-10.

35. Bell KJ, Barclay AW, Petocz P, Colagiuri S, Brand-Miller JC. Efficacy of carbohydrate counting in type 1 diabetes: a systematic review and meta-analysis. Lancet Diabetes Endocrinol. 2014;2(2):133-40.

36. Gilbertson HR, Thorburn AW, Brand-Miller JC, Chondros P, Werther GA. Effect of low-glycemic-index dietary advice on dietary quality and food choice in children with type 1 diabetes. Am J Clin Nutr. 2003;77(1):83-90.

10

Reliability of Thyroid Imaging Reporting and Data System (TI-RADS), and ultrasonographic classification of the American Thyroid Association (ATA) in differentiating benign from malignant thyroid nodules

Bruno Mussoi de Macedo[1], Rogério F. Izquierdo[1],
Lenara Golbert[1], Erika L. Souza Meyer[1]

ABSTRACT

Objective: Ultrasonography (US) is the best diagnostic tool for initial assessment of thyroid nodule. Recently, data reporting systems for thyroid lesions, such as the Thyroid Imaging Reporting and Data System (TI-RADS) and American Thyroid Association (ATA), which stratifies the risk for malignancy, have demonstrated good performance in differentiating malignant thyroid nodules. The purpose of this study is to determine the reliability of both data reporting systems in predicting thyroid malignancy in a tertiary care hospital. Materials and methods: We evaluated 195 thyroid nodules using modified TI-RADS and ATA risk stratification. The results were compared to the cyto-pathology analysis. Histopathological results were available for 45 cases after surgery, which is considered the golden standard for diagnosis of thyroid cancer. Results: When compared with cytological results, sensitivity, specificity, negative predictive value (NPV), and accuracy were 100, 61.1, 100, and 63%, respectively, for TI-RADS; and 100, 75, 100, and 76%, respectively, for ATA. When compared with histopathological results, sensitivity, specificity, NPV, and accuracy were 90, 51.4, 94.7, and 60% respectively, for TI-RADS; and 100, 60, 100, and 68%, respectively, for ATA. All patients with malignant nodules were classified in the categories 4 or 5 of TI-RADS and in the intermediate or high suspicion risk according to the ATA system. Conclusion: Both TI-RADS and the ATA guidelines have high sensitivity and NPV for the diagnosis of thyroid carcinoma. These systems are feasible for clinical application, allowing to better select patients to undergo fine-needle aspiration biopsies. Arch Endocrinol Metab. 2018;62(2):131-8

[1] Thyroid Section, Endocrine Division, Irmandade da Santa Casa de Misericórdia de Porto Alegre, Universidade Federal de Ciências da Saúde de Porto Alegre (UFCSPA), Porto Alegre, RS, Brazil

Correspondence to:
Erika L. Souza Meyer
Serviço de Endocrinologia
Irmandade da Santa Casa de Misericórdia de Porto Alegre
Rua Professor Annes Dias, 295
90020-090 – Porto Alegre, RS, Brasil
erikam@ufcspa.edu.br

Keywords
Thyroid nodules; US patterns; thyroid cancer

INTRODUCTION

Thyroid nodules are a common finding within the general population, and their detection is increasing with the widespread use of ultrasound (US) (1). Thyroid US is a widely accepted imaging modality for the initial assessment of thyroid nodules. It has been widely used to stratify the risk of malignancy in thyroid nodules and also in aiding with making decisions about whether fine-needle aspiration (FNA) is indicated. There are well-established ultrasound findings that differentiate benign and malignant thyroid nodules (2-8). A study by Kim and cols. (7) previously reported that hypoechogenicity, marked hypoechogenicity, microlobulated or irregular margins, microcalcifications, and taller than wide shape are the ultrasound features which best predicted the chance of

malignancy in thyroid nodules. Since the malignancy risk estimated by US is not determined by a single US predictor, it should be assessed by a combination of the US features (9-11). There are several classification systems which categorize thyroid nodules according to the risk of cancer (12-21). An interesting thyroid imaging reporting and data system (TI-RADS) derived from the breast imaging reporting and data system (BI-RADS) was prospectively tested in 4550 nodules where it demonstrated a high sensitivity and NPV for the diagnosis of thyroid carcinoma (21). One of the limitations of this recent version of TI-RADS was related to some significant US signs not considered for the flow chart, such as the halo sign, size and central flow by Doppler study. This way, the American Thyroid Association's (ATA) thyroid nodule guideline (20) proposed a new ultrasonographic pattern considering nodule margins. There has been no standardized malignancy risk stratification system for thyroid nodules. Thus, it is important to validate these classifications in different healthcare centers. We proposed to evaluate the diagnostic accuracy of a modified TI-RADS and 2015 ATA's ultrasound risk for the diagnosis of malignancy in thyroid nodules.

MATERIALS AND METHODS

Patients

Between July 2014 and August 2015, we prospectively analyzed data from 178 consecutive unselected patients with thyroid nodules attending the Endocrinology Division at *Santa Casa de Misericórdia de Porto Alegre*, a tertiary, university-based hospital located in an iodine-replete area in Southern Brazil. All patients underwent a complete clinical evaluation and thyroid ultrasonography. Patients with known thyroid cancer and/or patients with purely cystic nodules were excluded. This study was approved by the local ethics committees and participants provided written informed consent (CAAE:16398613.2.0000.5335).

Imaging technique and TI-RADS and ATA ultrasound classification

Thyroid Ultrasound Conventional B-mode and Doppler images of the neck and thyroid gland were obtained by ultrasound machine (ACUSON S2000™, Siemens and ACUSON Antares™, Siemens HealthCare, Erlangen, Germany) using a high-frequency probe (12 MHz). All US examinations were performed by the same radiologist (RFI) who has more than 10 years of experience in thyroid ultrasound. All images were examined on real-time two-dimensional gray-scale and Doppler imaging. All sonograms obtained were saved in a picture archive. Ultrasound features were assessed for each nodule characteristic like composition (solid, cystic, mixed), echogenicity (hyperechoic, isoechoic, hypoechoic, markedly hypoechoic), margins (well defined with or without halo sign, microlobulated, ill-defined, irregular), presence of calcification (microcalcification, macrocalcification), and shape of the nodule (round, oval). Also, the presence of cervical lymphadenopathy was evaluated. Findings that were considered in favor of a malignancy were hypoechoic or markedly hypoechoic in echogenicity; irregular, microlobulated, or ill-defined margins; presence of microcalcification; round shape

and the presence of lymphadenopathy. We performed a prospective evaluation using the modified Russ classification (21), each nodule was classified into a TI-RADS category (2, 3, 4 and 5) based on the US features (Figure 1). Differently from the Russ classification (21) in which mildly or moderately hypoechoic nodules (TI-RADS 4A) are categorized differently from markedly hypoechoic nodules (TI-RADS 4B), we have decided not to subdivide category 4 with the intention of simplifying this score for clinical practice. Posteriorly, the same radiologist (RFI) who was blind about the pathological results, scored all evaluated nodules of the saved pictures using a flowchart (Figure 1) based on new ATA thyroid nodule guideline of as previously published (20). Based on the number of features suspicious for malignancy we considered four different sonographic patterns: "very low suspicion"; "low suspicion"; "intermediate"; and "high suspicion". Pure cystic nodules were not included in the analyses. Figure 2 demonstrate representative US features in thyroid nodules.

The diagnostic performance of TI-RADS and ATA classification system was evaluated by comparison with the fine-needle aspiration cytology (FNA) reports and anatomopathological examination.

Thyroid FNA, thyroid cytology, and histology

All 195 nodules were submitted to FNA performed by using a capillary US-guided (FNA-US) technique with 23-gauge needle attached to a 10 mL disposable plastic syringe. There was no nodule size threshold for indicating FNA. In most of the cases, only one needle pass was made per lesion. Cytology smears were prepared on four to six slides. Slides were fixed immediately in 95% alcohol and stained with Papanicolaou stain. One cytopathologist from of our institution who has vast experience in thyroid pathology interpreted the smears. A thyroid FNA specimen was considered satisfactory if at least 6 groups of follicular cells were present, and each group comprised at least 10 cells (22). The Bethesda System for Cytological Classification of Thyroid Nodules was used to interpret smears (23) as: 1) non-diagnostic or unsatisfactory, 2) benign, 3) atypia of undetermined significance, 4) a follicular neoplasm or suspicious for a follicular neoplasm, 5) suspicious for malignancy, and 6) malignant. Surgery was indicated based on cytopathological results (Bethesda 4, 5 and 6), or when the nodule was benign (Bethesda 2) but larger than 3-4 cm and causing compressive symptoms.

	Suspect patterns		Benign patterns	
	Signs of High Suspicion: - Taller-than-wide - Irregular Borders - Microcalcifications - Markedly Hypoechoic		Very Probable - Isoechoic or Hyperechoic AND - No sign of high suspicion	Constantly - Simple cyst - Spongiform nodule - Isolated macrocalficication - Nodular hyperplasia
	Hypoechoic solid nodule with 3 to 5 signs of high suspicion	Hypoechoic solid nodule with 1 to 2 signs of high suspicion		
TI-RADS	SCORE 5	SCORE 4	SCORE 3	SCORE 2
ATA 2015	HIGH RISK	INTERMEDIATE RISK	LOW RISK	VERY LOW RISK
	Solid hypoechoic nodule or solid hypoechoic component of a partially cystic nodule	Hypoechoic solid nodule with smooth margins	Isoechoic or hyperechoic solid nodule Partially cystic nodule with eccentric solid areas, without any High Risk Features	Spongiform Partially cystic nodules Without any of the sonographic features described in low, intermediate, or high suspicion patterns Purely cystic nodules
	+ 1 ou more of HRF	without any of HRF		
	High Risk Features - irregular margins (infiltrative, microlobulated) - microcalcifications - taller than wide shape - rim calcifications with small extrusive soft tissue component - evidence of extrathyroidal extension			

Figure 1. Comparative chart: TI-RADS (modified from Russ and cols.) and American Thyroid Association (ATA) 2015 HRF: High Risk Features.

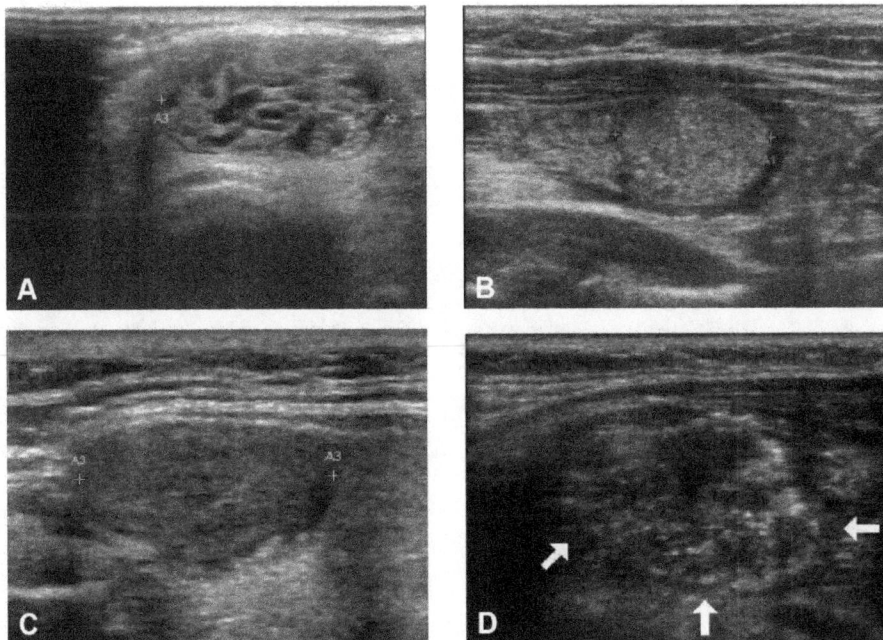

Figure 2. Representative images of TI-RADS and ATA systems in thyroid nodules. **A:** Spongiform nodule – TI-RADS 2 or ATA very low risk. **B:** Isoechoic solid nodule, regular-shaped and borders, without HRF - TI-RADS 3 or ATA low risk. **C:** Hypoechoic solid nodule with regular borders – TI-RADS 4 or ATA intermediate risk. **D:** Hypoechoic solid nodule with irregular borders and microcalcifications (arrows) – TI-RADS 5 or ATA high risk.

Anatomopathological examinations of tissue samples obtained at thyroidectomy were carried out according to the World Health Organization Guidelines (24), and the pathology reports pertaining to these samples were considered identical to the gold standard for the diagnosis of thyroid cancer.

Statistical analysis

Clinical, laboratory, ultrasonography and cytological data, which are reported as the mean – standard deviation (SD) values, or as the median with percentiles between 25 and 75 (continuous variables), or as absolute numbers and percentages (categorical variables), were compared using Mann-Whitney U-test or chi-squared test as appropriate. Specificity, sensitivity, positive and negative predictive value were calculated to evaluate the reliability of TI-RADS and ATA classification methods in differentiation between benign and malignant features. In all analyses, $P < 0.05$ was considered for statistical significance. Statistical analysis of the results was performed with SPSS software (Statistical Package for Social Sciences) version 18.0.

RESULTS

Demographic data and global results of 195 nodules by US features and scores

The clinical characteristics of the 178 patients (195 nodules) included in this study were as follow: the median age was 59 years (range 49-66) and 94.9% were female. The median size of nodules was 24 mm (range 15-37). Nodules were classified as TI-RADS 2, 3, 4 and 5 in 11, 43, 44, and 2% of cases, respectively. Posteriorly, nodules were re-classified by ATA scores as very low risk in 35.9%; low risk in 28.2%; intermediate in 30.8% and high in 5.1% of cases. There was no difference in the size of the nodules among the TI-RADS scores as well as among the ATA sonographic categories (p = 0.25 and 0.20, respectively).

The cytological descriptive statistics results are as follow: 15.9% (n = 31) nondiagnostic (Bethesda 1), 68.2% (n = 133) benign (Bethesda 2), 4.3% (n = 9) atypia of undetermined significance (Bethesda 3), 6.7% (n = 13); suspicious for a follicular neoplasm (Bethesda 4), 2.1% (n = 4) suspicious for malignancy (Bethesda 5) and 2.6% (n = 5) malignant (Bethesda 6).

Final histopathological results were available for 45 cases after surgery. Surgery was indicated based on cytopathological results (5 malignant, 4 suspect,

8 follicular neoplasm, and 3 atypia of indeterminate significance cases) or when the nodule was benign but larger than 3 cm and causing compressive symptoms (25 cases). There were 35 benign cases: 18 adenomatous goiters, and 17 adenomas. There were 10 malignant cases (5.13%), 9 classical papillary thyroid carcinomas, and 1 follicular thyroid variants of papillary carcinoma.

Diagnostic performance of TI-RADS and ATA scores compared with cytological results

By cytology, 77% of TI-RADS scores 2 and 3 were benign (Bethesda category 2), 8.6% were indeterminate (Bethesda categories 3 and 4), and 1.9% were suspicious of malignancy (Bethesda categories 5) and none were malignant (Bethesda 6). For ATA score, 79% of low and very low risk were benign; 8.9% were indeterminate, 0.8% were suspicious of malignancy and none were malignant. Interestingly, 100% of carcinomas (Bethesda 6) and 50% of suspicious lesions (Bethesda 5) were classified as TI-RADS scores 4 and 5, and 100% of carcinomas and 75% of suspicious lesions were classified as intermediate and high risk ATA score.

To compare TI-RADS and ATA score with cytological results, only Bethesda categories 2 and 6 were used (n = 138), as the probability of mistake of these two categories is < 3%. The sensitivity, specificity, NPV, and accuracy of the TI-RADS were 100, 61.6, 100, and 63% respectively. In same way, the sensitivity, specificity, NPV, and accuracy of the ATA score were 100, 75, 100, and 76% respectively. The estimated pretest probability of malignant nodule was at 3.6% for the cytology endpoint.

Diagnostic performance of TI-RADS and ATA scores compared with histopathological results (n = 45)

Distribution of carcinomas among TI-RADS categories 2, 3, 4 and 5 was 0, 5.5, 26 and 100%, respectively (Table 1). Among ATA score the percentage was 0, 0, 28, and 83% for "very low", "low", "intermediate suspicion" and "high suspicion", respectively (Table 2). When compared to histopathological results, sensitivity, specificity, NPV, and accuracy of the TI-RADS it was 90, 51.4, 94.7, and 60%, respectively. In addition, the sensitivity, specificity, NPV, and accuracy of the ATA score was 100, 60, 100, and 68%, respectively. The estimated pretest probability of malignant nodule was at 22.2% for the histology endpoint. The matched results of TI-RADS and ATA categories with final histopathological and cytological results are shown in Table 3.

Reclassification of thyroid nodules from TI-RADS to ATA score

Twenty-one nodules TI-RADS category 4 were reclassified according to ATA score as very low risk (10 cases) and low risk (11 cases). Of the ATA very low risk cases, 8 presented cytological results of Bethesda 2 (benign) and 2 cases were Bethesda 3, one of them being submitted to surgery and the histopathological

Table 1. TIRADS categories and risk of malignancy by final histopathological

TIRADS category	Benign	Malignant	Total	Risk of malignancy (%)
TIRADS 2 (n= 2)	1	0	1	0
TIRADS 3 (n= 18)	17	1	18	5.5
TIRADS 4 (n= 23)	17	6	23	26
TIRADS 5 (n= 3)	0	3	0	100
Total (n= 45)	35	10	45	

Table 2. ATA categories and risk of malignancy by final histopathological

ATA category	Benign	Malignant	Total	Risk of malignancy (%)
High suspicion (n= 6)	1	5	6	83.3
Intermediate suspicion (n= 18)	13	5	18	27.7
Low suspicion (n= 10)	10	0	10	0
Very low suspicion (n= 11)	11	0	11	0
Total	35	10	45	

diagnosis was follicular adenoma. Of the ATA low risk cases, 10 were classified by cytological analysis as Bethesda 2. One case was Bethesda category 3 and the outcome of the anatomopathological was follicular adenoma.

Performance of TI-RADS and ATA scores in thyroid nodules with indeterminate results on cytology

Of the 12 indeterminate nodules (Bethesda categories 3 and 4) examined, 10 (83.3%) were histologically benign. Sonographic classification of nodules by TI-RADS category 2 or 3, or as very low to low suspicion by ATA standards displayed negative predictive value of 100% for both systems. Positive predictive values for TI-RADS categories 4 and 5 and ATA intermediate and high risks were 54.5 and 40%, respectively.

DISCUSSION

The ultrasonography terminology of thyroid nodules should be feasible for clinical application, should be useful for malignancy risk stratification, and show a low inter observer variability. Here, we demonstrated a very high NPV and a high sensibility to cancer diagnosis of scores TI-RADS and ATA ultrasound risk.

The Thyroid Imaging Reporting and Data System (TI-RADS) was used by Park and cols. (12) and Horvath and cols. (13) and both systems appear to be difficult to use in routine clinical practice. In order to achieve a practical tool for analyzing thyroid nodules and to improve communication between radiologists and physicians, Russ and cols. (21) proposed a new TI-RADS classification that has a high sensitivity (95.7%) and NPV (99.7%) for diagnosis of thyroid carcinoma. Accordingly, we found NPV of 94.7% for scores TI-RADS 2 and 3.

Table 3. Matched results of TIRADS and ATA categories with final histopathological and cytological results

Ultrassonographic score	Benign histological results (N = 35)						Malignant histological results (N = 10)					
	I	II	III	IV	V	VI	I	II	III	IV	V	VI
TIRADS 2	0	1	0	0	0	0	0	0	0	0	0	0
TIRADS 3	0	12	2	2	1	0	0	0	0	0	1	0
TIRADS 4	4	5	3	4	1	0	0	1	0	2	0	3
TIRADS 5	0	0	0	0	0	0	0	0	0	0	1	2
ATA VERY LOW RISK	0	7	1	2	1	0	0	0	0	0	0	0
ATA LOW RISK	0	7	1	2	0	0	0	0	0	0	0	0
ATA INTERMEDIATE RISK	4	4	3	1	1	0	0	1	0	2	0	2
ATA HIGH RISK	0	0	0	1	0	0	0	0	0	0	2	3

Recently, the American Thyroid Association (ATA) proposed a classification of thyroid nodules into five categories based on US features (20). In the same way, the reassessment of ATA ultrasound classification of malignancy in our patients shows a very high NPV (100%) for very low and low ATA ultrasound risk. These results confirm a high probability of both systems to discard malignancy. In fact, TI-RADS 2 or 3, and ATA very low or low risk consider similar benign patterns like spongiform nodules, isoechoic or hyperechoic solid nodules without signs of high suspicion. Interestingly, isoechoic solid nodules with some suspicious finding are not included in any of the TI-RADS or ATA categories. The risk of malignancy found in previous studies was between 16 to 20%, similar to that observed for hypoechoic nodules without any suspicious finding (25-27). We observed a prevalence of malignancy of 5.5% of nodules categorized as TI-RADS 3, similarly observed by Russ and cols. (4.3%) (21). Also, no nodule classified as low suspicion by ATA was malignant in our sample, reinforcing data from Rosario and cols. (25) that demonstrated in a large number of nodules the risk of malignancy of only 1.7%, lower than suggested by ATA (5-10%) in this category. TI-RADS category 2 or 3 and ATA very low and low risk represented a significant proportion of patients, 54% and 64%, respectively. Therefore, proven high sensitivity and NPV of both systems could allow to ultrasonographically (without FNA) monitoring these nodules categories, especially nodules under 2 cm, unless they increase in volume or if there are new suspicious sonographic features.

TI-RADS proposed by Russ (21) categorize differently mild or moderate hypoechoic nodules (TI-RADS 4A) from markedly hypoechoic nodules (TI-RADS 4B) and unlike this system, we did not subdivide the category 4 of TI-RADS considering this category hypoechoic solid thyroid nodules. This was done to simplify the TI-RADS system for clinical practice minimizing discrepancies in the evaluation of the degree of hypoechogenicity. Also, to calculate the accuracy of TIRADS, it was necessary to group these categories. In addition, there is a general recommendation of US-PAAF of hypoechoic thyroid nodule especially above 1 cm, regardless of the degree of hypoechogenicity (20,28). Thus, TI-RADS 4 nodules were considered an intermediate suspicious for malignancy and were evaluated by cytology. In contrast to TI-RADS, hypoechogenicity associated with only one suspicious finding is sufficient for a nodule to be classified as "high suspicion" by ATA (20). Only 5.8% (5 of 86) of our TI-RADS 4 were reclassified to ATA "high suspicion", meaning that most of TI-RADS 4 nodules were hypoechoic solid thyroid nodules without sonographic patterns of high suspicion, considered by ATA as "intermediate suspicion". We believe this is due to a better definition of the nodule margins (smooth vs irregular margins) proposed by ATA (20). In addition, we found a similar prevalence of malignancy of 26% for TI-RADS 4 and 28% for ATA intermediate suspicion. In fact, the risk of malignancy estimated by ATA in the "intermediate suspicion" category is 10 to 20% and, unlike Rosario that demonstrated only 9.9% for intermediate suspicion, we found a significant frequency of carcinoma in this category.

We observed a malignancy risk of 100% of nodules TI-RADS 5. In fact, this category was composed of highly suspect nodules with more than 3 signs of high suspicion. For ATA "high risk" that included hypoechoic nodules with one or more signs of high suspicion, we found 83% of carcinomas, similar to risk estimated by ATA of 70-90% and a higher rate than what was observed by Rosario (54.8%) (25). Previous results of same author have been demonstrated that "high suspicion" category of ATA, markedly hypoechoic nodules with one or more suspicious findings and mildly or moderately hypoechoic with two or more suspicious findings had a similar risk of malignancy of 66% (95 % CI 57.6-73.7%) (25). These results reinforce that the degree of hypoechogenicity of nodules may not be so definitive in determining the suspicion pattern as the association of established features predictive of malignancy.

In our study, US reevaluation had some disagreements regarding nodules mildly hypoechoic without suspicious US features classified initially as TI-RADS 4 that were reclassified as very low or low by ATA risk. This could have happened due to the heterogeneity of the nodules (hypoechoic areas between iso- hyperechoic areas) and the characteristics of borders, a feature not well defined in TI-RADS score. Moreover, it is important to note that poorly defined margins are sometimes difficult to delineate, and are not equivalent to irregular margins. An irregular margin, which indicates the demarcation between nodule and parenchyma, is clearly visible but demonstrates an irregular, infiltrative or spiculated course. The reassessing of these nodules in a low suspicion category by ATA was strongly corroborated by cytology and/or histology confirming benign thyroid lesions.

The TI-RADS classification does not consider nodular size to indicate FNA-US (21). However, ATA risk score has recommended size threshold for biopsy (no biopsy in benign, > 2 cm in very low, > 1.5 cm in low, > 1 cm in intermediate, and > 1 cm in high risk, respectively) (20). In fact, the correlation between the nodule size and the risk for malignancy remains controversial. Although a recent systematic review suggested that the larger nodules present a higher pretest probability of malignancy (29). In addition, the growth of a nodule is not a reliable predictor of malignancy since many benign nodules can slowly grow over time (30-33). In our study, no correlation was found between the size of the nodules and sonographic risk assessments, reinforcing the importance of ultrasound findings more than the size of thyroid nodule in indicating FNAB-US. However, the increase of incidence of thyroid cancer in the last years, due to the diagnosis of microcarcinoma (25%), supports the ATA recommendation (20).

Even with few samples evaluated by histology, a good performance of TI-RADS and ATA ultrasound risk was observed in thyroid nodules with indeterminate cytology (Bethesda categories 3 and 4). Sonographic classification of nodules by TI-RADS category 2 or 3, or as very low to low suspicion by ATA displayed NPV of 100% for both systems. Positive predictive values for TI-RADS category 4 and 5 and ATA intermediate and high risk rose the cancer prevalence to 54.5 and 40%, respectively, compared to described prevalence of 5-15% (0% in our sample) of Bethesda 3 nodules and 15-30% (15.4% in our sample) for Bethesda 4. Previous studies have demonstrated that TI-RADS 3 and 4A scores led to 80% sensitivity and 90% NPV in Bethesda 3 cases. In contrast, for nodules scored as TI-RADS 4B and 5, the combined cytological results of Bethesda 4 and 5 resulted in a higher risk of malignancy (75% and 76 9%, respectively, P < 0.001) (34). More recently studies confirm a NPV values for ATA and TI-RADS were 91 and 74%, respectively, to rule out malignancy in cytologically indeterminate thyroid nodules (35). Further, taken together, these results suggest that cytological indeterminate nodules with TI-RADS 2 or 3 and ATA very low or low risk sonographic pattern have a higher likelihood of being benign.

This study has some limitations because we retrospectively evaluated thyroid nodules by ATA system. Also an inter-observer analysis was not possible, as only one radiologist with thyroid expertise evaluated the patients. The small number of histopathology examinations of nodules with indeterminate cytology, limited conclusions of this subgroup. In addition, this study represents a single specialized thyroid clinic's work with the intent to implement TI-RADS and/ or ATA diagnostic guidelines in our clinical practice; however, results have to be confirmed by other centers.

In conclusion, the sonographic patterns proposed by TI-RADS and the recently revised ATA's guidelines have high sensitivity and NPV for the diagnosis of thyroid carcinoma. Both systems are feasible for clinical application and have an excellent negative predictive value allowing the selection of patients to FNA-US.

REFERENCES

1. Cooper DS, Doherty MG, Haugen BR, Hauger BR, Kloos RT, Lee SL, et al. American Thyroid Association (ATA) Guidelines Taskforce on Thyroid Nodules and Differentiated Thyroid Cancer. Thyroid. 2009;19:1167-214.

2. Choi N, Moon WJ, Lee JH, Baek JH, Kim DW, Park SW. Ultrasonographic findings of medullary thyroid cancer: Differences according to tumor size and correlation with fine needle aspiration results. Acta Radiol. 2011;52:312-6.

3. Hong YJ, Son EJ, Kim EK, Kwak JY, Hong SW, Chang HS. Positive predictive values of sonographic features of solid thyroid nodule. Clin Imaging. 2010;34:127-33.

4. Kim DW, Lee EJ, Jung SJ, Ryu JH, Kim YM. Role of sonographic diagnosis in managing Bethesda class III nodules. Am J Neuroradiol. 2011;32:2136-41.

5. Kim DW, Lee YJ, Eom JW, Jung SJ, Ha TK, Kang T. Ultrasound-based diagnosis for solid thyroid nodules with the largest diameter < 5 mm. Ultrasound Med Biol. 2013;39:1190-6.

6. Kim DW, Park JS, In HS, Choo HJ, Ryu JH, Jung SJ. Ultrasound-based diagnostic classification for solid and partially cystic thyroid nodules. Am J Neuroradiol. 2012;33:1144-49.

7. Kim EK, Cheong SP, Woung YC, Ki KO, Dong IK, Jong TL, et al. New sonographic criteria for recommending fine-needle aspiration biopsy of nonpalpable solid nodules of the thyroid. Am J Roentgenol. 2002;178:687-91.

8. Moon WJ, Jung SL, Lee JH, Na DG, Baek JH, Lee YH, et al. Benign and malignant thyroid nodules: US differentiation--multicenter retrospective study. Radiology. 2008;247:762-70.

9. Campanella P, Ianni F, Rota CA, Corsello SM, Pontecorvi A. Quantification of cancer risk of each clinical and ultrasonographic suspicious feature of thyroid nodules: a systematic review and meta-analysis. Eur J Endocrinol. 2014;170(5):R203-11.

10. Remonti LR, Kramer CK, Leitão CB, Pinto LCF, Gross JL. Thyroid Ultrasound Features and Risk of Carcinoma: A Systematic Review and Meta-Analysis of Observational Studies. Thyroid. 2015;25:538-50.

11. Lee MJ, Kim EK, Kwak JY, Kim MJ. Partially cystic thyroid nodules on ultrasound: probability of malignancy and sonographic differentiation. Thyroid. 2009;19:341-6.

12. Park JY, Lee HJ, Jang HW, Kim HK, Yi JH, Lee W, et al. A proposal for a thyroid imaging reporting and data system for ultrasound features of thyroid carcinoma. Thyroid. 2009;19:1257-64.

13. Horvath E, Majlis S, Rossi R, Franco C, Niedmann JP, Castro A, et al. An ultrasonogram reporting system for thyroid nodules stratifying cancer risk for clinical management. J Clin Endocrinol Metab. 2009;94:1748-51.

14. Kwak JY, Jung I, Baek JH, Baek SM, Choi N, Choi YJ, et al. Image reporting and characterization system for ultrasound features of thyroid nodules: Multicentric Korean retrospective study. Korean J Radiol. 2013;14:110-17.

15. Kwak JY, Han KH, Yoon JH, Moon HJ, Son EJ, Park SH, et al. Thyroid Imaging Reporting and Data System for US Features of Nodules: A Step in Establishing Better Stratification of Cancer Risk. Radiology. 2011;260:892-99.

16. Hambly NM, Gonen M, Gerst SR, Li D, Jia X, Mironov S, et al. Implementation of evidence-based guidelines for thyroid nodule biopsy: a model for establishment of practice standards. AJR Am J Roentgenol. 2011;196:655-60.

17. Perros P, Boelaert K, Colley S, Evans C, Evans RM, Gerrard Ba G, et al. Guidelines for the management of thyroid cancer. Clin Endocrinol (Oxf). 2014;81:1-136.

18. Shin JH, Baek JH, Chung J, Ha EJ, Kim JH, Lee YH, et al. Ultrasonography diagnosis and imaging-based management of thyroid nodules: Revised Korean society of thyroid Korean J. Radiol. 2016;17:370.

19. Gharib H, Papini E, Garber JR, Duick DS, Harrell RM, Hegedus L, et al. American Association of Clinical Endocrinologists, American College of Endocrinology, and Associazione Medici Endocrinologi Medical Guidelines for Clinical Practice for the Diagnosis and Management of Thyroid Nodules--2016 Update. Endocr Pract. 2016;22:622-39.

20. Haugen BR, Alexander EK, Bible KC, Doherty G, Mandel SJ, Nikiforov YE, et al. 2015 American Thyroid Association Management Guidelines for Adult Patients with Thyroid Nodules and Differentiated Thyroid Cancer. Thyroid. 2016;26:1-133.

21. Russ G, Royer B, Bigorgne C, Rouxel A, Bienvenu-Perrard M, Leenhardt L. Prospective evaluation of thyroid imaging reporting and data system on 4550 nodules with and without elastography. Eur J Endocrinol. 2013;168:649-55.

22. Suen KC, Ahdul-Karim FW, Kaminsky DB, Layfield LJ, Miller TR, Spires SE, et al. Guidelines of the Papanicolaou Society of Cytopathology for fine-needle aspiration procedure and reporting. Diagn Cytopathol. 1997;17:239-47.

23. Cibas ES, Ali SZ. The Bethesda System for Reporting Thyroid Cytopathology. Am J Clin Pathol. 2009;132:658-65.

24. DeLellis RA, Lloyd RV, Heitz PU, Eng C. World Health Organization Classification Classification of Tumours: Pathology and Genetics of Tumours of Endocrine Organs. Lyon, Fr. IARC Press; 2004. p. 147-66, p. 147-166.

25. Rosario PW, Silva AL, Nunes MS, Ribeiro Borges MA, Mourão GF, Calsolari MR. Risk of malignancy in 1502 solid thyroid nodules >1 cm using the new ultrasonographic classification of the American Thyroid Association. Endocrine. 2017 May;56(2):442-5.

26. Yoon JH, Lee HS, Kim EK, Moon HJ, Kwak JY. Malignancy risk stratification of thyroid nodules: comparison between the thyroid imaging reporting and data system and the 2014 American thyroid association management guidelines. Radiology. 2016;278:917-24.

27. Na DG, Baek JH, Sung JY, Kim J, Kim JK, Choi YJ, et al. Thyroid imaging reporting and data system risk stratification of thyroid nodules: categorization based on solidity and echogenicity. Thyroid. 2016;26:562-72.

28. Rosario PW, Ward LS, Carvalho GA, Graf H, Maciel RMB, Maciel LMZ, et al. Thyroid nodule and differentiated thyroid cancer: update on the Brazilian Consensus. Arq Bras Endocrinol Metabol. 2013;57:240-64.

29. Shin JJ, Caragacianu D, Randolph GW. Impact of thyroid nodule size on prevalence and post-test probability of malignancy: a systematic review. Laryngoscope. 2015;125:263-72.

30. Kamran SC, Marqusee E, Kim MI, Frates MC, Ritner J, Peters H, et al. Thyroid nodule size and prediction of cancer. J Clin Endocrinol Metab. 2013;98:564-70.

31. McHenry CR, Huh ES, Machekano RN. Is nodule size an independent predictor of thyroid malignancy? Surgery. 2008;144:1062-68.

32. Shrestha M, Crothers BA, Burch HB. The impact of thyroid nodule size on the risk of malignancy and accuracy of fine-needle aspiration: a 10-year study from a single institution. Thyroid. 2012;22:1251-56.

33. Asanuma K, Kobayashi S, Shingu K, Hama Y, Yokoyama S, Fujimori M, et al. The impact of thyroid nodule size on the risk of malignancy and accuracy of fine-needle aspiration: a 10-year study from a single institution. Eur J Surg. 2001;167:102-5.

34. Maia FFR, Matos PS, Pavin EJ, Zantut-Wittmann DE. Thyroid imaging reporting and data system score combined with Bethesda system for malignancy risk stratification in thyroid nodules with indeterminate results on cytology. Clin Endocrinol (Oxf). 2015;82:439-44.

35. Grani G, Lamartina L, Ascoli V, Bosco D, Nardi F, D'Ambrosio F, et al. Ultrasonography scoring systems can rule out malignancy in cytologically indeterminate thyroid nodules. Endocrine. 2017;57(2):256-61.

11

Assessing endocrine and immune parameters in human immunodeficiency virus-infected patients before and after the immune reconstitution inflammatory syndrome

Liliana Rateni[1], Sergio Lupo[1,2], Liliana Racca[3], Jorge Palazzi[2], Sergio Ghersevich[3]

ABSTRACT

Objective: The present study compares immune and endocrine parameters between HIV-infected patients who underwent the Immune Reconstitution Inflammatory Syndrome (IRIS-P) during antiretroviral therapy (ART) and HIV-patients who did not undergo the syndrome (non-IRIS-P). Materials and methods: Blood samples were obtained from 31 HIV-infected patients (15 IRIS-P and 16 non-IRIS-P) before ART (BT) and 48 ± 2 weeks after treatment initiation (AT). Plasma Interleukin-6 (IL-6) and Interleukin-18 (IL-18) were determined by ELISA. Cortisol, dehydroepiandrosterone sulfate (DHEA-S) and thyroxin concentrations were measured using chemiluminescence immune methods. Results: Concentrations of IL-6 (7.9 ± 1.9 pg/mL) and IL-18 (951.5 ± 233.0 pg/mL) were significantly higher ($p < 0.05$) in IRIS-P than in non-IRIS-P (3.9 ± 1.0 pg/mL and 461.0 ± 84.4 pg/mL, respectively) BT. Mean T4 plasma level significantly decreased in both groups of patients after treatment ($p < 0.05$). In both groups cortisol levels were similar before and after ART ($p > 0.05$). Levels of DHEA-S in IRIS-P decreased AT (1080.5 ± 124.2 vs. 782.5 ± 123.8 ng/mL, $p < 0.05$) and they were significantly lower than in non-IRIS-P (782.5 ± 123.8 vs. 1203.7 ± 144.0 ng/mL, $p < 0.05$). IRIS-P showed higher values of IL-6 and IL-18 BT and lower levels of DHEA-S AT than in non-IRIS-P. Conclusion: These parameters could contribute to differentiate IRIS-P from non-IRIS-P. The significant decrease in DHEA-S levels in IRIS-P after ART might suggest a different adrenal response in these patients, which may reflect the severity of the disease. Arch Endocrinol Metab. 2018;62(1):57-64

Keywords

HIV; interleukins; immune reconstitution syndrome; cortisol; dehydroepiandrosterone sulfate

[1] Facultad de Ciencias Médicas, Universidad Nacional de Rosario, Santa Fe, Rosario, Argentina
[2] Center for Assistance and Comprehensive Clinical Research (CAICI), IICTlab, Mendoza, Rosario, Argentina
[3] Facultad de Ciencias Bioquímicas y Farmacéuticas, Universidad Nacional de Rosario, Rosario, Argentina

Correspondence to:
Liliana Rateni
Facultad de Ciencias Médicas,
Universidad Nacional de Rosario,
Santa Fe 3100, (2000)
Rosario, Argentina
lilirateni@yahoo.com.ar

INTRODUCTION

The immune reaction to different diseases elicits an endocrine response which influences the course of the process (1). In inflammatory processes, pro-inflammatory cytokines (besides their immunological effects) are known to affect the function of crucial neuroendocrine mechanisms, which, in turn, can modulate the immune response (2,3). Such mechanisms include the actions of cytokines on the hypothalamus-pituitary-adrenal (HPA), -gonadal and -thyroid axis (2,4).

Viral infections, in general, are physiologically stressful, as shown by the concomitant activation of the HPA axis, and it has become clear that cytokine-HPA axis interactions are fundamental for immune regulation during these infections (3,5). Among the pro-inflammatory cytokines, Interleukin-18 (IL-18)

was shown to have an important role in the immune response to intracellular pathogens in acute infections and it may participate in the regulation of the HPA axis (6). Another pro-inflammatory cytokine, interleukin-6 (IL-6), can activate the HPA axis, leading to the final production of steroid hormones by the adrenal gland (7).

Glucocorticoids have a critical role in maintaining the balance between the beneficial and detrimental effects of pro-inflammatory cytokines as part of the bidirectional communication between the immune system and the HPA axis (3,8). Regarding the adrenal steroids, glucocorticoids can promote Th2 cytokine acquisition profile, facilitating Th2 activities, whereas dehydroepiandrosterone (DHEA) is able to favor Th1 related cytokine production and interferes with Th2 associated cytokine synthesis (9,10).

Some human immunodeficiency virus (HIV)-infected patients undergo a clinical deterioration during the antiretroviral therapy (ART), which occurs regardless of the increase of CD4$^+$ T lymphocyte counts and the decrease of plasma HIV-1 viral loads. This clinical condition, known as immune reconstitution inflammatory syndrome (IRIS), reflects an exacerbated inflammatory response to opportunistic pathogens and/or tumor antigens in HIV-infected patients [11,12]. This disorder occurs after the initiation of ART and is temporally related to an increase in the host CD4$^+$ lymphocyte count [11,13]. The mechanisms involved in IRIS are not fully understood but they appear to be associated with the restoration of the immune response against pre-existent pathogens related to sub-clinical infections [14]. The HIV-infected patients that will undergo IRIS during their treatment could present a more marked unbalance in their immune endocrine regulation [1,15].

Based on the mentioned data, the aim of the study was to assess parameters of adrenal and thyroid responses and immune pro-inflammatory reaction in HIV-infected patients receiving highly active ART. The results obtained from patients who suffered from IRIS (IRIS-P) and the ones who did not undergo the syndrome (non-IRIS-P) during treatment were compared in order to evaluate potential differences of the studied parameters between both groups of patients.

MATERIALS AND METHODS

Patients and ethics

All patients signed a written consent to participate in the study, and the protocol was approved by the Ethical Committee of CAICI Institute (Center for Assistance and Comprehensive Clinical Research, Rosario, Argentina). Patients with endocrine pathologies and hormonal treatments were excluded from the study.

This was a case-control study including 31 HIV-infected patients: 16 patients with normal response to ART (non-IP; 48 ± 11 years old), and 15 patients who underwent IRIS during the treatment (IP; 52 ± 12 years old). Both groups did not differ in age and sex composition (p > 0.05).

The diagnosis of IRIS was based on the criteria proposed by French and cols. [16], in patients who were infected with HIV and underwent a rapid clinical deterioration shortly after starting ART, despite having effective viral suppression. This was associated with co-infections caused by a diverse array of pathogens, and by tumor development. The diagnosis of IRIS was made by exclusion, ruling out other possible causes of disease after starting ART.

Blood sample collection

Ethylenediaminetetra-acetic acid (EDTA)-treated blood samples were obtained from patients at 8:00 a.m, before treatment initiation and 48 ± 2 weeks after ART initiation. Following plasma separation and addition of aprotinin (100 U/mL, Sigma-Aldrich Inc, USA), samples were preserved at -20°C until used in the assays.

T lymphocyte subsets count

T lymphocyte subsets (CD4, CD8) in patients' blood samples were quantified by standard flow cytometry techniques. Fluorochrome-labelled antibodies (anti-CD8-fluorescein isothiocyanate isomer, anti-CD3-phycoerythrin, and anti-CD4-PE-Cy5, Becton Dickinson, Heidelberg, Germany) that specifically bind to lymphocyte surface antigens were added to aliquots of blood samples. After incubation, a fixative solution (Becton Dickinson) was added and sample analysis was performed on a Becton Dickinson FACSCALIBUR flow cytometer (Four-Colors; Becton Dickinson, Heidelberg, Germany). The analysis provided absolute counts of CD4$^+$, CD8$^+$, CD3$^+$ lymphocytes and the CD4$^+$/CD8$^+$ ratio.

The absolute lymphocyte count was generated by a SYSMEX 2000i hematology analyzer (dual platform method, Roche, Basel, Switzerland).

Viral load quantification

Total RNA was extracted from the patients' samples and analyzed by the Amplicor HIV-1 Monitor test (Roche, Branchburg, NJ, USA) following the manufacturer's instructions.

Assays of IL-6 and IL-18

Both IL-6 and IL-18 plasma concentrations were assayed by Quantitative Elisa Kits from R & D Systems (Minneapolis, MN, USA), following the manufacturer's instructions. The sensitivities of the assays were 0.7 pg/mL and 12.5 pg/mL, respectively. The intra-assay variation coefficients for IL-6 and IL-18 assays were 5.0 % and 8.0 %, respectively.

Hormone measurements

Plasma concentrations of cortisol, DHEA-sulfate (DHEA-S), and thyroxin (T4), were determined using an Immulite 1000 Immunoassay System (Siemens, USA). The intra-assay variation coefficients were always lower than 5.0%.

Statistical analysis

Results from patients with and without IRIS or before and after ART were compared using the Student t-test or the alternative nonparametric Mann-Whitney test when required. Pearson's correlation coefficient (r) was used to analyze relationships among paired data. The Receiver Operating Characteristics (ROC) curve analysis was used to compare IL-18 values between IRIS-P and non-IRIS-P before the treatment. Results were expressed as media ± standard error (SE). A $p < 0.05$ was considered statistically significant.

RESULTS

The following disorders were associated with the IRIS that suffered the IRIS-P: *Herpes zoster* infection, tuberculosis, hepatitis B, toxoplasmosis, polyarthritis, and Kaposi's sarcoma. These disorders appeared 5.0 ± 0.6 months after ART initiation and usually in a sequential rather than a concurrent way. No patient had an active disease or opportunistic infection at the time of testing for this study, i.e., before the treatment and after 48 ± 2 weeks of ART initiation.

Immune parameters

The results indicated that all patients achieved a significant increase in their CD4+ T cell counts after treatment. The values of CD4+ T lymphocytes increased significantly after ART both in IRIS-P ($p < 0.01$) and in those who did not suffer from the syndrome ($p < 0.01$), compared to pre-treatment values (Table 1). The CD4+/CD8+ ratio was also significantly higher 48 ± 2 weeks after treatment initiation both in IRIS-P ($p < 0.05$) and in non-IRIS-P ($p < 0.01$). There were no significant differences in CD4+ - CD8+ cell counts or CD4+/CD8+ ratio between IRIS-P and non-IRIS-P, neither before nor after the treatment (Table 1).

Before treatment, the mean values of viral load in IRIS-P (261333 ± 117474 copy number/mL) and in non-IRIS-P (159954 ± 35324 copy number/mL) were not significantly different (Table 1).

Statistical analysis showed a significant difference in IL-6 mean plasma concentrations between IRIS-P and non-IRIS-P, before ART ($p < 0.05$, Table 2 and Figure 1A). In addition, in IRIS-P, the IL-6 values were significantly reduced after 48 ± 2 weeks after ART initiation ($p < 0.01$, Figure 1A) with respect to the values before the treatment. In the other patients, the decrease in IL-6 after ART did not reach statistical significance.

Before ART, mean plasma IL-18 levels in IRIS-P were higher than those in patients who did not suffer from the syndrome ($p < 0.05$, Table 2, Figure 1B). Based on a ROC curve analysis, a IL-18 value of 695 pg/mL before ART would allow to differentiate IRIS-P from patients who did not undergo IRIS in the present study, with 80% of specificity and 57% of sensitivity ($p = 0.08$).

After 48 ± 2 weeks of ART initiation, the IL-18 values tended to be higher in IRIS-P than in the other patients ($p = 0.09$). Plasma concentrations of IL-18 before ART were significantly higher than those after treatment both in IRIS-P and non-IRIS-P ($p < 0.05$ and $p < 0.01$, respectively, Figure 1B).

Table 1. Measured parameters in HIV-infected patients, before ART or after 48 ± 2 weeks of treatment initiation

	BT		AT	
	IRIS-P SRI	Non-IRIS-P +/-SE	IRIS-P	Non-IRIS-P +/-SE
CD4+ (cel/mL)	221.4 ± 40.2[a]	262.3 ± 43.7[b]	447.5 ± 67.8[a]	429.8 ± 41.7[b]
CD8+ (cel/mL)	760.4 ± 152	919.0 ± 100.7	715.7 ± 107.1	965 ± 134.1
CD4+/CD8+	0.46 ± 0.22[c]	0.40 ± 0.15[d]	0.59 ± 0.11[c]	0.51 ± 0.06[d]
VL (copy number/mL)	261332 ± 117474	159954 ± 35324	167 ± 37	50 ± 0.0

The table shows the mean results of the measured parameters in IRIS-P and in non-IRIS-P, before treatment initiation (BT) or after 48 ± 2 weeks (AT) of ART initiation. Results were expressed as media ± SE. CD4+: CD4+ T lymphocytes counts. CD8+: CD8+ T lymphocytes counts.

VL: viral load.

The same letters indicate mean values which are significantly different: [a] $p < 0.01$; [b] $p < 0.01$; [c] $p < 0.05$; [d] $p < 0.01$.

Table 2. Measured parameters in HIV-infected patients, before treatment initiation (BT) or after 48 ± 2 weeks (AT) of ART initiation

	BT		AT	
	IRIS-P SRI	Non-IRIS-P +/-SE	IRIS-P	Non-IRIS-P +/-SE
IL-6 (pg/mL)	7.9 ± 1.9[a,b]	3.9 ± 1.0[a]	3.2 ± 0.6[b]	2,8 ± 0.6
IL-18 (pg/mL)	951.5 ± 233.0[a,b]	461.0 ± 84.4[a,c]	270.4 ± 72.7[b]	30.7 ± 36.5[c]
Cortisol (µg/dL)	20.1 ± 1.5	20.3 ± 2.3	21.4 ± 2.5	21.0 ± 2.3
DHEA-S (µg/mL)	1080.5 ± 124.2[a]	1222.4 ± 1.7	782.5 ± 123.8[a,b]	1203.7 ± 144.0[b]
T4 (µg/dL)	8.9 ± 0.4[a]	7.8 ± 0.5[b]	7.2 ± 0.3[a]	6.9 ± 0.2[b]
DHEA/Cortisol	53.7 ± 6.5	66.2 ± 9.7	41.3 ± 7.9[a]	72.2 ± 11.9[a]

The table shows the mean results of the measured parameters in IRIS-P and in non-IRIS-P, before treatment initiation (BT) or after 48 ± 2 weeks (AT) of ART initiation. Results were expressed as media ± SE.

The same letters indicate mean values which were significantly different: IL-6: interleukin 6 ([a] $p < 0.05$; [b] $p < 0.01$); IL-18: interleukin 18 ([a] $p < 0.05$, [b] $p < 0.05$, [c] $p < 0.01$); DHEA-S: dehydroepiandrosterone sulfate ([a] $p < 0.05$, [b] $p < 0.05$); DHEA-S/Cortisol ratio ([a] $p < 0.05$); T4: thyroxin ([a] $p < 0.05$, [b] $p < 0.05$).

Endocrine measurements

Mean plasma concentrations of T4 in patients from each group are shown in Table 2, before and after the initiation of ART. Despite a significant decrease in the mean T4 plasma level after 48 ± 2 weeks of treatment in both groups of patients ($p < 0.05$, Figure 1C), the T4 concentrations always remained within the normal range. In addition, the mean values of T4 between the two groups, before or after ART, were not significantly different.

Table 2 shows the mean plasma concentration values of cortisol found in IRIS-P and in the other patients. In both groups, cortisol levels were similar both before and after ART initiation (Figure 2A).

Before ART, a significant correlation ($r = 0.59$, $p < 0.05$) between the values of CD4+ lymphocytes count and cortisol plasma levels was observed in the patients who did not undergo IRIS. However, no association was found between CD4+ cell count and cortisol concentrations in IRIS-P before the treatment, nor between these parameters after ART initiation in both groups of patients.

The mean plasma DHEA-S concentrations significantly decreased after treatment in IRIS-P ($p < 0.05$; Table 2 and Figure 2B). Statistical analysis indicated a significant difference in mean plasma levels of DHEA-S between the IRIS-P and non-IRIS-P, after receiving ART ($p < 0.05$, Table 2 and Figure 2B). However, before ART, plasma levels of DHEA-S in IRIS-P were not different from the values in non-IRIS-P.

No significant correlation between the mean values of CD4+ cell count and DHEA-S plasma levels was found neither in IRIS-P nor in the other patients, neither before nor after ART initiation.

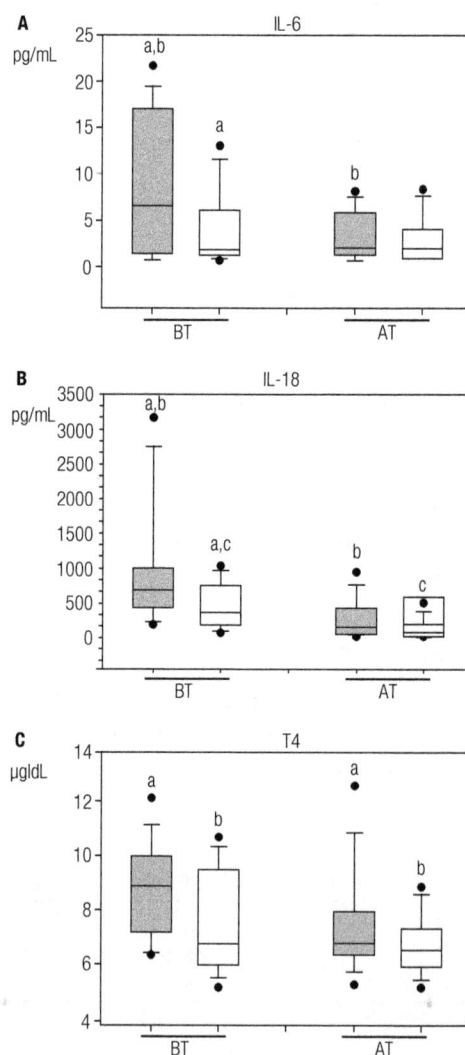

Figure 1. Box plots show plasma levels before (BT) or 48 ± 2 weeks after (AT) of ART initiation in IRIS-P (grey boxes) and non-IRIS-P (white boxes): A) interleukin 6 (IL-6, a: $p < 0.05$, b: $p < 0.01$); B) interleukin 18 (IL-18, a: $p < 0.05$, b: $p < 0.05$, c: $p < 0.01$); C) thyroxin (T4, a: $p < 0.05$, b: $p < 0.05$). The same letters indicate the groups that were compared statistically in the corresponding graph. Line inside box: median; limits of box: 75th and 25th percentiles.

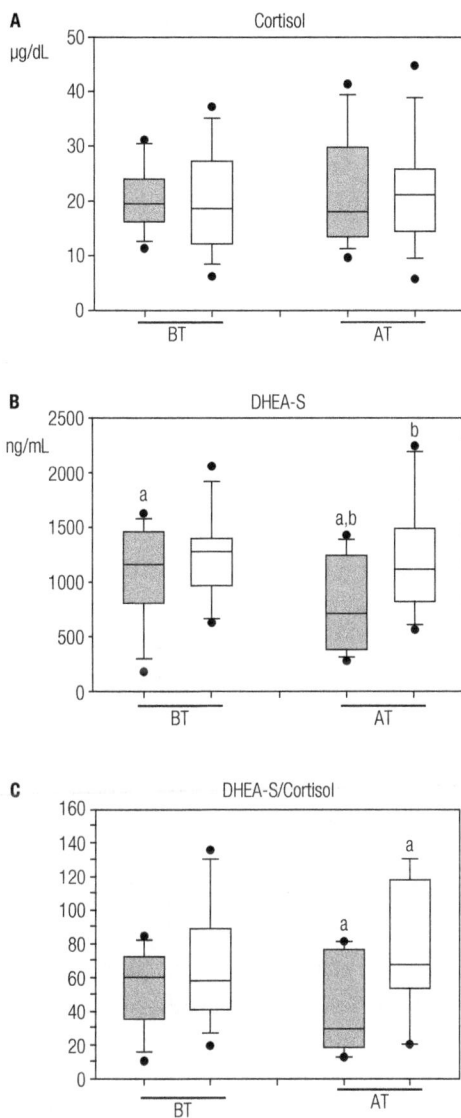

Figure 2. Box plots show plasma concentrations before (BT) or 48 ± 2 weeks after (AT) of ART initiation in IRIS-P (grey boxes) and non-IRIS-P (white boxes): A) cortisol; B) dehydroepiandrosterone sulfate (DHEA-S; a: p < 0.05, b: p < 0.05). C) Box plot indicates values of DHEA-S/Cortisol ratio before (BT) or after 48 ± 2 weeks (AT) of ART initiation in IRIS-P (grey boxes) and non-IRIS-P (white boxes, a: p < 0.05). The same letters indicate the groups that were compared statistically in the corresponding graph. Line inside box: median; limits of box: 75th and 25th percentiles.

The statistical analysis did not reveal a significant difference in the values of DHEA-S/Cortisol ratio between the two groups of patients before ART (Table 2 and Figure 2C). However, after ART initiation, the values of DHEA-S/Cortisol ratio were significantly lower in IRIS-P (p < 0.05; Table 2 and Figure 2C) than the values observed in the other patients studied.

DISCUSSION

It is known that treatment-induced immune improvement may increase the risk of an exacerbated immune response in some patients, worsening infections already present in the host, and leading to IRIS (12,17).

It has been reported that HIV-infected patients with a lower CD4+ cell count before ART initiation are at a higher risk of undergoing IRIS (18,19). However, in the present study there were no significant differences in CD4+ - CD8+ cell counts, CD4+/CD8+ ratio or in viral loads between IRIS-P and non-IRIS-P before treatment. This lack of difference in CD4+/CD8+ rate between the two groups may be due to the small sample size. The results indicated that all patients responded to ART, increasing CD4+ cell counts, which is in agreement with previous studies (20,21). It has been reported that the increase in CD4+ cell count with ART was not a risk factor for IRIS because it can occur without an appreciable CD4+ cell increase (22).

A previous study reported that a low CD4+/CD8+ ratio was an independent predictor for IRIS (23). They concluded that patients with a CD4+/CD8+ ratio less than 0.15 were more likely to have an IRIS event than were patients with a ratio greater than 0.30. However, in the present study CD4+/CD8+ ratios did not differ between IRIS-P and non-IRIS-P. In addition, 6 IRIS-P and 6 non-IRIS-P patients presented CD4+/CD8+ ratios less than 0.15 before ART.

The results showed that after one year of ART initiation, IL-6 plasma levels were significantly reduced in IRIS-P respect to pre-treatment values. Previous studies have also shown that ART decreases most markers of inflammation (24,25). The present study indicated that ART also caused a significant decrease in plasma levels of IL-18 in all the patients studied with respect to pretreatment values.

Before treatment, both IL-6 and IL-18 plasma concentrations in IRIS-P were significantly higher than in non-IRIS-P. Other authors also reported higher levels of inflammatory cytokines in IRIS-P than in non-IRIS-P previous to ART (24). The increased levels of these cytokines might be thought to be a characteristic of patients at risk of suffering from IRIS during ART. The higher values of IL-6 might reflect a resistance to glucocorticoids, which are normally involved in the decrease of the cytokine level and can promote a Th2 cytokine acquisition profile (15).

Interleukin-18 produced by macrophages is known to drive the differentiation of Th cells toward the Th1 type (6). It has been suggested that the higher levels of IL-18 in HIV-infected patients co-infected with TB may contribute to the sudden recovery of Th1 responses in those conditions (26). Thus, the higher IL-18 concentrations observed in IRIS-P before ART could also reflect this possibility. In the present study, an attempt to identify patients at potential risk of developing IRIS, a cut-off value of IL-18 ≥ 695 pg/mL before ART was chosen with 80% of specificity and 57% of sensitivity. Despite the fact that the study showed significant differences of IL-18 and IL-6 values between IRIS-P and non-IRIS-P, it would be necessary to carry out studies with larger number of patients to define cut-off values of both cytokines that could differentiate, with higher specificity and sensitivity, both types of patients from the general population of HIV patients prior to receiving ART, standardizing the pre-analytical and analytical variables.

Before ART, a positive correlation between CD4+ cell count and levels of cortisol was found in patients who did not suffer from IRIS. This correlation was suggested to indicate a more controlled clinical response of the HIV-infected patients (27). The results showed that plasma cortisol concentrations were similar before and after ART in all the patients studied. It was suggested that patients experiencing IRIS could present an inadequate HPA axis response (1). Previous reports have suggested an intra-adrenal shift from DHEAS towards the cortisol production during critical illness (28-30), as could be the case of HIV infected patients who suffered IRIS. It has been proposed that an exacerbated proinflammatory response could result from the suppression of the HPA axis and of adrenal failure or reflect glucocorticoid tissue resistance as well (31,32). This clinical disorder is known as critical illness-related corticosteroid insufficiency resulting from an inadequate corticosteroid production or action for such severe disease (32,33). In agreement with the previous idea, patients with adrenal insufficiency could present an altered regulation of the immune system, which has been linked to IRIS (34). The fact that plasma levels of DHEA-S, which are mainly of adrenal origin, did not significantly change in non-IRIS-P after ART, but rather decreased more than 20% in IRIS-P with respect to values before treatment, could reflect a more impaired adrenal function in IRIS-P than in non-IRIS-P. These results are consistent with

other studies in chronic diseases, such as tuberculosis, suggesting that the decrease in DHEA-S levels were associated with worse prognosis of the disease (35). An inadequate adrenal steroid production could be thought to aggravate the inflammatory process, and to contribute to the development of IRIS in HIV-infected patients. Supporting this idea, the DHEA-S/Cortisol ratios were significantly lower in IRIS-P after ART than in the other patients. This decrease has been associated with the altered metabolic pathways of adrenocorticoids synthesis (33,34,36).

It has been reported that acquired immune deficiency syndrome patients with decreased levels of DHEA-S show excessive cytokine production by Th2 cells (IL-4, IL-5, IL-6, and IL-10) and suppression of other cytokines (IL-2, IFN-γ, IL-12) (37). This would negatively affect these patients' evolution.

Abnormal thyroid function tests are more frequent in HIV-infected patients than in the general population (38). In the present study, the results showed that the plasma concentrations of T4 decreased significantly after ART, but the levels always remained within the normal range in all the patients.

Despite an intense search for hormonal or immune markers, which could predict which HIV-infected patients may be at risk of suffering IRIS after ART initiation, no reliable markers have been reported so far. The results of this study indicated that mean levels of IL-6 and IL-18 in IRIS-P almost duplicate the respective values in non-IRIS-P before ART. In addition, the decreased DHEA-S plasma levels and DHEA-S/cortisol ratio in IRIS-P with respect to values in non-IRIS-P, after ART initiation, could suggest a mild but critical adrenal deficiency in HIV-infected patients who undergo IRIS during ART. Based on these results, it could be useful to test the adrenal function of patients before they receive ART, in order to correlate the results with the potential development of IRIS.

In recent years, the enormous progress of ART has changed the survival expectations of HIV-infected patients. However, around 10% of the patients treated will suffer from IRIS during ART (18,39). Since the syndrome represents an important clinical problem, more studies on risk factors involving a larger number of patients, as well as the development of strategies for detection of patients at higher risk for IRIS are needed.

Acknowledgements: the authors thank Gustavo Dip and Alicia Pelizani for their laboratory assistance. We would like to thank the staff from the English Department of Facultad de Ciencias Bioquímicas y Farmacéuticas, UNR, for the language correction of the manuscript.

Funding statement: the study was partially supported by a training grant from Fogarty International Center to L. Rateni.

REFERENCES

1. George MM, Bhangoo A. Human immune deficiency virus (HIV) infection and the hypothalamic pituitary adrenal axis. Rev Endocr Metab Disord. 2013;14:105-12.

2. Webster JI, Sternberg EM. Role of the hypothalamic-pituitary-adrenal axis, glucocorticoids and glucocorticoid receptors in toxic sequelae of exposure to bacterial and viral products. J Endocrinol. 2004;181:207-21.

3. Silverman MN, Pearce BD, Biron CA, Miller AH. Immune modulation of the hypothalamic-pituitary-adrenal (HPA) axis during viral infection. Viral Immunol. 2005;18:41-78.

4. Mebis L, van den Berghe G. The hypothalamus-pituitary-thyroid axis in critical illness. Neth J Med. 2009;67:332-40.

5. Bhangoo A, Desai N. Endocrinopathies in HIV, AIDS and HAART. Rev Endocr Metab Disord. 2013;14:101-3.

6. Maxwell JR, Yadav R, Rossi RJ, Ruby CE, Weinberg AD, Aguila HL, et al. IL-18 bridges innate and adaptive immunity through IFN-gamma and the CD134 pathway. J Immunol. 2006;177:234-45.

7. Päth G, Scherbaum WA, Bornstein SR. The role of interleukin-6 in the human adrenal gland. Eur J Clin Invest. 2000;30:91-5.

8. Bellavance M-A, Rivest S. The HPA-immune axis and the immunomodulatory actions of glucocorticoids in the brain. Front Immunol. 2014;5:1-13.

9. Elenkov IJ. Glucocorticoids and the Th1/Th2 balance. Ann N Y Acad Sci. 2004;1024:138-46.

10. Hazeldine J, Arlt W, Lord JM. Dehydroepiandrosterone as a regulator of immune cell function. J Steroid Biochem Mol Biol. 2010;120:127-36.

11. Breton G, Duval X, Estellat C, Poaletti X, Bonnet D, Mvondo Mvondo D, et al. Determinants of immune reconstitution inflammatory in HIV type I-infected patients with tuberculosis after initiation of antiretroviral therapy. Clin Infect Dis. 2004;39:1709-12.

12. Barber D, Andrade B, Sereti I, Sher A. Immune reconstitution inflammatory syndrome: the trouble with immunity when you had none. Nat Rev Microbiol. 2012;10:150-6.

13. Shelburne SA, Visnegarwala F, Darcourt J. Incidence and risk factors for immune reconstitution inflammatory syndrome during highly active antiretroviral therapy. Aids. 2005;19:399-406.

14. Achenbach CJ, Harrington RD, Dhanireddy S, Crane HM, Casper C, Kitahata MM. Paradoxical Immune Reconstitution Inflammatory Syndrome in HIV-infected patients treated with combination antiretroviral therapy after AIDS-defining opportunistic infection. Clin Infect Dis. 2012;54:424-33.

15. Chrousos GP, Zapanti ED. Hypothalamic-pituitary-adrenal axis in HIV infection and disease. Endocrinol Metab Clin North Am. 2014;43:791-806.

16. French MA, Lenzo N, John M, Mallal SA, McKinnon EJ, James IR, et al. Immune restoration disease after the treatment of immunodeficient HIV-infected patients with highly active antiretroviral therapy. HIV Med. 2000;1:107-15.

17. Sereti I, Rodger AJ, French MA. Biomarkers in immune reconstitution inflammatory syndrome. signals from pathogenesis. Curr Opin HIV AIDS. 2010;5:504-10.

18. Grant PM, Komarow L, Andersen J, Sereti I, Pahwa S, Lederman MM, et al. Risk factor analyses for immune reconstitution inflammatory syndrome in a randomized study of early vs. deferred ART during an opportunistic infection. PLoS ONE. 2010;5:e11416.

19. Chang CC, Sheikh V, Sereti I, French MA. Immune reconstitution disorders in patients with HIV infection: from pathogenesis to prevention and treatment. Curr HIV/AIDS Rep. 2014;11:223-32.

20. Hart JE, Jeon CY, Ivers LC, Behforouz HL, Caldas A, Drobac PC, et al. Effect of directly observed therapy for highly active antiretroviral therapy on virologic, immunologic, and adherence outcomes: a meta-analysis and systematic review. J Acquir Immune Defic Syndr. 2010;54:167-79.

21. Krebs SJ, Ananworanich J. Immune activation during acute HIV infection and the impact of early antiretroviral therapy. Curr Opin HIV AIDS. 2016;11:163-72.

22. French MA. The immunopathogenesis of mycobacterial immune restoration disease. Lancet Infect Dis. 2006;6:461-2.

23. Ratnam I, Chiu C, Kandala NB, Easterbrook PJ. Incidence and risk factors for immune reconstitution inflammatory syndrome in an ethnically diverse HIV type-1-infected cohort. Clin Infect Dis. 2006;42:418-27.

24. Ledwaba L, Tavel JA, Khabo P, Maja P, Qin J, Sangweni P, et al.; Project Phidisa Biomarkers Team. Pre-ART levels of inflammation and coagulation markers are strong predictors of death in a South African cohort with advanced HIV disease. PLoS One. 2012;7:e24243.

25. Hattab S, Guiguet M, Carcelain G, Fourati S, Guihot A, Autran B, et al. Soluble biomarkers of immune activation and inflammation in HIV infection: impact of 2 years of effective first-line combination antiretroviral therapy. HIV Med. 2015;16:553-62.

26. Tan HY, Yong YK, Andrade BB, Shankar EM, Ponnampalavanar S, Omar SF, et al. Plasma interleukin-18 levels are a biomarker of innate immune responses that predict and characterize tuberculosis-associated immune reconstitution inflammatory syndrome. AIDS. 2015;29:421-31.

27. Patterson S, Moran P, Epel E, Sinclair E, Kemeny M, Deeks S, et al. Cortisol patterns are associated with T cell activation in HIV. PLoS ONE. 2013;8:e63429.

28. Vermes I, Beishuizen A. The hypothalamic-pituitary-adrenal response to critical illness. Best Pract Res Clin Endocrinol Metab. 2001;15:495-511.

29. Beishuizen A, Thijs LG, Vermes I. Decreased levels of dehydroepiandrosterone sulphate in severe critical illness: a sign of exhausted adrenal reserve? Crit Care. 2002;6:434-8.

30. Mueller C, Blum CA, Trummler M, Stolz D, Bingisser R, Mueller C, et al. Association of adrenal function and disease severity in community-acquired pneumonia. PLoS One. 2014;9(6):e99518.

31. Marik PE. Critical illness-related corticosteroid insufficiency. Chest. 2009;135:181-93.

32. Levy-Shraga Y, Pinhas-Hamiel O. Critical illness-related corticosteroid insufficiency in children. Horm Res Paediatr. 2013;80:309-17.

33. Moraes RB, Czepielewski MA, Friedman G, de Borba EL. Diagnosis of adrenal failure in critically ill patients. Arq Bras Endocrinol Metabol. 2011;55:295-302.

34. Charmandari E, Nicolaides NC, Chrousos GP. Adrenal insufficiency. Lancet. 2014;383:2152-67.

35. Quiroga MF, Angerami MT, Santucci N, Ameri D, Luis Francos JL, Wallach J, et al. Dynamics of Adrenal Steroids Are Related to Variations in Th1 and treg populations during mycobacterium tuberculosis infection in HIV positive persons. PLoS ONE. 2012;7:e33061.

36. Chittiprol S, Kumar AM, Shetty KT, Kumar HR, Satishchandra P, Rao RS, et al. HIV-1 clade C infection and progressive disruption in the relationship between cortisol, DHEAS and CD4 cell numbers: a two-year follow-up study. Clin Chim Acta. 2009;409(1-2):4-10.

37. Maingat F, Polyak M, Paul A, Vivithanaporn P, Noorbakhsh F, Ahboucha S, et al. Neurosteroid-mediated regulation of brain innate immunity in HIV/AIDS: DHEA-S suppresses neurovirulence. Front Endocrinol. 2013;27:725-37.

38. Hoffmann CJ, Brown TT. Thyroid function abnormalities in HIV-infected patients. Clin Infect Dis. 2007;45:488-94.

39. Novak RM, Richardson JT, Buchacz K, Novaka RM, Richardsonb JT, Buchaczc K, et al.; HIV Outpatient Study (HOPS) Investigators. Immune reconstitution inflammatory syndrome: incidence and implications for mortality. AIDS. 2012;26:721-30.

12

Liver metabolic changes induced by conjugated linoleic acid in calorie-restricted rats

Camila de Moraes[1], Camila Andrea de Oliveira[1], Maria Esméria
Corezola do Amaral[1], Gabriela Arcurio Landini[1], Rosana Catisti[1]

ABSTRACT

Objective: Complexes like conjugated linoleic acid (CLA) reduce the percentage of body fat by increasing energy expenditure, fat oxidation, or both. The aim of this study was to verify if CLA is able to mimic caloric restriction (CR), and determine the effects of CLA on liver metabolic profile of young adult male Wistar rats. **Materials and methods**: We divided 36 animals into the following groups: 1) Control; 2) CLA (1% of daily food intake, 21 days, orogastric intubation); 3) Restr (fed 60% of the diet offered to controls); and 4) CLA Restr. Liver tissues were processed for biochemical and molecular or mitochondrial isolation (differential centrifugation) and blood samples were collected for biochemical analyses. **Results**: Treatment of the animals for 21 days with 1% CLA alone or combined with CR increased liver weight and respiration rates of liver mitochondria suggesting significant mitochondrial uncoupling. We observed a decrease in adipose tissue leading to insulin resistance, hyperinsulinemia, and hepatic steatosis due to increased liver cholesterol and triacylglycerol levels, but no significant effects on body mass. The expression of hepatic cellular connexins (43 and 26) was significantly higher in the CLA group compared with the Control or Restr groups. **Conclusion**: CLA does not seem to be a safe compound to induce mass loss because it upregulates the mRNA expression of connexins and induces hepatic mitochondrial changes and lipids disorders. Arch Endocrinol Metab. 2017;61(1):45-53

Keywords
Trans10cis12-conjugated linoleic acid; mitochondria, liver; restriction, caloric; metabolism, liver; metabolism, connexins

[1] Programa de Pós-Graduação
de Ciências Biomédicas, Centro
Universitário Hermínio Ometto,
Uniararas, Araras, SP, Brazil

Correspondence to:
Rosana Catisti
Av. Maximiliano Baruto, 500
13607-339 – Araras, SP, Brazil
rosanacatisti@uniararas.br

INTRODUCTION

Studies on the reduction of dietary caloric intake without lack of essential nutrients, called caloric restriction (CR), have shown that this intervention can modulate biochemical pathways and prevent molecular diseases (1). In mammals, CR stimulates respiration rates (1), increases biogenesis and mitochondrial density in tissues (2), and decreases the coupling between oxygen uptake and oxidative phosphorylation (3). CR promotes mitochondrial biogenesis through a pathway signaled by lower insulin levels, increased nitric oxide production, and activation of the transcriptional coactivator PGC-1α. In addition, CR is associated with lower mitochondrial reactive oxygen species (ROS) generation, possibly due to enhanced uncoupling promoted by this dietary intervention (4). The broad spectrum of actions and marked metabolic and hormonal changes induced by CR have encouraged the identification of natural and synthetic compounds that mimic the effects of CR.

The discovery of compounds that attenuate diseases of old age could have a profound impact on public health, reducing the incidence of diseases, increasing quality of life, and extending longevity. One of these compounds that has been extensively studied is conjugated linoleic acid (CLA, dienoic isomers of linoleic acid).

Some studies (5) but not all (6) have shown that CLA may reduce adiposity and suppress weight gain in humans. The health benefits attributed to CLA include anticarcinogenic activity (7), antiatherosclerotic effects (8), modification of the composition and metabolism of adipose tissue (9), immune response modulation (10), and increased glucose and insulin tolerance (11). Some investigators have proposed that CLA reduces body fat percentage by increasing energy expenditure in AKR/J mice without increasing the uncoupling protein gene expression (12), fat oxidation, or both (13). However, the cause of increased fat oxidation remains unknown, and it is still unclear whether it affects ingested or endogenous fat. Some studies suggest that mitochondrial oxidative capacity is altered in liver disease (14,15). Substantial published data have reported the effect in liver mitochondria of CLA not associated with CR (16-18). In skeletal muscle cells, CLA increases mitochondrial biosynthesis (19), a similar effect promoted by CR.

Previous studies have determined the occurrence of upregulation and redistribution of beta-catenin and E-cadherin in MCF-7 breast cancer cells (20) with CLA treatment. The coordinated integration of extracellular, intracellular, and intercellular mechanisms promotes the maintenance of homeostasis in higher organisms. The establishment of communicative networks between the different liver cell types is, therefore, indispensable. Hepatocytes, the most prominent liver cell population, communicate directly with each other through gap junctions (connexins) and adhesion molecules (cadherins) (21). An issue that has been investigated is whether treatment with CLA and/or CR could interfere with the cellular integrity of the liver tissue through modulation of connexins and cadherins that may impair important cellular functions, such as migration, adhesion, and cell cycle.

The objective of the present study was to investigate the role of CLA alone or combined with CR on liver metabolism. We first analyzed the mitochondrial oxidative stress to verify if CLA, as a mitochondrial uncoupler, would mimic CR. We specifically studied energy parameters measured by mitochondrial swelling and oxygen uptake in hepatic mitochondria isolated from control rats and rats submitted to 40% CR supplemented or not with CLA. We also measured serum glucose, insulin, total protein and lipid levels, muscle and liver glycogen, and weight changes in hepatic and periepididymal adipose tissues, and investigated the integrity and homeostasis maintenance in liver tissue by analyzing the expression of connexins and cadherins transcripts.

MATERIALS AND METHODS

Animal care

All experiments were conducted in strict agreement with the Guide for the Care and Use of Laboratory Animals and were approved by the local Animal Care and Use Committee (Permit No. 313/2009). Eight-week-old male Wistar rats were maintained in individual metabolic cages on a 12-h light/12-h dark cycle at a controlled temperature ($21 \pm 1°C$), with free access to food and water. After an adaptation period of 24 h, we measured the food and water intake of the animals for an additional 24 h. No differences in food and water intake between the treated and untreated groups were observed at any time. Thirty-six animals were randomly divided into four groups of nine animals each: 1) Control group; animals fed a standard diet (Nuvilab CR-1, Nuvital, Colombo, PR, Brazil) and water by orogastric intubation; 2) CLA group; animals fed a standard diet and treated with CLA; 3) Restr group; animals fed 60% of the diet consumed by control animals and water by orogastric intubation; 4) CLA Restr group; animals fed 60% of the diet consumed by control animals and treated with CLA. The groups received the commercial CLA mixture 75% AdvantEdge® CLA (EAS™ Golden, CO, USA) or water at a concentration corresponding to 1% of daily food intake. The fatty acid composition of the commercial mixture 75% AdvantEdge® CLA, expressed in g/100 g of fatty acids, is detailed in (22). Briefly, fatty acid composition of CLA (g/100 g of fatty acids): 0.75 of C18:2 *cis*-9, *cis*-12; 40.12 of C18:2 *cis*-9, *trans*-11 CLA; 39.15 C18:2 *trans*-10, *cis*-12 CLA. The animals were supplemented daily by orogastric intubation using disposable 1-mL syringes and gavage needles. The amount of supplement administered was calculated every 2 days based on the mean daily food intake in each group. The density of each supplement was taken into account for the calculation of the quantity in milliliters (approximately 0.1 to 0.6 mL). Body weight and food intake were recorded weekly.

Experimental procedures

Rectal temperature was measured with a digital thermometer (BD Basic, Becton Dickinson, São Paulo, Brazil). Temperatures were recorded between 2 and 3 pm once a week. In addition, the animals were weighed individually once a week. After 21 days of treatment, the four groups of six animals were sacrificed for mitochondrial isolation after a 12-h fast by cervical dislocation performed by a technician experienced in the procedure. For biochemical analysis (four groups of three animals), blood samples were obtained after anesthesia by heart puncture and sera were stored at -20°C. Liver tissues were collected and weighed, and fragments were processed for histological and biochemical analysis. Serum glucose, total protein, cholesterol, and triacylglycerol levels were measured using commercial kits according to the manufacturer's instructions (Laborlab, São Paulo, Brazil). Insulin was measured by ELISA (Linco Research, St. Charles, MO, USA). Hepatic and muscle glycogen were determined as described elsewhere (23). Liver total lipids were extracted according to the method of Folch and cols. (24).

Histology

Livers were removed and their fragments were immersed in a fixative solution containing 10% formaldehyde in Millonig buffer, pH 7.4, for 24 h at room temperature. Next, the specimens were washed in buffer and submitted to standard procedures for embedding in Paraplast® (Merck, Darmstadt, Germany). Longitudinal 6-μm thick sections were stained with hematoxylin-eosin. The slides were analyzed and documented under a Leica DM2000 photomicroscope at the Laboratory of Micromorphology/Uniararas.

Intraperitoneal glucose tolerance test

After 21 days of treatment, the four groups of three animals were fasted overnight (16-18 h), weighed, and injected intraperitoneally with d-glucose (Sigma-Aldrich, St. Louis, MO, USA) at a dose of 2 g/kg of body weight. Blood samples were collected by cutting the tip of the tail at 0, 30, 60, and 120 min after glucose injection. Serum glucose was determined using test tapes (MediSense Optium Xceed, Abbott Laboratories, CA, USA). The glucose response was calculated by estimating the total area under the curve using the trapezoidal method (25). Liver mitochondria were not isolated from these animals.

Isolation of rat liver mitochondria

The livers were weighed immediately after sacrifice. Rat liver mitochondria (RLM) were isolated from the livers of overnight-fasted adult Wistar rats by conventional differential centrifugation according to (26). RLM samples were homogenized for the determination of protein content. All experiments using isolated mitochondria were conducted within 1 h of isolation.

Standard incubation procedure

The RLM experiments were carried out at 28°C in a reaction medium containing 125 mM sucrose, 65 mM KCl, 10 mM HEPES buffer, pH 7.2, 1 mM inorganic phosphate, 2 mM sodium succinate, 5 μM rotenone, and 10 μM $CaCl_2$. Rotenone, sodium succinate, and HEPES were purchased from Sigma-Aldrich (St. Louis, MO, USA).

Determination of mitochondrial swelling and oxygen uptake

Mitochondrial swelling and oxygen uptake were performed according to established protocol (27). The variation in absorbance at 540 nm was measured with a Genesys 10UV spectrophotometer (Thermo Electron Corporation, Madison, WI, USA), and oxygen uptake was monitored with a Clark-type electrode (Oxytherm System, Hansatech Instruments, Norfolk, UK). Briefly, RLM (0.5 mg/mL) were incubated in standard reaction medium. Inorganic phosphate (2 mM) was added after 1 min of mitochondrial preincubation and absorbance was recorded over a period of 10 min. The mitochondrial swelling and oxygen uptake experiments were performed simultaneously using the same preparation of isolated RLM under the same experimental conditions. Mitochondrial respiration (oxygen uptake) was recorded over a period of 10 min, assuming a solubility of 210 μmol/mL at 28°C.

RNA isolation and semiquantitative reverse transcriptase-PCR (RT-PCR)

Total RNA was isolated from approximately 100 mg of rat liver with the TRIzol® reagent (Invitrogen, CA, USA) and digested with DNAse I, Amplification Grade (Invitrogen) according to the manufacturer's instructions. RNA concentration was determined by measuring UV absorbance at 260 nm using a spectrophotometer, and integrity was confirmed by formaldehyde gel electrophoresis. The total RNA samples were stored at -80°C until further use for analysis. cDNA was synthesized from 2 μg of RNA in the presence of dithiothreitol, dNTP, random primers, RNAseOUT, and SuperScript™ II Reverse Transcriptase (Invitrogen) in a final volume of 20 μL. The mRNA levels of the E-cad, N-cad, Cx26, Cx32, and Cx43 genes were investigated by semiquantitative RT-PCR. Primer sequences used in the PCR reactions were chosen based on the sequences available in GenBank. E-cad was amplified using gene-specific forward (5'-GCAGTTCTGCCAGAGAAACC-3') and reverse (5'-AATCCTGCTTCCAGGGAGAT-3') primers with an expected amplicon of 315 bp (Tm

55°C). The primers for N-cad (forward primer 5'-TGTTGCTGCAGAAAACCAAG-3' and reverse primer 5'-GGCGACTCTCTGTCCAGAAC-3') amplified a predicted amplicon of 309 bp (Tm 53°C) while the primers used for Cx26 (forward primer 5'-GGTGTGGGGAGATGAGCAAG-3' and 5'-GACTTCCCTGAGCAATACCT-3') had an expected amplicon of 540 bp (Tm 62°C). Cx32 was amplified using gene-specific primers (Tm 57°C; forward primer 5'-AATGAGGCAGGATGAACTGG-3' and reverse primer 5'-CCTCAAGCCGTAGCATTTTC-3') and resulted in the amplification of the predicted 339 bp product. Cx43 was amplified using gene-specific forward (5'-GATTGAAGAGCACGGCAAGG-3') and reverse (5'-GTGTAGACCGCGCTCAAG-3') primers with an expected amplicon of 144 bp (Tm 58°C). ACTB (β-actin) was used as a housekeeping gene (Tm 57°C; forward primer 5'-AGAGGGAAATCGTGCGTGACA-3' and reverse primer 5'-CGATAGTGATGACCTGACCGTCA-3') yielding an amplification product of 178 bp that was used to normalize connexins and cadherins mRNA levels.

The amplified products were separated on 1.5% agarose gel stained with ethidium bromide, visualized, and photographed by the gel documentation system Syngene G: Box®. Signal intensities of the bands were measured densitometrically using the Scion Image software. Each value was determined as the mean of three densitometric readings. The results are expressed as average ratios of the relative optical densities of E-cad, N-cad, Cx26, Cx32, and Cx43 PCR products in relation to β-actin.

Data analysis

Figures 1-3 report the mean ± standard deviation (SD) of measurements from six different animals. Data were compared by one-way ANOVA followed by Tukey's *post hoc* test performed using GraphPad Prism software (GraphPad Software, Inc., La Jolla, CA, USA) adopting a level of significance of 5% ($p < 0.05$).

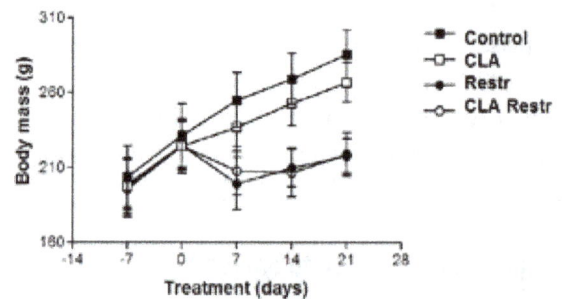

Figure 1. CLA treatment had no effect on body mass. Body mass was recorded weekly in Control (full square symbols), Restricted (Restr, full circle symbols), CLA-treated (CLA, empty square symbols), and restricted CLA-treated (CLA Restr, empty circle symbols) animals. Time 0 represents the start of treatment (* $p < 0.05$ versus Control group, $n = 9$).

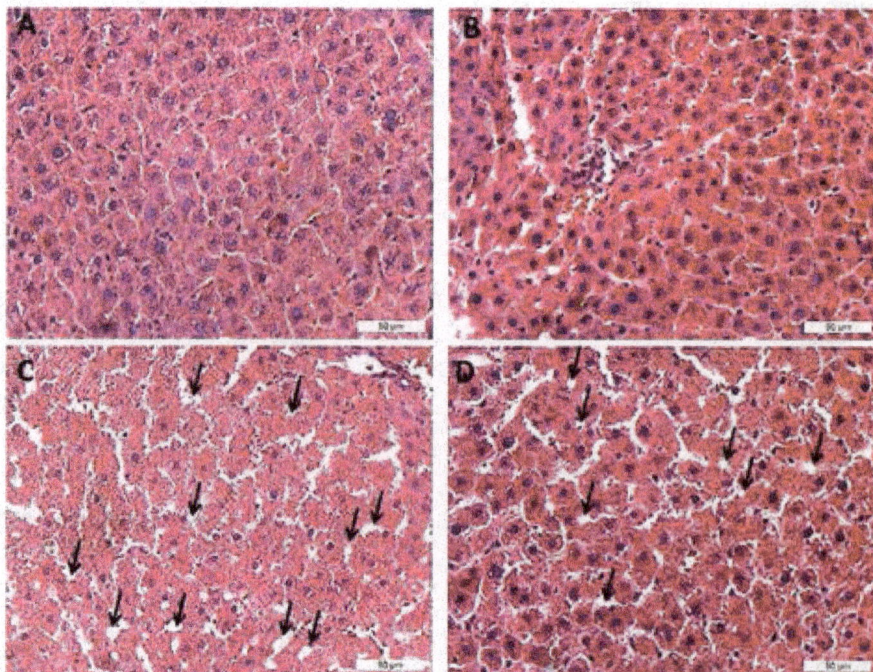

Figure 2. Photomicrographs of sagittal liver sections stained with hematoxylin-eosin. Tissue sections of 4.0 mm are shown in panels **A** (Control), **B** (Restr), **C** (CLA), and **D** (CLA Restr). Magnification X50. Arrows indicate fat vesicles.

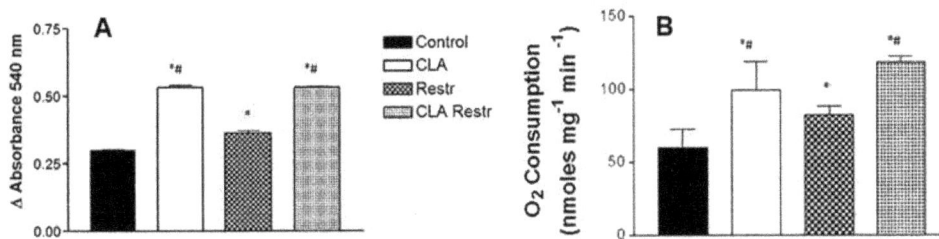

Figure 3. CLA increased mitochondrial swelling and oxygen consumption. Rat liver mitochondria (RLM; 0.5 mg/mL) were added to a standard reaction medium containing 125 mM sucrose, 65 mM KCl, 10 mM HEPES buffer, pH 7.2, 10 μM CaCl2, 1 mM iP, 2 mM succinate, 5 μM rotenone, at 28°C, and the (**A**) variation in 540-nm absorbance (**B**) and oxygen uptake were measured over a period of 10 min, as described in the Materials and Methods section. Inorganic phosphate (1 mM) was added after 1 min of mitochondrial preincubation ($p < 0.05$; * versus Control, # versus Restr, $n = 6$).

RESULTS

Characteristics of the animals

The body weight gain of the animals was analyzed weekly (0, 7, 14, and 21 days) during the treatment period (Figure 1). The results of the Restr and CLA Restr groups showed a significant reduction in body mass from day 7 to 21 of treatment compared with the CLA and Control groups. The ratio of liver weight and body weight (LW/BW) (Table 1A) showed that CLA treatment significantly increased the liver mass. The ratio of gonadal adipose tissue weight and body weight (AW/BW) showed a significant reduction promoted by CLA treatment. There were no differences in total protein, liver glycogen, or area under the glucose curve in the intraperitoneal glucose tolerance test between groups. Glucose, insulin, liver cholesterol, and triacylglycerol levels were lower in rats exposed to CR when compared with control animals. Treatment for 21 days resulted in an increase in insulin and total liver cholesterol, and a decrease in muscle glycogen and AW/BW index in the CLA and CLA Restr groups compared with the Control group. Serum triacylglycerol and cholesterol levels did not differ between the CLA and CLA Restr groups.

Liver histology

Photomicrographs of livers of Control (A), Restr (B), CLA (C), and CLA Restr (D) rats are shown in Figure 2. The normal structure of the hepatocytes ducts, with visible improvement in tissue organization, can be seen in Figure 2B when compared with 2A. Some pyknotic nuclei and loss of cell and tissue definition, suggestive of mild steatosis (black arrows), were observed in the liver of control rats treated with CLA (Figure 2C). Discrete cell and structural organization were noted in the liver of CLA Restr (Figure 2D compared with 2C).

CLA-stimulated mitochondrial swelling and oxygen uptake

As seen in Figure 3A, Ca^{2+}-induced mitochondrial swelling, measured by variation of absorbance in arbitrary units, was stimulated in RLM isolated from CLA (0.5340#* ± 0.012), Restr (0.3754* ± 0.004), and CLA Restr (0.5330#* ± 0.003) animals compared with those in the Control group (0.2970 ± 0.004) (* versus Control; # versus Restr, $p < 0.05$, $n = 6$). Under the same conditions, CR increased respiration in isolated mitochondrial preparations (Figure 3B). The results of liver oxygen uptake were 72.96 ± 3.154 nmol O_2 mg^{-1} min^{-1} in the Control group, 109.5* ± 9.509 nmol O_2 mg^{-1} min^{-1} in CLA-treated animals, 87.02* ± 2.171 nmol O_2 mg^{-1} min^{-1} in the Restr group, and 137.42*# ± 2.602 nmol O_2 mg^{-1} min^{-1} in the CLA Restr group.

Modulation of connexins and cadherins in the liver

Compared with the Control group, the CLA Restr group showed significant increases in mRNA expression levels of connexin 43 (0.65 ± 0.026 versus 1.4 ± 0.019, respectively), connexin 26 (0.61 ± 0.07 versus 0.98 ± 0.022, respectively), connexin 32 (0.85 ± 0.003 versus 1.39 ± 0.07, respectively), N-cad (0.67 ± 0.03 versus 1.25 ± 0.06, respectively), and E-cad (0.89 ± 0.07 versus 1.33 ± 0.08, respectively) (Figure 4). Similarly, hepatic mRNA expressions of connexins 43 (1.06 ± 0.025) and 26 (0.95 ± 0.05) were significantly increased in the CLA group compared with the Control group (0.65 ± 0.026 and 0.61 ± 0.07, respectively). In contrast, CR caused a significant reduction in connexins 43 (0.49 ± 0.030) and 32 (0.6 ± 0.03) mRNA and an increase in N-cad (1.2 ± 0.06) and E-cad (1.25 ± 0.1) levels compared with the Control group.

Table 1. Serum levels of fasting glucose, insulin, cholesterol, triacylglycerol, total protein; liver cholesterol, triacyglycerol, glycogen, and glycogen muscle and adipose tissue of control and of rats maintained on CR (Restr) or CLA treated (CLA and CLA Restr) for 21 days

Parameter	Control	Restr	CLA	CLA Restr
Body weight BW (g)	277.4 ± 42.06	215.40* ± 35.53	257.00 ± 53.28	215.2* ± 44.53
Liver weight LW (g)	10.12 ± 0.3481	6.565* ± 0.3951	11.41*# ± 1.285	7.685* ± 0.09152
LW/BW (%)	3.65 ± 0.02	3.05* ± 0.03	4.44* ± 0.03	3.57# ± 0.02
Gonadal adipose tissue weight AW (g)	1.1 ± 0.11	0.77* ± 0.11	0.85 ± 0.26	0.62* ± 0.15
AW/BW (%)	0.39 ± 0.02	0.35 ± 0.03	0.33* ± 0.01	0.28*# ± 0.02
Glucose (mmol/L)	5.39 ± 0.5	3.84* ± 0.23	5.11# ± 0.21	4.12 ± 0.22
Insulin (U/mL)	0.39 ± 0.12	0.21* ± 0.05	1.4* ± 0.22	1.7* ± 0.5
Cholesterol (mg/dL)	168.00 ± 9.3	129.01* ± 21.00	171.00# ± 19.00	179.00# ± 20.00
Triacylglycerol (mg/dL)	91.00 ± 18.00	70.00* ± 6.00	125.00# ± 15.01	121.01# ± 7.00
Total protein (g/dL)	8.66 ± 0.66	9.64 ± 0.56	9.02 ± 0.62	8.91 ± 0.34
Liver cholesterol (mg/g tissue)	16.9 ± 2.5	10.8* ± 2	22.7*# ± 3.9	31.4*# ± 2.6
Liver triacylglycerol (mg/g tissue)	20.01 ± 6.5	9.35* ± 3.2	27.5*# ± 3.5	23.00# ± 4.3
Muscle glycogen (g/100 g tissue)	0.44 ± 0.02	0.45 ± 0.03	0.35*# ± 0.17	0.32*# ± 0.08
Liver glycogen (g/100 g tissue)	3.34 ± 0.33	2.45 ± 0.24	3.39 ± 0.7	2.09 ± 0.9
Area under glucose curve	15830 ± 127	16100 ± 179	15480 ± 132	15840 ± 156

p < 0.05 * vs Control; # vs Restr (Mean ± SD; n = 6-9).

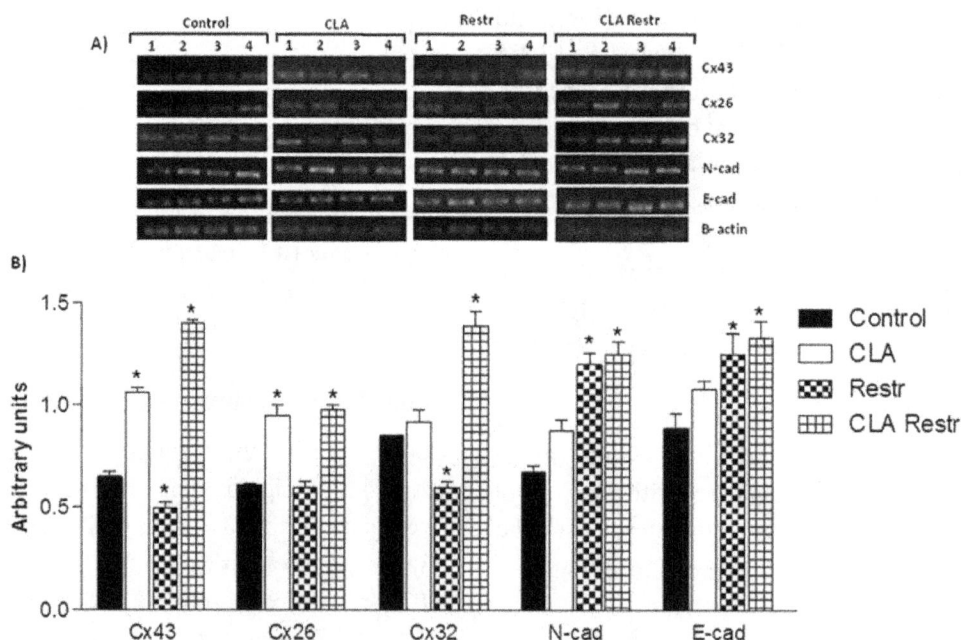

Figure 4. Liver mRNA levels of connexins (Cx) and cadherins (cad). (**A**) Representative semiquantitative RT-PCR of mRNA expression of *Cx43*, *Cx32*, *Cx26*, *N-cad*, and *E-cad*. (**B**) Bars represent densitometric analyses of connexins and cadherins mRNA expression in control and treated animals. Changes in mRNA are expressed as normalized densitometric units relative to *β-actin* mRNA. Values are represented as mean ± standard error of the mean (SEM). * *P* < 0.05 indicates statistical significance.

DISCUSSION

Body weight gain analysis of the animals in our study showed that those in the Restr groups lost weight during the treatment period. These results validate the CR model: Restr animals presenting lower weight gain compared with Control ones, but with upward curves indicating animal growth. Body weight gain was similar in Control and CLA animals during the 3-week monitoring period. Weight gain was lower in Restr and CLA Restr animals. These results show that CLA had no effect on the body weight of the animals under the present experimental conditions. Biochemical analysis findings agree with the literature and suggest that CLA-treated animals had hyperinsulinemia in the presence of normoglycemia and presented no changes in plasma cholesterol or triacylglycerol, features of insulin resistance (28). A small reduction in liver glycogen and a significant reduction in muscle glycogen were observed in CLA-treated animals. This glycogen reduction is usually seen in hyperinsulinemic animals (29).

The significant increase in the LW/BW index found in rats treated with CLA may indicate physiological changes consistent with hepatic steatosis. These data were demonstrated by photomicrographs of sagittal sections of liver stained with hematoxylin-eosin (Figure 2). In fact, these were confirmed by the results in Sprague-Dawley rats suggesting that CLA accelerates the decomposition of storage lipids, resulting in lipid peroxidation and morphological change in the liver (30). The presence of fat and liver cell alterations suggests hepatic steatosis and intoxication by CLA (30,31). In contrast, liver cells were intact in Restr animals, and CLA Restr animals showed less cell damage than CLA ones, suggesting a protective effect of CR. Our results show that the LW/BW ratio decreased in Restr, increased in CLA, and remained the same in CLA Restr animals compared with those in the Control group. Conversely, we observed a decrease in the AW/BW ratio in the CLA group, an effect enhanced by the CR. The body weight reduction in the Restr group can be explained by the reduction in liver weight, and in the CLA Restr group, by the reduction in adipose tissue weight. Taken together, these data may explain the liver damage caused by treatment with CLA.

The study of inner mitochondrial membrane permeability (MMP) induced by Ca^{2+} can be associated with a nonspecific increase in membrane permeability that stimulates respiratory rates and decreases the coupling between oxygen consumption and oxidative phosphorylation (32). The results suggest that the RLM CLA, Restr, and CLA Restr groups were more susceptible to the same MMP transition conditions than animals in the Control group. With the same stimulus to induce oxidative damage (10 μM $CaCl_2$ and 2 mM inorganic phosphate), RLM from CLA, Restr, and CLA Restr animals exhibited a higher respiration rate. The uncoupling effect of CLA treatment on mitochondrial respiration was confirmed by the results of liver oxygen uptake (Figure 2). As expected, CR increased respiration in isolated mitochondrial preparations, promoting mild mitochondrial uncoupling and proportional swelling, an effect that was enhanced in the CLA-treated groups. Kowaltowski and cols. have elegantly demonstrated that mild mitochondrial uncoupling is a highly effective *in vivo* antioxidant strategy, and that murine lifespan can be extended by low doses of the mitochondrial uncoupler 2,4-dinitrophenol in a manner accompanied by weight loss and lower serum levels of glucose, insulin, and triacylglycerol, as well as a pronounced decrease in biomarkers of oxidative damage and tissue ROS release (33). In the present study, the CLA-induced mitochondrial uncoupling activity was probably promoted by hepatic steatosis due to increased liver lipids content and had no effect on weight loss.

The increased hepatic cholesterol observed in CLA and CLA Rest animals may also explain the increases in connexin 43 and 26 mRNA expression in these groups. Also, the reduction in connexin 43 and 32 may be related to a decrease in cholesterol in the Restr group. Specific phospholipids are associated with different connexin isoforms, which suggests connexin-specific regulatory and/or structural interactions with lipid membranes and a potential role of membrane cholesterol in gap junction assembly and function (34). Cadherins are a superfamily of calcium-dependent adhesion molecules that play multiple roles in morphogenesis. A reduction in E-cadherin, in particular, is associated with invasion, increased cell proliferation, and metastasis (35). Expression levels of N-cadherin and E-cad mRNA were increased in Restr and CLA Restr animals compared with Control ones. This fact may suggest an antiproliferative effect of hepatocytes mediated by E-cadherin induced by CR, with no effect of CLA treatment. Therefore, our data are consistent with the literature and suggest that the increase in cadherins in animals undergoing CR contributes to decrease hepatic cell damage. Taken together, the present results suggest that CLA supplementation stimulates the accumulation of fat in the liver and increases insulin levels. CLA does not seem to be a safe mass loss compound because it induces hepatic mitochondrial and plasma lipid disorders, and upregulates the mRNA expression of connexins. The understanding of the biochemical mechanisms underlying the effect of CLA is important for the correct formulation of dietary interventions and adequate administration of food supplements.

Author contributions: Camila de Moraes isolated the mitochondria and performed the mitochondrial respiration measurements. Camila Andrea de Oliveira performed the RT-PCR. Maria Esméria Corezola do Amaral performed the biochemical analysis. Gabriela Arcurio Landini performed the mitochondrial swelling. Camila de Morae and Gabriela Arcurio Landini nursed and treated animals. Rosana Catisti designed the study. Camila Andrea de Oliveira, Maria Esméria Corezola do Amaral and Rosana Catisti wrote the paper. All authors approved the final version of the manuscript.

Acknowledgments: the authors thank Armindo A. Alves for helpful suggestions, and José R. Passarini, Renata Barbieri and Lia M. G. Neves for excellent technical assistance. Rosana Catisti was the recipient of a fellowship from Fundação de Amparo à Pesquisa do Estado de São Paulo (Fapesp, 2008, 52140-2) and PROPESq/Uniararas. Camila de Moraes was a student supported by a fellowship from Pibic/CNPq and Coordenação de Aperfeiçoamento de Pessoal de Nível Superior (Capes, Prosup).

Fundings: this work was partly supported by Conselho Nacional de Pesquisa (Pibic/CNPq), Fundação de Amparo à Pesquisa do Estado de São Paulo (Fapesp, 2008, 52140-2), Coordenação de Aperfeiçoamento de Pessoal de Nível Superior (Capes, Prosup) and Centro Universitário Hermínio Ometto (PROPESq/Uniararas).

REFERENCES

1. Guarente L. Mitochondria – A nexus for aging, calorie restriction and sirtuins? Cell. 2008;132:171-6.

2. Lambert AJ, Wang B, Yardley J, Edwards J, Merry BJ. The effect of aging and caloric restriction on mitochondrial protein density and oxygen consumption Exp Gerontol. 2004;39:289-95.

3. Lambert AJ, Merry BJ. Effect of caloric restriction on mitochondrial reactive oxygen species production and bioenergetics: reversal by insulin. Am J Physiol Regul Integr Comp Physiol. 2004;286: R71-9.

4. López-Lluch G, Hunt N, Jones B, Zhu M, Jamieson H, Hilmer S, et al. Calorie restriction induces mitochondrial biogenesis and bioenergetic efficiency. Proc Natl Acad Sci USA. 2006;103: 1768-73.

5. Gaullier JM, Halse J, Hoye K, Kristiansen K, Fagertun H, Vik H, et al. Supplementation with conjugated linoleic acid for 24 months is well tolerated by and reduces body fat mass in healthy, overweight humans. J Nutr. 2005;135:778-84.

6. Zambell KL, Keim NL, Van Loan MD, Gale B, Benito P, Kelley DS, et al. Conjugated linoleic acid supplementation in humans: effects on body composition and energy expenditure. Lipids. 2000,35:777-82.

7. Ip C, Briggs SP, Haegele AD, Thompson HJ, Storkson J, Scimeca JA. The efficacy of conjugated linoleic acid in mammary cancer prevention is independent of level or type of fat in the diet. Carcinogenesis. 1996;17:1045-50.

8. Nicolosi RJ, Rogers EJ, Kritchevsky D, Scimeca JA, Huth PJ. Dietary conjugated linoleic acid reduces plasma lipoproteins and early aortic atherosclerosis in hypercholesterolemic hamsters. Artery. 1997;22:266-77.

9. Zhong W, Jiang Z, Zheng C, Lin Y, Yang L, Zou S. Relationship between proteome changes of Longissimus muscle and intramuscular fat content in finishing pigs fed conjugated linoleic acid. Br J Nutr. 2011;105(1):1-9.

10. Whigham LD, Higbee A, Bjorling DE, Park Y, Pariza MW, Cook ME. Decreased antigen-induced eicosanoid release in conjugated linoleic acid-fed guinea pigs. Am J Physiol Regul Integr Comp Physiol. 2002;282:R1104-12.

11. Liu LF, Purushotham A, Wendel AA, Belury MA. Combined effects of rosiglitazone and conjugated linoleic acid on adiposity, insulin sensitivity, and hepatic steatosis in high-fat-fed mice. Am J Physiol Gastrointest Liver Physiol. 2007;292:G1671-8.

12. West DB, Blohm FY, Truett AA, DeLany JP. Conjugated linoleic acid persistently increases total energy expenditure in AKR/J mice without increasing uncoupling protein gene expression. J Nutr. 2000;130:2471-7.

13. Azain MJ, Hausman DB, Sisk MB, Flatt WP, Jewell DE. Dietary conjugated linoleic acid reduces rat adipose tissue cell size rather than cell number. J Nutr. 2000;130:1548-54.

14. Mantena SK, King AL, Andringa KK, Eccleston HB, Bailey SM. Mitochondrial dysfunction and oxidative stress in the pathogenesis of alcohol- and obesity-induced fatty liver diseases. Free Radic Biol Med. 2007;44:1259-72.

15. Szendroedi J, Roden M. Ectopic lipids and organ function. Curr Opin Lipidol. 2009;20:50-6.

16. Choi JS, Koh IU, Jung MH, Song J. Effects of three different conjugated linoleic acid preparations on insulin signalling, fat oxidation and mitochondrial function in rats fed a high-fat diet. Br J Nutr. 2007;98:264-75.

17. Yamasaki M, Miyamoto Y, Chujo H, Nishiyama K, Tachibana H, Yamada K. Trans10, cis12-conjugated linoleic acid induces mitochondria-related apoptosis and lysosomal destabilization in rat hepatoma cells. Biochim Biophys Acta. 2005;15;1735:176-84.

18. Palacios A, Piergiacomi V, Catalá A. Antioxidant effect of conjugated linoleic acid and vitamin A during non-enzymatic lipid peroxidation of rat liver microsomes and mitochondria. Mol Cell Biochem. 2003;250:107-13

19. Vaughan RA, Garcia-Smith R, Bisoffi M, Conn CA, Trujillo KA. Conjugated linoleic acid or omega 3 fatty acids increase mitochondrial biosynthesis and metabolism in skeletal muscle cells. Lipids Health Dis. 2012;11:142.

20. Bocca C, Bozzo F, Francica S, Colombatto S, Miglietta A. Involvement of PPAR gamma and E-cadherin/beta-catenin pathway in the antiproliferative effect of conjugated linoleic acid in MCF-7 cells. Int J Cancer. 2007;121(2):248-56.

21. Bauer R, Valletta D, Bauer K, Thasler WE, Hartmann A, Müller M, et al. Downregulation of P-cadherin expression in hepatocellular carcinoma induces tumorigenicity. J Clin Exp Pathol. 2014;7(9):6125-32.

22. Santos-Zago LF, Botelho AP, de Oliveira AC. Supplementation with commercial mixtures of conjugated linoleic acid in association with vitamin E and the process of lipid autoxidation in rats. Lipids. 2007;42:845-54.

23. Lo S, Russell JC, Taylor AW. Determination of glycogen in small tissue samples. J Appl Physiol. 1970;28:234-36.

24. Folch J, Lees M, Sloane-Stanley GH. A simple method for the isolation and purification of total lipids from animal tissues. J Biol Chem. 1957;226:497-509.

25. Le Floch JP, Escuyer P, Baudin E, Baudon D, Perlemuter L. Blood glucose area under the curve Methodological aspects. Diabetes Care. 1990;13:172-5.

26. Schneider WC, Hogeboom GH. Intracellular distribution of enzymes V Further studies on the distribution of cytochrome C in rat liver homogenates. J Biol Chem. 1950;183:123-8.

27. Moraes C, Rebelato HJ, Amaral ME, Resende TM, Silva EV, Esquisatto MA, et al. Effect of maternal protein restriction on liver metabolism in rat offspring. J Physiol Sci. 2014;64(5):347-55.

28. Ingelsson E, Risérus U. Effects of trans10 cis12CLA-induced insulin resistance on retinol-binding protein 4 concentrations in abdominally obese men Diabetes Res Clin Pract. 2008;82:e23-4.

29. Ueno M, Carvalheira JB, Tambascia RC, Bezerra RM, Amaral ME, Carneiro EM, et al. Regulation of insulin signalling by hyperinsulinaemia: role of IRS-1/2 serine phosphorylation and the mTOR/p70 S6K pathway Diabetologia. 2005;48:506-18.

30. Yamasaki M, Mansho K, Mishima H, Kimura G, Sasaki M, Kasai M, et al. Effect of dietary conjugated linoleic acid on lipid peroxidation and histological change in rat liver tissues. J Agric Food Chem. 2000,48:6367-71.

31. Vyas D, Kadegowda AK, Erdman RA. Dietary conjugated linoleic acid and hepatic steatosis: species-specific effects on liver and adipose lipid metabolism and gene expression J Nutr Metab. 2012;2012:932928.

32. Kowaltowski AJ, Castilho RF, Vercesi AE. Opening of the mitochondrial permeability transition pore by uncoupling or inorganic phosphate in the presence of Ca2+ is dependent on mitochondrial-generated reactive oxygen species. FEBS Lett. 1996;378:150-2.

33. Caldeira da Silva CC, Cerqueira FM, Barbosa LF, Medeiros MH, Kowaltowski AJ. Mild mitochondrial uncoupling in mice affects energy metabolism, redox balance and longevity Aging Cell. 2008;7:552-60.

34. Locke D, Harris AL. Connexin channels and phospholipids: association and modulation. BMC Biol. 2009;7:52.

35. Ohta T, Elnemr A, Yamamoto M, Ninomiya I, Fushida S, Nishimura G, et al. Thiazolidinedione, a peroxisome proliferator-activated receptor-gamma ligand, modulates the E-cadherin/beta-catenin system in a human pancreatic cancer cell line, BxPC-3. Int J Oncol. 2002;21(1):37-42.

13

Dynamic changes of central thyroid functions in the management of Cushing's syndrome

Sema Ciftci Dogansen[1], Gulsah Yenidunya Yalin[1],
Bulent Canbaz[1], Seher Tanrikulu[1], Sema Yarman[1]

ABSTRACT

Objective: The aim of this study was to determine the frequency of central thyroid dysfunctions in Cushing's syndrome (CS). We also aimed to evaluate the frequency of hyperthyroidism due to the syndrome of the inappropriate secretion of TSH (SITSH), which was recently defined in patients with insufficient hydrocortisone replacement after surgery. Materials and methods: We evaluated thyroid functions (TSH and free thyroxine [fT4]) at the time of diagnosis, during the hypothalamo-pituitary-adrenal axis recovery, and after surgery in 35 patients with CS. The patients were separated into two groups: ACTH-dependent CS (group 1, n = 20) and ACTH-independent CS (group 2, n = 15). Patients' clinical and laboratory findings were evaluated in five visits in the outpatient clinic of the endocrinology department. Results: The frequency of baseline suppressed TSH levels and central hypothyroidism were determined to be 37% (n = 13) and 26% (n = 9), respectively. A negative correlation was found between baseline cortisol and TSH levels (r = -0.45, p = 0.006). All patients with central hypothyroidism and suppressed TSH levels showed recovery at the first visit without levothyroxine treatment. SITSH was not detected in any of the patients during the postoperative period. No correlation was found between prednisolone replacement after surgery and TSH or fT4 levels on each visit. Conclusion: Suppressed TSH levels and central hypothyroidism may be detected in CS, independent of etiology. SITSH was not detected in the early postoperative period due to our adequate prednisolone replacement doses. Arch Endocrinol Metab. 2018;62(2):164-71

[1] Istanbul University, Istanbul
Faculty of Medicine, Department
of Internal Medicine, Division
of Endocrinology and
Metabolism, Istanbul, Turkey

Correspondence to:
Sema Ciftci Dogansen
Istanbul University,
Istanbul Faculty of Medicine,
Department of Internal Medicine,
Division of Endocrinology and
Metabolism,
Capa, 34090 – Istanbul, Turkey
sdogansen@gmail.com

Keywords
Cushing's syndrome; thyroid dysfunction; syndrome of inappropriate secretion of TSH; endogenous hypercortisolemia; central hypothyroidism

INTRODUCTION

The major regulators of TSH secretion are commonly known as the stimulation effect of TRH and the negative feedback of the fT4 and fT3. However several factors such as dopamine and somatostatin, also play a role in the modulation of TSH secretion and the secretion pattern demonstrates a diurnal rhythm via these regulators (1). The hypothalamus-pituitary-thyroid (HPT) axis may be altered in Cushing's syndrome (CS). Both endogenous CS and exogenous hypercortisolism suppress serum TSH levels (2-10). Hypercortisolemia decreases the TSH pulse amplitude and nocturnal surge without causing any changes in the TSH pulse frequency (4-6,8). Furthermore, many studies have indicated that hypercortisolemia blunts the TSH response to TRH (2,4,10-12). TSH suppression in hypercortisolemia is most likely related to decreased TRH gene expression

(13). However, the presence of hypercortisolemia may also decrease TSH secretion by having a direct effect on the pituitary thyrotropin cells through annexin-1, somatostatin, leptin, and dopamine (4,14-17). Another possible mechanism in the TSH suppression of glucocorticoids is the type 2 deiodinase enzyme activity that converts T4 to T3 in the hypothalamus and pituitary. The local T3 levels in the hypothalamus and pituitary are also important in the regulation of the HPT axis. Increased type 2 deiodinase activity due to glucocorticoids causes increased local T3 levels which eventually leads to the suppression of TRH and TSH secretion (18,19). In addition, central hypothyroidism with reduced fT4 may be present in patients with hypercortisolism (6,7). Mathioudakis and cols. (7) reported that central hypothyroidism can be seen in patients with ACTH-secreting pituitary microadenomas with a prevalence as high as 18%.

Recently, the syndrome of the inappropriate secretion of TSH (SITSH) was reported as a clinical condition with the presence of normal or elevated TSH secretion despite inappropriately high levels of thyroid hormones in patients who receive insufficient hydrocortisone replacement following surgery for CS (19). Furthermore, SITSH is considered as the main cause of steroid withdrawal syndrome (SWS) (20).

In light of these reports, we aimed to determine the frequency of central thyroid dysfunctions in patients who underwent endogenous hypercortisolism. We evaluated thyroid function tests at baseline in the time of CS diagnosis and during the period of hypothalamo-pituitary-adrenal (HPA) axis recovery following surgery for CS and at remission.

MATERIALS AND METHODS

This is a retrospective observational study from a university hospital outpatient clinic. We identified the patients (n = 35) with a confirmed diagnosis of CS who had a record of thyroid function tests during the past 10 years. All of the procedures were applied in accordance with the Declaration of Helsinki. The diagnosis of CS was based on the clinical and radiological findings (pituitary adenoma, adrenal adenoma, or bronchial carcinoid tumor confirmed by sellar or abdominal magnetic resonance imaging [MRI], lung computed tomography [CT] or ocreotide scintigraphy) and laboratory tests. The diagnosis of CS was confirmed by failure to suppress plasma cortisol levels after the administration of 1-mg-overnight and low-dose dexamethasone suppression tests (48 hours, 2 mg/day) in accordance with the current guideline (21). A definitive diagnosis of Cushing's disease (CD) was made with positive immunostaining for the ACTH of the pituitary adenoma and clinical cortisol dependency for several months after adenomectomy. The diagnosis of ectopic ACTH syndrome (EAS) was based on high plasma ACTH levels, the presence of a lung lesion on high-resolution CT scanning or ocreotide scintigraphy, histological confirmation of the tumor with positive immunostaining for ACTH, and clinical cortisol dependency during the follow-up period after tumor resection. The diagnosis of primary adrenal CS was based on the absence or diminished dexamethasone suppression of serum cortisol, a low or undetectable plasma ACTH concentration, the presence of a unilateral adrenal adenoma on CT or MRI scanning, and histological confirmation of the adenoma.

Patients with known thyroid disease at the time of CS diagnosis, patients who developed thyroid disease (including autoimmune thyroid disease) during follow-up, and patients who were on drugs known to alter thyroid functions were excluded. Macroadenoma ($\geq$ 10 mm) of the pituitary, a history of conventional radiotherapy (RT) for the pituitary, and the development of hypopituitarism after pituitary surgery were also among the exclusion criteria of the study.

Among the patients who underwent pituitary surgery, adrenalectomy, or bronchial carcinoid resection, those who fulfilled the initial surgical remission criteria were included. Patients with a residual tumor after an unsuccessful initial operation or late relapse were excluded.

Initial surgical remission was defined as morning serum cortisol levels less than 2 µg/dL within a week of cortisol-secreting tumor resection. Late remission was defined as cortisol suppression with a 1-mg-overnight dexamethasone test following HPA axis recovery and the discontinuation of a glucocorticoid (prednisolone) replacement. HPA axis recovery was evaluated by using morning cortisol and/or ACTH stimulation tests. Prednisolone replacement was discontinued when morning plasma cortisol levels were $\geq$ 10 µg/dL or stimulated cortisol levels were approximately $\geq$ 18 µg/dL with ACTH stimulation test (22). Prednisolone replacement was gradually tapered and discontinued following HPA axis recovery.

We analyzed the correlation of serum cortisol with TSH and fT4 levels with in patients who had hypercortisolism due to CD (n = 17); EAS (n = 3); or primary-adrenal CS (n = 15). Comparisons were conducted before and after the remission with surgical treatment to evaluate the changes in TSH and fT4 due to the aberrations in the HPT axis.

Serum cortisol, TSH (0.27-4.2 µU/Ml, intra-assay CV = 3.8%, inter-assay CV = 1.4%) and fT4 (12-22 pmol/L, intra-assay CV = 2.1%, inter-assay CV = 1.7%) levels were measured using an electrochemiluminescent immunoassay (Roche Hitachi). Serum ACTH (0-46 pg/mL, intra-assay CV: < 10%, inter-assay CV: < 10%) levels were measured using a chemiluminescence immunoassay (Immulite 2000).

Sex, age at diagnosis, mean duration of CS, duration of follow-up, baseline cortisol, ACTH, TSH, and fT4 levels, and the baseline adenoma diameter were evaluated retrospectively for each patient. Serum cortisol levels were recorded in the early postoperative period. Patients' clinical findings and laboratory tests were evaluated in a total of five visits; the first visit was between the first and the third month; the second visit was at the sixth month; the third visit was at the 12th month; the fourth visit was at the time of HPA axis recovery; and the fifth visit was the last visit of the follow-up period. Cortisol, TSH, fT4, and the prednisolone replacement dose (for patients who were on prednisolone replacement) were recorded during each visit.

ACTH-dependent (group 1) and ACTH-independent (group 2) CS patients were compared in terms of the baseline characteristics and thyroid function tests during follow-up.

Statistical analyses were performed using SPSS version 21.0. Categorical variables were defined by frequency and percentage rate, and numeric variables by mean ± standard deviation (SD). In dual independent group comparisons, the student's t test was used for normally distributed continuous variables, and the Mann-Whitney U test for non-normally distributed data. Categorical variables were compared using the chi-square test. Correlation analyses were performed using the Pearson correlation test. Statistical significance was set at $p < 0.05$. Ranges of the correlation r value were accepted as 0-0.24 weak, 0.25-0.49 moderate, 0.50-0.74 strong, and 0.74-1.00 very strong.

RESULTS

Thirty-five patients (28 female and seven male; mean age at diagnosis of 37.2 ± 11.4 years; range of 17-61 years) were included in the study. The mean follow-up time was 57.1 ± 27.6 months (range of, 21-114 months). The mean duration of CS was 2.7 ± 1.5 years (range of, 1-7 years). Group 1 consisted of bronchial

carcinoid tumors (n = 3, 8%) and CD (n = 17, 49%) and group 2 consisted of cortisol-secreting adrenal adenomas (n = 15, 43%).

The mean cortisol, TSH, and fT4 levels at the initial assessment are shown in Table 1. The frequencies of baseline-suppressed TSH levels and central hypothyroidism were determined to be 37% (13/35) and 26% (9/35), respectively. The diagnosis of patients with central hypothyroidism were CD (n = 3), EAS (n = 2), and primary adrenal CS (n = 4). The baseline cortisol levels correlated negatively with the baseline TSH levels (r = -0.45, p = 0.006). However, no correlation was found between the baseline cortisol and fT4 levels (p = 0.183). In addition, no differences were found between the baseline cortisol levels of patients with and without central hypothyroidism (p = 0.218).

The mean postoperative early cortisol levels of the patients were 0.7 ± 0.6 µg/dL (range of, 0.1-1.8 µg/dL). Thus, all of the patients achieved remission after surgery, and prednisolone replacement was initiated. All of the patients with central hypothyroidism were recorded as euthyroid on the first visit without the replacement of levothyroxine. The mean cortisol, TSH, and fT4 levels and prednisolone replacement dose (for patients who were on prednisolone replacement) during each visit are shown in Table 1. No correlation was found between prednisolone replacement and TSH or fT4 levels during each visit (p > 0.05). The mean HPA axis recovery time was 16.2 ± 13.2 months (range of 7-60 months). TSH levels during the last visit were significantly higher than the baseline TSH levels, and no differences in the fT4 levels were found between baseline and the last visit (p = 0.003, p = 0.295, respectively). Changes in the TSH and FT4 levels during follow-up are shown in Figure 1.

In group 1, the mean diameter of the pituitary adenoma was 5.9 ± 1.6 mm (range, of 3-9 mm), and the

Table 1. The mean cortisol, TSH, fT4 levels and prednisolone replacement dose* on each visit

	Cortisol levels (µg/dL) mean ± SD (range)	TSH levels (µU/mL) mean ± SD (range)	fT4 levels (pmol/L) mean ± SD (range)	Prednisolone replacement dose* (mg/day) mean ± SD (range)
Baseline	26.3 ± 8.7 (13-46)	0.8 ± 0.7 (0.1-2.9)	13.8 ± 2.7 (9.3-19.7)	-
First visit	0.9 ± 1.1 (0.1-4.7)	2.1 ± 1.2 (0.5-4.7)	15.9 ± 2.2 (12.8-20.7)	7.3 ± 1.5 (5-10)
Second visit	2.9 ± 2.8 (0.1-8.3)	2.4 ± 1.3 (0.3-1.8)	15.1 ± 1.8 (12.4-18.6)	4.6 ± 1.5 (2.5-7.5)
Third visit	8.9 ± 5.8 (0.3-18.6)	2.7 ± 1.2 (0.5-4.8)	15.2 ± 1.3 (12.5-18.1)	3.6 ± 1.1 (2.5-5)
Fourth visit	13.2 ± 1.7 (10.4-16.9)	2.5 ± 1.2 (0.7-4.8)	15.1 ± 1.6 (12.7-19.1)	-
Fifth visit	15.3 ± 2.9 (10.7-21)	2.3 ± 1.1 (0.9-4.7),	15.6 ± 1.8 (12.1-20)	-

*: Prednisolone replacement doses were revised for patients who were receiving prednisolone replacement after surgical treatment. Baseline: at initial assessment, First visit: Between the 1st and the 3rd months; Second visit: On the 6th month; Third visit: On the 12th month; Fourth visit: At the time of HPA axis recovery; Fifth visit: Last visit of the follow-up period.

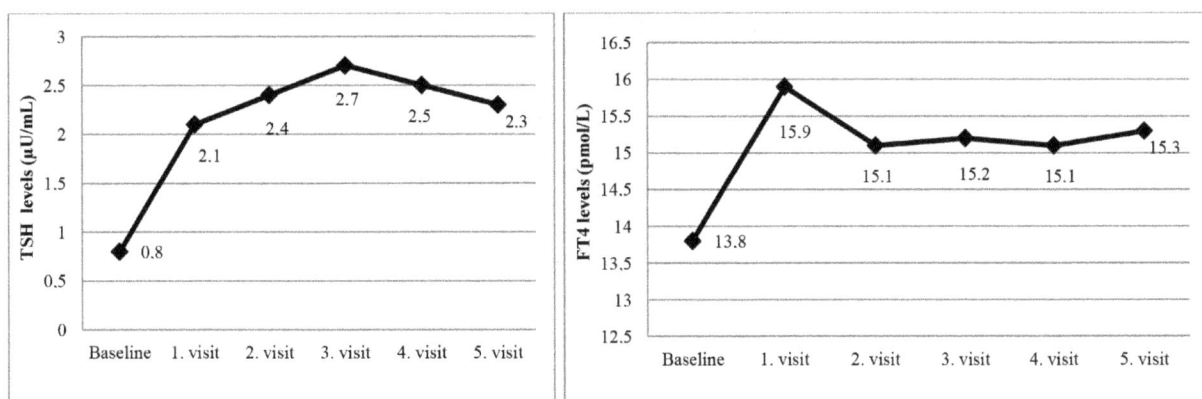

Figure 1. Changes in TSH and FT4 levels during folliw-up. First visit: Between the 1st and the 3rd months; Second visit: On the 6th month; Third visit: On the 12th month; Fourth visit: At the time of HPA axis recovery; Fifth visit: Last visit of the follow-up period.

mean baseline ACTH level was 66.6 ± 33.8 pg/mL (range of, 16-155 pg/mL). No correlation was found between the baseline TSH and ACTH levels or the diameter of the pituitary adenoma (p = 0.268, p = 0.813, respectively). In group 2, the mean diameter of the adrenal adenomas was 32 ± 11 mm (range of, 20-54 mm).

Patients in group 1 were found to be younger than those in group 2 (p = 0.03). Although baseline cortisol levels were higher in group 1, the difference was not statistically significant (p = 0.645). The frequency of central hypothyroidism at the initial assessment, and the baseline TSH and fT4 levels were not statistically different between the two groups (p = 0.912, p = 0.242, p = 0.631, respectively). The frequency of baseline-suppressed TSH levels were higher in group 1, but the difference was not statistically significant (p = 0.069). As for the TSH and fT4 levels, the TSH levels of group 2 were higher only at the second visit (p = 0.035). No statistically significant difference was found between the two groups in terms of the HPA axis recovery time and the plasma TSH; and fT4 levels (p = 0.825, p = 0.761, p = 0.841, respectively). In addition, no difference was observed between the two groups regarding the change in plasma TSH levels (Δ TSH) at the last visit (p = 0.257). The comparisons of the two groups are shown in Table 2.

DISCUSSION

In this study, we demonstrated the effect of hypercortisolism on thyroid functions in patients with CS. Because it is common knowledge that plasma T3 levels decrease through peripheral type 1 deiodinase enzyme inhibition, we aimed to show the central

effects of hypercortisolism on thyroid functions (23). Furthermore, glucocorticoids are used in the treatment of hyperthyroidism due to these peripheral effects (24). We have shown suppressed baseline TSH levels in patients with active CS, which is also compatible with a number of studies in the literature (2,3,5-7,10). In this study, a very selective population was evaluated to detect merely the effect of hypercortisolism on thyroid functions, contrary to the studies in the literature. Patients who had secondary conditions that could affect thyroid function tests, such as autoimmune thyroid disease, the presence of pituitary macroadenoma or RT were not included in the study population. Although the most important factor affecting TSH secretion in CS is considered to be hypercortisolism itself, various other factors associated with CS have been investigated as well, such as severe additional disease, goiter, and diabetes mellitus (10). Similarly in this study we observed an inverse relationship between cortisol levels and TSH levels which was compatible with many other studies (6,10-12). Furthermore, it is known that glucorticoid administration in healthy individuals also may cause dose-dependent TSH suppression (9). However, one study in the literature indicated that serum cortisol levels and TSH and fT4 levels did not show a significant correlation. That study indicated that TSH suppression in CS might be related to high cumulative cortisol levels and it is rather difficult to detect such an effect. The authors suggested that high ACTH levels in CD patients might have an effect on thyroid function tests independent of plasma cortisol levels. However, such a relationship was not proved in their study (7). Therefore, we also included an evaluation of the association between ACTH and TSH

Table 2. Comparison of ACTH-dependent and ACTH-independent Cushing's syndrome

	Group 1 (ACTH-dependent Cushing's syndrome) (n =20)	Group 2 (ACTH-independent Cushing's syndrome) (n = 15)	p
Age at diagnosis (years) Mean ± SD	33.8 ± 11.7 (17-61)	41.8 ± 9.6 (25-58)	**0.03**
Sex (F/M)	14/6	14/1	0.08
Duration of follow-up (months) Mean ± SD	63.7 ± 26.7 (25-114)	46.5 ± 23.8 (21-90)	0.06
Baseline cortisol levels (μg/dL) Mean ± SD	28.9 ± 9.6 (14.2-46)	22.8 ± 5.9 (13.3-32)	0.645
Baseline TSH levels (μU/mL) Mean ± SD	0.6 ± 0.6 (0.1-2.6)	1.2 ± 0.8 (0.2-2.9)	0.242
Frequency of baseline suppressed TSH levels [n, (%)]	10 (50)	3 (20)	0.069
Baseline FT4 levels (pmol/L) Mean ± SD	13.9 ± 2.8 (9.3-19.3)	13.6 ± 2.4 (10.3-19.7)	0.631
Patients with central hypothyroidism atinitial assessment (n; %)	5 (25)	4 (27)	0.912
Early postoperative cortisol levels (μg/dL) Mean ± SD	0.6 ± 0.4 (0.1-1.3)	0.8 ± 0.7 (0.1-1.9)	0.194
First visit (Mean ± SD)			
TSH levels (μU/mL)	2.1 ± 1.2 (0.5-4.7)	2.1 ± 1.3 (0.6-4.7)	0.950
FT4ˈ levels (pmol/L)	15.6 ± 2.2 (12.8-20.7)	16.5 ± 2.2 (13.4-19.5)	0.903
Second visit (Mean ± SD)			
TSH levels (μU/mL)	2.2 ± 1.1 (0.3-4)	2.7 ± 1.4 (0.8-4.8)	**0.035**
FT4 levels (pmol/L)	14.9 ± 1.6 (12.4-17.7)	15.1 ± 2.3 (12.5-18.6)	0.752
Third visit (Mean ± SD)			
TSH levels (μU/mL)	2.6 ± 1.4 (0.5-4.5)	2.8 ± 1.2 (0.8-4.8)	0.317
FT4 levels (pmol/L)	15.2 ± 1.1 (13.4-17.8)	15.2 ± 1.5 (12.5-18.1)	0.747
HPA axis recovery time (months) Mean ± SD	13.6 ± 5.1 (7-25)	19.6 ± 19.3 (7-60)	0.825
Fourth visit (Mean ± SD)			
TSH levels (μU/mL)	2.4 ± 1.2 (0.7-4.5)	2.7 ± 1.3 (0.8-4.8)	0.761
FT4 levels (pmol/L)	14.9 ± 1.7 (12.7-19.1)	15.3 ± 1.4 (13.5-17.1)	0.841
Fifth visit (Mean ± SD)			
Cortisol levels (μg/dL)	15.1 ± 2.9 (10.7-20)	15.7 ± 3.1 (10.7-21)	0.472
TSH levels (μU/mL)	1.9 ± 1.1 (0.5-4.5)	2.8 ± 1.2 (0.5-4.7)	0.458
FT4 levels (pmol/L)	16.1 ± 1.8 (13.2-20)	14.9 ± 1.5 (12.1-17.1)	0.554
Δ TSH levels° (μU/mL) Mean ± SD	1.3 ± 1.1 (0.2-3.4)	1.7 ± 0.9 (-0.1-3)	0.257

Bold values are statistically significant (p < 0.05), °Δ TSH: The change in TSH levels between baseline and the last visits. First visit: Between the 1st and the 3rd months; Second visit: On the 6th month; Third visit: On the 12th ; Fourth visit: At the time of HPA axis recovery; Fifth visit: Last visit of the follow-up period.

levels in our patients with ACTH-dependent CS, which has not been previously mentioned in the literature. However, we did not find any significant correlation between ACTH and TSH levels. A comparison between the isolated effects of local pituitary ACTH secretion and the ectopic secretion of ACTH would be possible only with the selective classification of two groups with either EAS or CD. However, due to

the low number of EAS patients, we were unable to design such a comparison in our study. Even though our study population included only microadenoma lesions, we also evaluated the mass effect of pituitary adenoma on TSH levels and found no significant correlation between adenoma size and TSH levels.

Lower plasma T4 levels due to supressed TSH levels may be expected in hypercortisolism. However, in our study we observed central hypothyroidism in only 26% of patients and normal plasma fT4 levels in most of the patients during hypercortisolism. Mathioudakis and cols. (7) reported an even lower prevalance of central hypothyroidism (18%). Relatively normal plasma fT4 levels in hypercortisolism may be explained with the increased biological activity of TSH through posttranslational processes (25). Although the baseline fT4 levels were lower than fT4 levels during the last visit; no statistically significant difference was found. Furthermore, the cortisol levels were similar in patients with or without central hypothyroidism, and also, no correlation was found between the baseline cortisol and fT4 levels. Thus, the presence of hypercortisolemia essentially affects plasma TSH levels, and as fluctuations in fT4 levels are independent of serum cortisol, predicting which patients will develop low fT4 levels or central hypothyoridism is difficult. The factors effective in this process may be related to the sensitivity of thyrotrop cells for TSH or the iodine status of the body. Even though the iodinization of household salt has been mandatory since 1999, a recent study demonstrated urinary iodine defficiency in the 23% of the adult population in our country (26). This may be the reason for the higher prevalence of central hypothyroidism in our study compared with Mathioudakis and cols. (7). Nevertheless, even patients with central hypothyroidism generally do not have clinically evident hypothyroidism. As the clinical presentation is silent and thyroid dysfunction is assumed to recover with the improvement of hypercortisolism, levothyroxine replacement in the preoperative period is not recommended (7,22). In the literature, only a few patients received levothyroxine replacement before surgery, all of whom presented with hypothyroidism as the first finding of CS (27,28). In our series levothyroxine replacement was not given to any of the patients.

Altough the effect of CS on thyroid function tests is widely studied, studies involving the long time clinical course of these patients after surgery are limited (6,7,10,19,20,29). It has been demonstrated that TSH and thyroid hormone levels start to recover in the first six months after surgery, and these changes may take place as early as two weeks, especially in the first month following surgery (7,10,20,30). In addition, in our series we observed the most significant increase in TSH levels in the first visit, with the levels gradually increasing until the 12th month of follow-up. Likewise,

Roelfsema and cols. (6) assessed TSH and thyroid functions for a mean of 6.8 years after surgery for CD and found increased basal TSH secretion compared with the control group.

To evaluate tyroid function changes according to the etiologies, we divided our patients into two groups: ACTH-dependent and ACTH-independent. No significant difference was found between the hormone levels at baseline and the clinical findings at the initial assessment. However the patients with ACTH-dependent CS were younger. The presence of central hpothyroidism and low fT4 levels are more frequently reported in CD (6,7). However, we found a similar frequency of central hypothyroidism in both groups. At the follow-up visits, the mean TSH levels were slightly higher in group 2 in the second visit, which we interpreted as an incidental finding. The results of our study showed that changes in thyroid function tests in CS are the result of hypercortisolism itself independent of the etiology of CS. No significant difference was found between the two groups in terms of cortisol levels during the baseline and follow-up visits. Bartalena and cols. (12) demonstrated similar results in thyroid function tests between ACTH-dependent or ACTH-independent groups.

Even though CS and TSH supression have been well known for a long time, hyperthyroidism due to TSH secretion after surgery for CS was recently defined in the literature. This situation is described as a novel cause of SITSH (19). A TSH-secreting pituitary adenoma and resistance to the thyroid hormone are the primary causes of SITSH (31). First, Tamada and cols. (19) reported two patients who presented with SITSH caused by a decrease in the hydrocortisone replacement dose after surgery for CS. Especially the rapid decreases in the hydrocortisone replacement doses in the early postoperative period were held responsible for this process. The study also discussed that sypmtoms of hyperthyroidism due to SITSH might have overlapped with symptoms of SWS. Because of this knowledge in literature, we evaluated the prednisolone replacement doses of all patients during each visit and did not detect the presence of SITSH. This may be explained with the higher glucocorticoid replacement doses in our study compared with the series in Tamada and cols. (19). In that study, hyperthyroidism was especially detected in the first month of follow-up when the daily hydrocortisone replacement doses were ≤ 20 mg. In our study patients received a mean of 7.3 mg/day of prednisolone replacement during the first visit. In light of these findings we suspect that a relationship might exist between glucocorticoid replacement doses and plasma TSH and fT4 level, a subject on which we could not find any comments in the current literature. However we could not demonstrate a significant correlation between the prednisolone replacement and the concurrent plasma TSH and fT4 levels until HPA axis recovery in the postoperative period. Our comment regarding this is that the mechanisms leading to SITSH may not be triggered as long as the glucocorticoid replacement doses are sufficient. Tamada and cols. also reported that hypocortisolemia was responsible for the onset of the syndrome (19). Because hypocortisolemia leads to decreased type 2 deiodinase activity resulting with declining in the local hypotalamo-pituitary T3 levels, the TSH levels are elevated independent of the peripheral thyroid hormone status (18-20). However this theory is not the only explanation because presence of hyperthyroidism would then be expected in all hypocortisolemic patients. Although baseline TSH levels are elevated in patients with adrenal defficiency, hyperthyroidism is not defined in these patients (32). Our explanation is that in patients with CS plasma deiodinase activity which is sensitive to local T3 levels develops new set-points in the active hypercortisolemic period of CS, and a certain amount of time is needed for the recovery of the initial set points. Glucocorticoid replacement should be decreased gradually until the initial set points are recovered as Tamada and cols. (20) demonstrated in another prospective study that hyperthyroidism due to SITSH was also triggered by SWS after the treatment of CS. Thus, gradual reductions in steroid replacement doses are important in the prevention of both SWS and hyperthyroidism due to SITSH.

In conclusion, plasma TSH or T4 levels may be affected in CS independent of etiology. The primary cause of this finding is hypercortisolism itself. However, the particular mechanism of these processes is not clear and needs to be further evaluated. Furthermore, central hypothyroidism may be detected in these patients. Treatment recommendations need to be evaluated individually for each patient. In contrast to the general belief that TSH levels are initially suppressed in CS, which eventually recover after CS treatment and that the follow-up of thyroid function tests is not mandatory, we suggest that patients should be monitored in the postoperative period especially

concerning hyperthyroidism due to SITSH. To prevent such an effect, we suggest avoiding rapid decreases in glucocorticoid replacement doses especially in the early postoperative period. The recovery of the HPT axis which was affected from glucocorticoid excess, may require some time, just as a certain period of time is necessary for the recovery HPA axis.

Ethical approval: for this type of study formal consent is not required.

Funding: there was no funding received for this study.

REFERENCES

1. Mariotti S. Normal physiology of the hypothalamo-pituitary-thyroidal system and relation to the neural system and other endocrine gland. 2006. Chapter 4 in Thyroid Disease Manager.

2. Duick DS, Wahner HW. Thyroid axis in patients with Cushing's syndrome. Arch Intern Med. 1979;139(7):767-72.

3. Nicoloff JT, Fisher DA, Appleman MD Jr. The role of glucocorticoids in the regulation of thyroid function in man. J Clin Invest. 1970;49(10):1922-9.

4. Samuels MH, McDaniel PA. Thyrotropin levels during hydrocortisone infusions that mimic fasting-induced cortisol elevations: a clinical research center study. J Clin Endocrinol Metab. 1997;82(11):3700-4.

5. Adriaanse R, Brabant G, Endert E, Wiersinga WM. Pulsatile thyrotropin secretion in patients with Cushing's syndrome. Metabolism 1994; 43(6):782-6.

6. Roelfsema F, Pereira AM, Biermasz NR, Frolich M, Keenan DM, Veldhuis JD et al. Diminished and irregular TSH secretion with delayed acrophase in patients with Cushing's syndrome. Eur J Endocrinol 2009; 161:695-703.

7. Mathioudakis N, Thapa S, Wand GS, Salvatori R. ACTH-secreting pituitary microadenomas are associated with a higher prevalence of central hypothyroidism compared to other microadenoma types. Clin Endocrinol (Oxf). 2012;77(6):871-6.

8. Samuels MH, Luther M, Henry P, Ridgway EC. Effects of hydrocortisone on pulsatile pituitary glycoprotein secretion. J Clin Endocrinol Metab. 1994;78(1):211-5.

9. Brabant A, Brabant G, Schuermeyer T, Ranft U, Schmidt FW, Hesch RD, et al. The role of glucocorticoids in the regulation of thyrotropin. Acta Endocrinol (Copenh). 1989;121(1):95-100.

10. Benker G, Raida M, Olbricht T, Wagner R, Reinhardt W, Reinwein D. TSH secretion in Cushing's syndrome: relation to glucocorticoid excess, diabetes, goitre, and the 'sick euthyroid syndrome'. Clin Endocrinol (Oxf). 1990;33(6):777-86.

11. Visser TJ, Lamberts SW. Regulation of TSH secretion and thyroid function in Cushing's disease. Acta Endocrinol (Copenh). 1981;96(4):480-3.

12. Bartalena L, Martino E, Petrini L, Velluzzi F, Loviselli A, Grasso L, et al. The nocturnal serum thyrotropin surge is abolished in patients with adrenocorticotropin (ACTH)-dependent or ACTH-independent Cushing's syndrome. J Clin Endocrinol Metab. 1991;72(6):1195-9.

13. Alkemade A, Unmehopa UA, Wiersinga WM, Swaab DF, Fliers E. Glucocorticoids decrease thyrotropin-releasing hormone messenger ribonucleic acid expression in the paraventricular nucleus of the human hypothalamus. J Clin Endocrinol Metab. 2005;90(1):323-7.

14. Saane LM, Carro E, Tovar S, Casanueva FF, Dieguez C. Regulation of in vivo TSH secretion by leptin. Regul Pept. 2000;92:25-9.

15. Lewis BM, Dieguez C, Lewis MD, Scanlon MF. Dopamine stimulates release of thyrotrophin-releasing hormone from perfused intact rat hypothalamus via hypothalamic D2-receptors. J Endocrinol. 1987;115:419-24.

16. Taylor AD, Flower RJ, Buckingham JC. Dexamethasone inhibits the release of TSH from the rat anterior pituitary gland in vitro mechanisms dependent on de novo protein synthesis and lipocortin 1. J Endocrinol. 1995;147:533-44.

17. Estupina C, Belmar J, Tapia-Arancibia L, Astier H, Arancidia S. Rapid and opposite effects of dexamethasone on in vivo and in vitro hypothalamic somatostatin release. Exp Brain Res. 1997;113:337-42.

18. St Germain DL, Galton VA, Hernandez A. Minireview: defining the roles of the iodothyronine deiodinase: current concepts and challenges. Endocrinology. 2009;150:1097-107.

19. Tamada D, Onodera T, Kitamura T, Yamamoto Y, Hayashi Y, Murata Y, et al. Hyperthyroidism due to thyroid-stimulating hormone secretion after surgery for Cushing's syndrome: a novel cause of the syndrome of inappropriate secretion of thyroid-stimulating hormone. J Clin Endocrinol Metab. 2013;98(7):2656-62.

20. Tamada D, Kitamura T, Onodera T, Hamasaki T, Otsuki M, Shimomura I. Clinical significance of fluctuations in thyroid hormones after surgery for Cushing's syndrome. Endocr J. 2015;62(9):805-10.

21. Nieman LK, Biller BM, Findling JW, Newell-Price J, Savage MO, Stewart PM, et al. The diagnosis of Cushing's syndrome: An Endocrine Society Clinical Practice Guideline. J Clin Endocrinol Metab. 2008;93(5):1526-40.

22. Nieman LK, Biller BM, Findling JW, Murad MH, Newell-Price J, Savage MO, et al. Endocrine Society. Treatment of Cushing's Syndrome: An Endcorine Society Clinical Practice Guideline. J Clin Endocrinol Metab. 2015;100(8):2807-31.

23. Chopra IJ, Williams DE, Orgiazzi J, Solomon DH. Opposite effects of dexamethasone on serum concentrations of 3,3',5'-triiodothyronine (reverse T3) and 3,3'5-triiodothyronine (T3). J Clin Endocrinol Metab. 1975;41(5):911-20.

24. Bahn RS, Burch HB, Cooper DS, Garber JR, Greenlee MC, Klein I, et al. American Thyroid Association; American Association of Clinical Endocrinologists. Hyperthyroidism and other causes of thyrotoxicosis: management guidelines of the American Thyroid Association and American Association of Clinical Endocrinologists. Endocr Pract. 2011;17(3):456-520.

25. Persani L. Hypothalamic thyrotropin-releasing hormone and thyrotropin biological activity. Thyroid. 1998;8:941-6.

26. Idiz C, Kucukgergin C, Yalin GY, Onal E, Yarman S. Iodine Status of Pregnant Women in the Apparently Iodine-Sufficient in Istanbul Province: At Least Thirteen Years After Iodization of Table Salt Became Mandatory. Acta Endocrinol (Buc). 2015;11(3):407-12.

27. Katahira M, Yamada T, Kawai M. A case of cushing syndrome with both secondary hypothyroidism and hypercalcemia due to postoperative adrenal insufficiency. Endocr J. 2004;51(1):105-13.

28. Hara Y, Sekiya M, Suzuki M, Hiwada K, Kato I, Kokubu T. A case of isolated thyrotropin deficiency with Cushing's syndrome. Jpn J Med. 1989;28(6):727-30.

29. Hashimoto K. The pituitary ACTH, GH, LH, FSH, TSH and prolactin reserves in patients with Cushing's syndrome. Endocrinol Jpn. 1975;22(1):67-77.

30. Stratakis CA, Mastorakos G, Magiakou MA, Papavasiliou E, Oldfield EH, Chrousos GP. Thyroid function in children with Cushing's disease before and after transsphenoidal surgery. J Pediatr. 1997;131(6):905-9.

31. Weintraub BD, Gershengorn MC, Kourides IA, Fein H. Inappropriate secretion of thyroid-stimulating hormone. Ann Intern Med. 1981;95:339-51.

32. Samuels MH. Effects of Variations in Physiological Cortisol Levels on Thyrotropin Secretion in Subjects with Adrenal Insufficiency: A Clinical Research Center Study. J Clin Endocrinol Metab. 2000;85(4):1388-93.

14

Metabolic syndrome components are associated with oxidative stress in overweight and obese patients

Nayara Rampazzo Morelli[1], Bruna Miglioranza Scavuzzi[1],
Lucia Helena da Silva Miglioranza[2], Marcell Alysson Batisti Lozovoy[3],
Andréa Name Colado Simão[3], Isaias Dichi[4]

ABSTRACT

Objective: The aim of this study is to evaluate the influence of the body mass index (BMI) and the metabolic syndrome (MetS) parameters on oxidative and nitrosative stress in overweight and obese subjects. **Subjects and methods:** Individuals were divided into three groups: the control group (G1, n = 131) with a BMI between 20 and 24.9 kg/m², the overweight group (G2, n = 120) with a BMI between 25 and 29.9 kg/m² and the obese group (G3, n = 79) with a BMI ≥ 30 kg/m². **Results:** G3 presented higher advanced oxidation protein products (AOPPs) in relation to G1 and G2 (p = 0.001 and p = 0.011, respectively) whereas G2 and G3 had lower levels of nitric oxide (NO) (p = 0.009 and p = 0.048, respectively) compared to G1. Adjusted for the presence of MetS to evaluate its influence, the levels of AOPPs did not differ between the groups, whereas NO remained significantly lower. Data adjusted by the BMI showed that subjects with higher triacylglycerol levels had higher AOPPs (p = 0.001) and decreased total radical-trapping antioxidant parameter/uric Acid (p = 0.036). Subjects with lower high-density lipoprotein (HDL) levels and patients with higher blood pressure showed increased AOPPs (p = 0.001 and p = 0.034, respectively) and lower NO levels (p = 0.017 and p = 0.043, respectively). Subjects who presented insulin resistance had higher AOPPs (p = 0.024). **Conclusions:** Nitrosative stress was related to BMI, and protein oxidation and nitrosative stress were related to metabolic changes and hypertension. MetS components were essential participants in oxidative and nitrosative stress in overweight and obese subjects. Arch Endocrinol Metab. 2018;62(3):309-18

Keywords
Overweight; obesity; metabolic syndrome; oxidative stress; nitrosative stress

[1] Departamento de Pós-Graduação em Ciências da Saúde, Universidade Estadual de Londrina (UEL), Londrina, PR, Brasil
[2] Departamento de Ciência e Tecnologia de Alimentos, Universidade Estadual de Londrina (UEL), Londrina, PR, Brasil
[3] Departamento de Patologia, Análises Clínicas e Toxicológicas, Universidade Estadual de Londrina (UEL), Londrina, PR, Brasil
[4] Departamento de Medicina Interna, Universidade Estadual de Londrina (UEL), Londrina, PR, Brasil

Correspondence to:
Isaias Dichi
Departamento de Medicina Interna,
Universidade Estadual de Londrina
Av. Robert Koch, 60
86038-440 – Londrina, PR, Brasil
dichi@sercomtel.com.br

INTRODUCTION

Obesity and overweight are chronic disorders of multifactorial origin, which can be defined as an increase in the accumulation of body fat (1). Changes in lifestyle and diet have resulted in an increased number of overweight and obese subjects in developed and developing countries (2). This trend has been verified in practically all ages, genders and ethnicities (2). Therefore, overweight and obesity have emerged as two of the largest public health problems worldwide. Excess body weight is associated with an increased risk of developing metabolic syndrome (MetS). MetS is a complex disorder that is represented by a cluster of cardiovascular risk factors that are associated with central fat deposition, abnormal plasma lipid levels, elevated blood pressure, insulin resistance and a low-grade inflammatory state. MetS has also been associated with increased oxidative and nitrosative stress (3).

The harmful effects of free radicals, which are mainly represented by reactive oxygen species (ROS) or reactive nitrogen species, have been implicated in the physiopathology of overweight, obesity, hypertension, endothelial dysfunction, and MetS (4,5), suggesting that oxidative stress can be the underlying mechanism of this dysfunctional metabolic picture in obese subjects (6). In addition, high ROS production and the decrease in antioxidant capacity leads to various abnormalities. These abnormalities include endothelial dysfunction – which is characterized by a reduction in the bioavailability of vasodilators, particularly nitric oxide (NO) (7), and an increase in endothelium-derived contractile factors, favoring atherosclerotic disease (1).

Although markers of oxidative stress have been studied in obese and overweight patients with and without MetS, we are not aware to date of studies evaluating the influence of body weight on oxo-nitrosative stress in the other components of MetS.

In a previous study performed by our group, we verified that an increase in oxidative stress is mostly attributable to obesity in patients with MetS (8), but this is not the case in overweight subjects without MetS. It is therefore unclear whether metabolic changes of obesity, referred to as metabolic obesity, are independent risk factors for increased oxo-nitrosative stress than the other components of MetS. In order to extend the data of the mentioned study, the objective of the present study was to evaluate the influence of the body mass index (BMI) on oxidative and nitrosative stress in overweight and obese subjects and to verify whether the presence of the components of MetS would modify the results.

SUBJECTS AND MATERIALS

Subjects

Patients from the Internal Medicine Ambulatory of the University Hospital of Londrina, Paraná, Brazil were chosen to participate in this cross-sectional study. Three hundred and thirty patients agreed to participate in the study. Inclusion criteria were patients (both genders) aged from 18 to 65 years. Exclusion criteria were thyroid, renal, hepatic, gastrointestinal, infectious or oncological diseases and the use of lipid-lowering drugs, drugs for hyperglycemia, anti-inflammatory drugs, hormone replacement therapy, and antioxidant supplements. For ethical reasons, patients who were taking antihypertensive drugs were not excluded and were allowed to continue taking the same dose of the drugs.

The patients were divided into three groups: the control group included 131 subjects with a BMI between 20 and 24.9 kg/m². The overweight group consisted of 120 subjects with a BMI between 25 and 29.9 kg/m², and the group with obesity consisted of 79 subjects with a BMI ≥ 30. MetS was defined following the Adult Treatment Panel III criteria. A diagnosis of MetS was arrived at for subjects with at least three of the following five characteristics: (1) abdominal obesity, which was defined as a waist circumference (WC) ≥ 102 cm in men and ≥ 88 cm in women; (2)

hypertriglyceridemia, which was defined as triglycerides ≥ 150 mg/dL; (3) low levels of high-density lipoprotein (HDL) cholesterol, which was defined as HDL ≤ 40 mg/dL in men and ≤ 50 mg/dL in women; (4) high blood pressure, which was defined as blood pressure ≥ 130/85 mmHg; and (5) high-fasting glucose, which was defined as glucose ≥ 100 mg/dL.

Ethics, consent, health and safety

The research was conducted in an ethical and responsible manner and is in full compliance with all relevant codes of experimentation. In addition, the Ethical Committee of the University of Londrina – Paraná, Brazil – approved all procedures involving human participants (185/2013). This clinical investigation was conducted according to the principles expressed in the Declaration of Helsinki.

Written informed consent was obtained from all the participants, who acknowledged that they cannot be identified via the paper and that they are fully anonymized.

All mandatory laboratory health and safety procedures have been complied.

Anthropometric and blood pressure measurements

Anthropometric measurements and laboratorial parameters were assessed. Body weight was measured to the nearest 0.1 kg in the morning through the use of an electronic scale, with individuals wearing light clothing and no shoes; height was measured to the nearest 0.1 cm through the use of a stadiometer. BMI was calculated as weight (kg) divided by height (m) squared. WC was measured on standing subjects midway between the lowest rib and the iliac crest. Three blood pressure measurements taken with a 1-min interval after the participant had been seated were recorded on the left arm. The mean of these measurements was used in the analysis. We considered the current use of antihypertensive medication as an indication of high blood pressure.

Biochemical, immunological, and hematological biomarkers

After fasting for 12 hours, the subjects underwent the following laboratory blood analysis evaluated through a biochemical auto-analyzer (Dimension Dade AR Dade Behring, Deerfield, IL, USA) using Dade Behring® kits: total cholesterol, HDL, low-density lipoprotein (LDL), triacylglycerol (TG), glucose and uric acid (UA). Plasma insulin level was determined by chemiluminescence microparticule immunoassay (Architect, Abbott Laboratory, Abbott Park, IL, USA). The homeostasis model assessment insulin resistance (HOMA-IR) was used as a surrogate measurement of insulin sensitivity. HOMA-IR = fasting insulin (U/ml) x fasting glucose (mmol/L)/22.5. IR was considered when HOMA-IR $\geq$ 2.5 (9).

Oxidative and nitrosative stress measurements

Samples for evaluating oxidative stress and total antioxidant capacity were analyzed with ethylenediamine tetraacetic acid as an anticoagulant and antioxidant. All samples were centrifuged at 3,000 rpm for 15 minutes, and plasma aliquots were stored at -70°C until assayed. All stress measurements were performed in triplicate.

Tert-butyl hydroperoxide-initiated chemiluminescence (CL-LOOH)

CL-LOOH in plasma was evaluated as described previously by Gonzales Flecha and cols. (10). CL-LOOH is considered to be much more sensitive and specific than the thiobarbituric acid reactive substances method, the usual method to determine lipid oxidation. For the CL measurement, reaction mixtures were placed in 20-mL scintillation vials (low-potassium glass) containing final concentrations of plasma (250 uL), 30 mM KH_2PO_4/K_2HPO_4 buffer (pH 7.4), and 120 mM KCl with 3 mM of LOOH in a final volume of 2 mL. CL-LOOH was measured in a Beckman LS 6000 liquid scintillation counter set to the out-of-coincidence mode, with a response of 300 to 620 nm. The vials were kept in the dark until the moment of assay, and determination was carried out in a dark room at 30°C. The results were expressed in counts per minute.

Determination of advanced oxidation protein products (AOPPs)

AOPPs were determined in the plasma using the semi-automated method described by Witko-Sarsat and cols. (11). AOPP concentrations were expressed as micromoles per liter (μmol/L) of chloramines-T equivalents.

Total radical-trapping antioxidant parameter (TRAP)

TRAP was determined as reported by Repetto and cols. (12). This method detects hydrosoluble and liposoluble plasma antioxidants by measuring the chemiluminescence inhibition time induced by 2,2-azobis (2-amidinopropane). The system was calibrated with the vitamin E analog TROLOX, and the values of TRAP were expressed in the equivalent of μM Trolox/mg UA. TRAP measurements in conditions associated with hyperuricemia, such as MetS, may be inaccurate because the UA concentration accounts for 60% of the total plasma antioxidant capacity. Some reports have verified an unexpected increase in TRAP in MetS subjects (13). Thus, a correction of TRAP based on UA concentration was performed (13).

Determination of sulfhydryl (SH) groups of proteins

SH groups of proteins were evaluated in plasma samples through a spectrophotometric assay based on 2,2-dithiobisnitrobenzoic acid (DTNB), as reported previously (14), and the results are expressed in μM.

Evaluation of nitric oxide metabolites (NOx)

The NO concentration in a sample was estimated by measuring the NOx in nitrites ($NO2^-$) and nitrates ($NO3^-$) using cadmium beads for the reduction of nitrate to nitrite. The concentrations of these metabolites were later determined according to the method proposed by Griess (15). The values were expressed in μM.

Statistical analysis

Categorical data were analyzed through a chi-squared test or, when appropriate, through Fisher's exact test, and data were expressed in absolute values. The Kolmogorov-Smirnov test was used to assess the normality of distribution. All continuous variables presented non-parametric distribution, even after logarithmic transformation. The comparisons of the three groups categorized by BMI were performed through the use of the non-parametric Kruskal-Wallis test with the *post-hoc* Dunn test. The variables that presented significance in the univariate analysis of variance were included in the multinomial logistic regression to verify which oxidative stress parameters were associated with BMI. The Mann-Whitney test was used to compare two groups, and a logistic binary regression analysis was performed to adjust for age, sex, ethnicity and BMI. The results were considered significant when $P < 0.05$. A statistical analysis program, SPSS version 20.0, was used for evaluations.

RESULTS

There was no statistically significant difference in ethnicity between the three groups (Table 1). Overweight (G2) and obese subjects (G3) did not differ regarding sex and age. However, the control group (G1) had a higher frequency of women compared to the subjects in G2 ($p < 0.0001$) and G3 ($p < 0.05$), and they were younger ($p < 0.0001$) than those in the G2 and G3 groups. The presence of MetS was higher ($p < 0.0001$) in G3 compared to G1 and G2 and in G2 compared to G1 (Table 1 and Figure 1). G3 presented higher WC ($p < 0.0001$, $p < 0.0001$), glucose ($p < 0.0001$, $p < 0.05$), insulin ($p < 0.001$, $p < 0.001$), HOMA-IR ($p < 0.001$, $p < 0.001$), and TG ($p < 0.001$, $p < 0.01$) and decreased HDL–cholesterol ($p < 0.001$, $p < 0.05$) levels compared to G1 and G2, respectively (Table 1). Meanwhile, G2 had higher WC ($p < 0.0001$), glucose ($p < 0.001$), insulin, HOMA-IR, and TG and decreased ($p < 0.001$) HDL-cholesterol levels compared to G1. G2 and G3 showed higher total cholesterol ($p < 0.05$) and LDL cholesterol ($p < 0.01$) levels compared to those of G1 (Table 1).

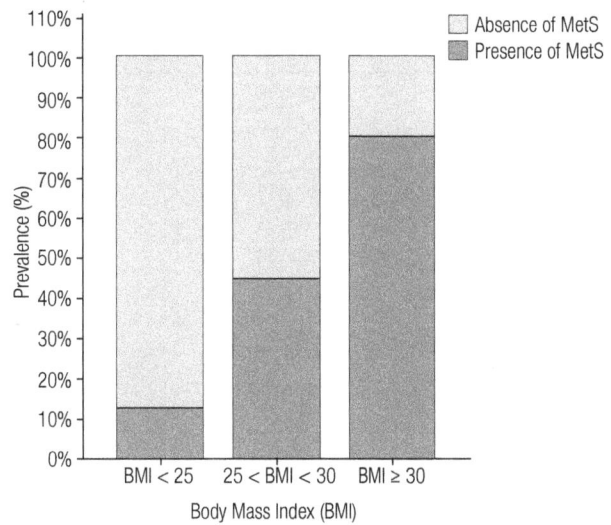

Figure 1. Prevalence of the metabolic syndrome across body mass index categories. Normal weight, < 25 kg/m^2; overweight, 25-30 kg/m^2; and obese, ≥ 30 kg/m^2.

Table 2 shows the results of oxidative stress in the three studied groups with p values adjusted for sex and age. G3 presented higher AOPP values in relation to

Table 1. Clinical and laboratory characteristics of controls (G1), overweight (G2) and obese subjects (G3)

	G1 (n = 131)	G2 (n = 120)	G3 (n = 79)	G1 X G2	G1 X G3	G2 X G3
Gender (% men)	18	43	32	**< 0.0001**	**< 0.05**	0.1231
Ethnicity (% caucasians)	80	78	82	0.8420	0.8525	0.6180
MetS (Y/N)	12/119	65/55	72/7	**< 0.0001**	**< 0.0001**	**< 0.0001**
Age	32.0 (25.0-43.0)	43.0 (34.5-53.0)	43.0 (34.0-50.0)	**< 0.001**	**< 0.001**	NS
BMI (kg/m^2)	22.04 (20.90-23.57)	27.12 (25.98-28.33)	32.25 (31.04-34.99)	**<0.001**	**< 0.001**	**< 0.001**
WC (cm)	82.0 (77.0-88.0)	97.0 (91.0-101.0)	108.0 (103.0-115.0)	**< 0.0001**	**< 0.0001**	**< 0.0001**
Fating glucose (mg/dL)	86.0 (83.0-92.0)	92.0 (85.0-98.0)	98.0 (88.0-107.0)	**< 0.001**	**< 0.001**	**< 0.05**
Insulin (U/mL)	6.4 (4.65-8.80)	8.10 (5.90-12.90)	14.5 (10.9-17.4)	**< 0.001**	**< 0.001**	**< 0.001**
HOMA-IR	1.338 (1,020-1,940)	1.989 (1.285-3.238)	3.234 (2.696-4.781)	**< 0.001**	**< 0.001**	**< 0.001**
Total cholesterol (mg/dL)	186.0 (152.5-209,0)	197.0 (168.0-226.0)	198.0 (180.0-224.0)	**< 0.050**	**< 0.010**	NS
HDL-cholesterol (mg/dL)	56.5 (48.5-67.0)	46.5 (38.0-59.5)	42.0 (37.0-51.0)	**< 0.001**	**< 0.001**	**< 0.05**
LDL-cholesterol (mg/dL)	109.8 (83.8-130.2)	121.0 (95.2-141.1)	125.3 (100.5-142.0)	**< 0.050**	**< 0.010**	NS
Triacylglycerol (mg/dL)	74.5 (48.5-107.5)	124.0 (90.0-183.0)	175.0 (127.0-231.0)	**< 0.001**	**< 0.001**	**< 0.01**

MetS: metabolic syndrome; BMI: body mass index; WC: waist circumference; IR: insulin resistance; HOMA: homeostasis model assessment; HDL: high-density lipoprotein; LDL: low-density lipoprotein; NS: nonsignificant; WC: waist circumference.

Table 2. Oxidative stress evaluation in controls (G1), overweight (G2) and obese subjects (G3)

	G1 (n = 131)	G2 (n = 120)	G3 (n = 79)	G1 X G2*	G1 X G3*	G2 X G3*
Hydroperoxides (cpm)	13900 (10740-17010)	14120 (10950-17350)	13540 (10250-16260)	NS	NS	NS
AOPP (µmol/L)	127.2 (98.2-174.4)	159.5 (124.7-230.3)	195.2 (157.3.257.1)	NS	**0.001**	**0.011**
NO (µM)	25.67 (13.67-40.45)	13.83 (8.17-42.84)	12.10 (7.96-27.63)	**0.009**	**0.048**	NS
TRAP/UA (µM Trolox/mg/dL)	177.1 (147.2-207.5)	158.8 (126.9-190.0)	138.0 (115.3-164.9)	NS	NS	NS

AOPP: advanced oxidation protein products; NO: nitric oxide; TRAP: total radical-trapping antioxidant parameter; UA: uric acid; NS: nonsignificant.

* Adjusted p value for sex and age. AOPP was not significant after adjusting for the presence of MetS, whereas NO maintained its significance.

Table 3. Stepway analysis for oxidative stress evaluation in controls (G1), overweight (G2) and obese subjects (G3) BMI

Parameters		Wald	p*	Odds-Ratio	Confidence interval
Gender	G1 x G2	14.294	**< 0.0001**	3.635	1.862 – 7.098
	G1 x G3	0.944	0.331	1.501	0.662 – 3.404
	G2 x G3	6.174	**0.013**	2.422	1.205 – 4.868
Age	G1 x G2	20.998	**< 0.0001**	1.067	1.038 – 1.097
	G1 x G3	5.46	**0.019**	1.040	1.006 – 1.074
	G2 x G3	3.211	0.073	1.026	0.998 – 1.056
MetS	G1 x G2	13.538	**< 0.0001**	4.308	1.979 – 9.378
	G1 x G3	53.367	**< 0.0001**	29.759	11.974 – 73.956
	G2 x G3	21.823	**< 0.0001**	0.145	0.064 – 0.326
AOPP	G1 x G2	0.080	0.777	0.999	0.995 – 1.004
	G1 x G3	0.102	0.750	1.001	0.996 – 1.005
	G2 x G3	0.491	0.483	0.999	0.995 – 1.002
NO	G1 x G2	7.377	**0.007**	1.018	1.005 – 1.031
	G1 x G3	3.440	0.064	1.016	0.99 – 1.032
	G2 x G3	0.065	0.799	1.002	0.987 – 1.017

MetS: metabolic syndrome; AOPP: advanced oxidation protein products; NO: nitric oxide. * Adjusted p value for sex, age and presence of MetS.
AOPP was not significant after adjusting for sex and age, whereas NO maintained its significance when comparing controls and overweight subjects.

G1 and G2 (p = 0.001 and p = 0.011, respectively), whereas significantly lower NOx values were found in G2 and G3 when compared to those of G1 (p = 0.009 and p = 0.048, respectively). The groups were then adjusted for the presence of MetS to evaluate its influence on the results. In this new analysis, AOPPs did not differ between the groups, whereas significant lower NO maintained its significance. Lipid hydroperoxides and TRAP/UA did not have any significant change in the groups. Table 3 shows the results obtained after performing multiple regressive stepwise analyses to clarify the importance of body weight on oxidative and nitrosative stress; AOPPs were not significant after adjusting for sex, age and the presence of MetS when comparing controls and overweight, controls and obese and overweight and obese (0.777; 0.750; 0.483, respectively). NO maintained its significance when comparing controls and overweight subjects (0.007; 0.064; 0.799, respectively).

To verify the association between oxidative stress biomarkers and the presence of MetS, a binary logistic regression was performed and was adjusted for sex and age. The AOPP levels were directly associated with the presence of MetS (Wald = 16.039, df = 1, OR = 1.009, 95% CI = 1.005-1.009, p < 0.0001), and the NO values were inversely associated (Wald = 18.941, df = 1, OR = 0.958, 95% CI = 0.940-0.977, p < 0.0001) with the presence of MetS (data not shown).

The association between the oxidative stress parameters and the individual components of MetS was measured, and the values were adjusted by BMI, sex, age

and ethnicity; the results are shown in Table 4. Subjects with higher TG levels had higher AOPPs (p = 0.001) and decreased TRAP/UA levels (p = 0.036) compared to individuals without hypertriacylglycerolemia. Subjects with lower HDL cholesterol and patients with higher blood pressure levels showed increased AOPPs (p = 0.001 and p = 0.034, respectively) and lower NO levels (p = 0.017 and p = 0.043, respectively) compared to individuals without low HDL-cholesterol levels and with normal blood pressure. Subjects who presented insulin resistance had higher AOPP levels (p = 0.024) compared to those without insulin resistance.

Multiple regressive stepwise analyses were performed (Table 5). After adjusting for sex, age and the presence of MetS, AOPPs maintained their significance for TG, HDL, blood pressure and HOMA-IR (< 0.0001, < 0.0001, 0.017, and 0.024, respectively); NO maintained its significance for HDL (0.025), and TRAP maintained its significance for TG (0.034).

DISCUSSION

The redox state was similar in healthy, overweight and obese subjects when controlled for the presence of MetS, and therefore, the principal finding of the present study was that oxidative stress evaluated through lipid and protein oxidation in patients with obesity is mainly related to the presence of MetS and is less related to BMI. However, nitrosative stress with decreased NO bioavailability was associated with BMI, independently of the presence of MetS. In addition,

Table 4. Oxidative stress evaluation according to the components of the metabolic syndrome

	Gender (%men)	Ethnicity (% cauc)	Age	BMI (Kg/m²)	LOOH (cpm)	AOPP (µmol/L)	NO (µM)	TRAP/UA (µM Trolox/mg/dL)
TG < 150 mg/dL n = 218	22	81	36.0 (28.0-47.0)	24.42 (21.74-27.68)	14120 (10900-17730)	134.2 (101.2-174.7)	23.72 (12.29-42.84)	170.7 (138.4-204.1)
TG ≥ 150 mg/dL n = 108	46	78	46.0 (37.0-53.0)	29.75 (26.63-32.10)	13570 (8549-18750)	225.1 (160.1-275-89)	11.19 (6.60-27.63)	137.8 (118.0-173.0)
p	< 0.001	0.6321	< 0.0001	< 0.0001	NS	< 0.0001	< 0.0001	< 0.0001
* Adjusted p	----	----	----	----	NS	**0.001**	NS	**0.036**
Normal HDL n = 186	26	80	38.5 (30.0-47.0)	24.36 (21.91-28.04)	14290 (10800-18110)	136.8 (102.9-181.2)	25.78 (12.38-43.93)	163.9 (138.0-205.1)
Reduced HDL n = 137	35	80	42.0 (30.5-50.0)	27.99 (25.44-31.60)	13650 (11480-16720)	183.8 (131.4-256.5)	12.37 (7.53-29.91)	149.6 (122.4-186.3)
p	NS	NS	NS	< 0.0001	NS	< 0.0001	< 0.0001	0.0011
* Adjusted p	----	----	----	----	----	**0.001**	**0.017**	NS
Normotensive n = 217	27	80	35.0 (27.0-44.0)	24.80 (21.83-28.04)	13750 (11130-17650)	134.4 (100.4-183.8)	22.84 (11.90-40.23)	166.3 (137.8-200.9)
Hypertensive n = 112	36	79	47.0 (39.0-55.0)	28.60 (26.17-31.70)	14550 (10010-18190)	195.7 (154.3-274.2)	11.95 (6.80-33.73)	145.7 (119.5-184.8)
p	0.1414	0.9926	< 0.0001	< 0.0001	0.7971	< 0.0001	0.0010	0.0010
* Adjusted p	----	----	----	----	NS	**0.034**	**0.043**	NS
Without IR n = 163	7	23	38 (29.0-47.0)	24.22 (21.76-26.67)	14200 (11070-17890)	137.4 (104.0-184.9)	23.5 (11.91-41.00)	169.6 (138.0-203.2)
With IR n = 115	36	22	42 (30.0-53.0)	30.05 (27.21-32.92)	13550 (9291-16690)	182 (127.9-256.5)	11.78 (7.07-27.74)	146.3 (116.3-179.6)
p	0.0781	NS	0.023	< 0.0001	NS	< 0.0001	< 0.0001	< 0.0001
* Adjusted p	----	----	----	----	----	**0.024**	NS	NS

Cauc: Caucasian; BMI: body mass index; IR: insulin resistance; LOOH: hydroperoxides; AOPP: advanced oxidation protein products; NO: nitric oxide; TRAP: total radical-trapping antioxidant parameter; UA: uric acid; TG: tryacylglycerols; NS: nonsignificant.
* Binary logistic regression adjusted for sex, age, ethnicity and BMI.

this study verified that protein oxidation was associated with several individual components of MetS, including insulin resistance.

The present data are partially in agreement with our previous study, which showed that increases in oxidative stress markers in overweight subjects were only verified in the presence of MetS (8). However, in that study, obese subjects and nitrosative stress were not evaluated, which differs from the conditions of the present study. Thus, the impact of this original work lays in the observation that only nitrosative stress was related to BMI, whereas protein oxidation was related to each component of MetS.

Although an increase in oxidative stress in patients with obesity is an undisputed issue and can be caused by several factors (16), the present study is in line with others, which pointed out the utmost importance of the presence of MetS to reinforce this association. Skalicky and cols. (17) verified in obese subjects and Krzystek-

Korpacka and cols. (18) verified in overweight and obese adolescents that oxidative stress seemed to be increased through a combination of risk factors associated with MetS rather than by obesity per se. Fujita and cols. (19) demonstrated that values of oxidative stress increased with the number of components of MetS. Taken together, these data suggest that – although weight gain or visceral fat may contribute, to some extent, to an increase in oxidative stress – the presence of MetS is fundamental in showing ROS augmentation in overweight and obese subjects.

Our data are also in accordance with that of previous studies, which showed that hypertriacylglycerolemia, hypertension, lower HDL cholesterol values and insulin resistance are essential factors in provoking oxidative stress (13,19,20). Obesity and IR are considered key factors for the development of MetS. There is mounting evidence that oxidative stress is involved in the development of insulin resistance and that, once IR

Table 5. Multiple regressive stepwise analysis for oxidative stress evaluation in different components of the metabolic syndrome

	Parameters	Wald	p	Odds-Ratio	Confidence interval
TG	Sex	8.613	**0.003**	0.289	0.126 – 0.662
	Age	0.098	0.755	1.005	0.972 – 1.040
	BMI	21.695	< 0.0001	1.212	1.118 – 1.314
	AOPP	20.380	< 0.0001	1.011	1.006 – 1.016
	NO	1.082	0.298	0.992	0.977 – 1.007
	SH	0.104	0.748	1.949	0.033 – 113.506
	TRAP-UA	4.495	**0.034**	0.990	0.980 – 0.999
HDL	BMI	13.434	**< 0.0001**	1.113	1.051 – 1.179
	AOPP	14.431	**< 0.0001**	1.006	1.003 – 1.010
	NO	5.006	**0.025**	0.987	0.975 – 0.998
	TRAP-UA	0.062	0.803	0.999	0.993 – 1.005
Blood Pressure	Age	20.787	**< 0.0001**	1.086	1.048 – 1.125
	BMI	16.929	**< 0.0001**	1.167	1.084 – 1.256
	AOPP	5.683	**0.017**	1.005	1.001 – 1.009
	NO	3.509	0.061	1.013	0.999 – 1.028
	SH	0.737	0.391	4.993	0.127 – 196.458
	TRAP-UA	1.586	0.208	0.995	0.987 – 1.003
HOMA-IR	Age	4.753	**0.029**	0.969	0.0942 – 0.997
	BMI	57.168	**< 0.0001**	1.463	1.325 – 1.614
	AOPP	5.092	**0.024**	1.004	1.001 – 1.008
	NO	1.574	0.210	0.991	0.977 – 1.005
	TRAP-UA	0.370	0.543	0.998	0.990 – 1.005

TG: triacylglycerol; HDL: high-density lipoprotein; HOMA-IR: homeostasis model assessment-insulin resistance; BMI: body mass index; AOPP: advanced oxidation protein products; NO: nitric oxide; Sulfhydryl (SH) groups of proteins; TRAP-UA: total radical-trapping antioxidant parameter-uric acid.
After adjusting for sex and age AOPP maintained its significance for TG, HDL, hypertension and HOMA-IR, NO maintained its significance for HDL and TRAP-AU maintained its significance for TG. Whereas the other oxidative and nitrosative stress markers lost significance.

is acquired, all the other components of MetS could be developed as a result (21,22). Hypertriacylglycerolemia and hypertension lead to an increased production of superoxide anion (O_2^-) via the nicotinamide adenosine diphosphate oxidase pathway. This anion reacts rapidly with NO to form peroxynitrite ($ONOO^-$) – thus inactivating NO and leading to endothelial dysfunction, one of the mechanisms responsible for hypertension in these patients (23) – whereas HDL cholesterol antioxidant activity, a major mechanism mediating its cardioprotective effect, is impaired (20). Of note, in the current study, hypertriacylglycerolemia showed the highest degree of redox imbalance, as it was the only MetS component, and it concomitantly increased protein oxidation and decreased antioxidant capacity.

Our results show an association between the presence of insulin resistance and increased levels of protein oxidation. Although several reports have established the importance of insulin resistance and

oxidative stress in the development of both diabetes and cardiovascular disease (24,25), the precise role of oxidative stress as a cause or consequence of insulin resistance is still debated. Furukawa and cols. (26) demonstrated in cultured adipocytes that elevated levels of fatty acids increased oxidative stress via NADPH oxidase activation, and oxidative stress caused dysregulated production of adipocytokines – including adiponectin, plasminogen activator inhibitor-1, IL-6, and monocyte chemotactic protein-1. In addition, in mice with obesity, treatment with an NADPH oxidase inhibitor reduced ROS production in adipose tissue; attenuated the dysregulation of adipocytokines; and improved diabetes, hyperlipidemia, and hepatic steatosis. NADPH oxidase inhibitors could improve insulin sensitivity via the suppression of the effects induced through chronic exposure to ROS. These results suggested that increased oxidative stress in accumulated fat is an early instigator of MetS and that the redox state in adipose tissue is a potentially useful therapeutic target for obesity-associated MetS. In addition, hydrogen peroxide impairs insulin signaling and inhibits glucose transport, two cardinal features of insulin resistance (27). On the other hand, insulin itself promotes hydrogen peroxide formation in human fat cells (4). Altogether, it is tempting to speculate that oxidative stress can be both cause and consequence of insulin resistance (16,28).

It has been suggested that AOPPs are an early marker of MetS and are the most appropriate parameter for the determination of oxidative stress in MetS patients (29). AOPPs are formed during oxidative stress through the action of chlorinated oxidants, mainly hypochlorous acid and chloramines, produced by myeloperoxidase in activated neutrophils (11). AOPPs are structurally similar to advanced glycation end products (AGEs) and exert similar biological activities to those of AGEs – i.e., induction of pro-inflammatory cytokines and adhesion molecules (11). The present study showing that AOPPs were associated with metabolic changes and hypertension is in line with the importance of protein oxidation in patients with these components of MetS, independent of BMI, and confirm our previous finding that protein oxidation is more related to MetS parameters than lipid oxidation (30). Of note, BMI does not participate in the definition of the MetS and does not have a robust association verified between WC and insulin resistance. Although some studies have reported an association between AOPPs and BMI (13,30), the current study only presented this finding when the groups were not adjusted for the presence of MetS.

Changes in NOx levels have been linked with disorders of metabolic and cardiovascular homeostasis that can culminate in obesity-induced IR and endothelial dysfunction. Serum NOx were shown to be increased in MetS and be associated with other metabolic components such as BP, BMI, waist-to-hip ratio, and fasting plasma glucose in cluster analyses (31). In addition to overproduced NO, reduced levels of NO may also be a risk factor for the development of cardiometabolic disease (32). Although endothelial dysfunction has been considered an important issue in patients with obesity, the results of studies on NOx levels have been contradictory. Whereas some reports have shown higher NO levels (33), others have found the opposite results, similarly to the present study (34). NO is synthesized in endothelial cells by endothelial nitric oxide synthase (eNOS) activity, and it is responsible for vasodilatation and the maintenance of endothelial function; eNOS is expressed constitutively and synthesizes NO in only small amounts under basal conditions. In contrast, oxidative stress provokes inducible nitric oxide synthase (iNOS) expression even in low-grade inflammatory conditions, such as obesity, and consequently increases NO – which would be consumed in a reaction with superoxide anion, yielding peroxynitrite (35). This hypothesis is supported by some authors who demonstrated an increase in nitrotyrosine, a marker of endogenous peroxinitrite generation (36). Thus, the balance between eNOS and iNOS could explain NO increases or decreases in obese subjects. Although oxidative stress may induce NO production, the NO decrease associated with BMI found in the present study is probably related to higher NO consumption through oxidative stress, reducing NO bioavailability. Furthermore, previous investigations have shown that HDL induces a variety of signaling events – involving scavenger receptor B type I, cholesterol efflux and the stimulation of the phosphorylation of eNOS – that lead to the activation and increased expression of eNOS and the subsequent production of NO. Thus, the decreased NO levels in the present study may be related to the HDL cholesterol reduction (37,38).

Overweight is highly associated with arterial hypertension, independently from the occurrence of MetS, and a BMI of 25 kg/m^2 or greater accounted for approximately 34% and 62% of hypertension in men and in women, respectively (35). NO plays a major role in regulating blood pressure, and its deficient bioactivity is an important component of hypertension (37). Hypertensive subjects have increased generation of ROS – which scavenge NO, thereby reducing NO bioavailability (23). This study confirms the well-established relationship between NO decreases and hypertension, independent of whether BMI is considered.

The following limitations have to be considered in the present study. The first limitation is the small number of participants. Second, the food pattern and physical activities of the individuals were not measured. Third, the antihypertensive drugs the patients were taking, such as angiotensin-converting enzyme inhibitors, may elevate plasma adiponectin levels, which in turn can increase NO levels (23). Fourth, additional tests to evaluate oxidative and, especially, nitrosative stress would make our data more consistent. Nevertheless, the present study also has several strengths. First, to our knowledge, this is the first study to evaluate concomitantly oxidative and nitrosative stress in overweight and obese subjects. Second, we adjusted the results of oxidative stress measurements for the presence of MetS to evaluate its influence on the results.

In conclusion, only nitrosative stress was related to BMI, whereas protein oxidation was related to each component of MetS. In addition, both NO and advanced oxidative protein products were related to hypertension. In general, MetS components were essential participants in overweight and obese subjects, but hypertriacylgcerolemia was the parameter that showed the highest degree of redox imbalance. Although more studies are warranted to confirm the present data, this study reinforces the importance of concomitantly analyzing oxidative and nitrosative stress to obtain a more complete picture of overweight, obesity and associated conditions.

REFERENCES

1. Fernández-Sánchez A, Madrigal-Santillán E, Bautista M, Esquivel-Soto J, Morales-González A, Esquivel-Chirino C, et al. Inflammation, oxidative stress, and obesity. Int J Mol Sci. 2011;12:3117-32.

2. Wang Y, Monteiro C, Popkin BM. Trends of obesity and underweight in older children and adolescents in the United States, Brazil, China, and Russia. Am J Clin Nutr. 2002;75:971-7.

3. Wildman RP, McGinn AP, Kim M, Muntner P, Wang D, Cohen HW, et al. Empirical derivation to improve the definition of the Metabolic Syndrome in the evaluation of cardiovascular disease risk. Diabetes Care. 2011;34(3):746-8.

4. Ohmori K, Ebihara S, Kuriyama S, Ugajin T, Ogata M, Hozawa A, et al. The relationship between body mass index and plasma lipid peroxidation biomarker in an older, healthy Asian community. Ann Epidemiol. 2005;15:80-4.

5. Van Guilder GP, Hoetzer GL, Greiner JJ, Stauffer BL, Desouza CA. Influence of metabolic syndrome on biomarkers of oxidative stress and inflammation in obese adults. Obesity (Silver Spring). 2006;14:2127-31.

6. Ceriello A, Motz E. Is oxidative stress the pathogenic mechanism underlying insulin resistance, diabetes, and cardiovascular disease? The common soil hypothesis revisited. Arterioscler Thromb Vasc Biol. 2004;24:816-23.

7. Singh VP, Aggarwal R, Singh S, Banik A, Ahmad T, Patnaik BR, et al. Metabolic syndrome is associated with increased oxo-nitrative stress and asthma-like changes in lungs. PLoS One. 2015;10(6):e0129850.

8. Venturini D, Simão ANC, Scripes NA, Bahls LD, Melo PA, Belinetti FM, et al. Oxidative stress evaluation in overweight subjects with or without metabolic syndrome. Obesity (Silver Spring). 2012;20:2361-6.

9. Oliveira EP; Lima MD, Souza MLA. Síndrome metabólica, seus fenótipos e resistência à insulina pelo HOMA-RI. Arq Bras Endocrinol Metab. 2007;51:1506-15.

10. Gonzalez Flecha B, Llesuy S, Boveris A. Hydroperoxide-initiated chemiluminescence: an assay for oxidative stress in biopsies of heart, liver, and muscle. Free Radic Biol Med. 1991;10:93-100.

11. Witko-Sarsat V, Friedlander M, Capeillère-Blandin C, Nguyen-Khoa T, Nguyen AT, Zingraff J, et al. Advanced oxidation protein products as a novel marker of oxidative stress in uremia. Kidney Int. 1996;49:1304-13.

12. Repetto M, Reides C, Gomez Carretero ML, Costa M, Griemberg G, Llesuy S. Oxidative stress in blood of HIV infected patients. Clin Chim Acta. 1996;255:107-17.

13. Simão ANC, Dichi JB, Barbosa DS, Cecchini R, Dichi I. Influence of uric acid and gamma-glutamyltransferase on total antioxidant capacity and oxidative stress in patients with metabolic syndrome. Nutrition. 2008;24:675-81.

14. Hu ML. Measurement of protein thiol groups and glutathione in plasma. In: Abelson JN, Simon MI, editors. Methods in enzymology. San Diego, CA: Academic Press; 1994. p. 380-2.

15. Navarro-Gonzálvez JA, García-Benayas C, Arenas J. Semiautomated measurement of nitrate in biological fluids. Clin Chem. 1998;44:679-81.

16. Simão ANC, Lovozoy MAB, Dichi I. Oxidative stress in overweight and obesity. In: Dichi I, Breganó JW, Simão ANC, Cecchini R (eds). Oxidative Stress in Chronic Diseases. Boca Raton: CRC Press; 2014. p. 121-36.

17. Skalicky J, Muzakova V, Kandar R, Meloun M, Rousar T, Palicka V. Evaluation of oxidative stress and inflammation in obese adults with metabolic syndrome. Clin Chem Lab Med. 2008;46:499-505.

18. Krzystek-Korpacka M, Patryn E, Boehm D, Berdowska I, Zielinski B, Noczynska A. Advanced oxidation protein products (AOPPs) in juvenile overweight and obesity prior to and following weight reduction. Clin Biochem. 2008;41:943-9.

19. Fujita K, Nishizawa H, Funahashi T, Shimomura I, Shimabukuro M. Systemic oxidative stress is associated with visceral fat accumulation and the metabolic syndrome. Circ J. 2006;70:1437-42.

20. Hansel B, Giral P, Nobecourt E, Chantepie S, Bruckert E, Chapman MJ, et al. Metabolic syndrome is associated with elevated oxidative stress and dysfunctional dense high-density lipoprotein particles displaying impaired antioxidative activity. J Clin Endocrinol Metab. 2004;89:4963-71.

21. Barnard RJ, Roberts CK, Varon SM, Berger JJ. Diet-induced insulin resistance precedes other aspects of the metabolic syndrome. J Appl Physiol (1985). 1998;84(4):1311-5.

22. Simão ANC, Lozovoy MAB, Dichi I. Oxidative Stress in Metabolic Syndrome. Role of Oxidative Stress in Chronic Diseases, 1st ed., vol. 1. CRC Press; 2014. p. 246-59.

23. Simão ANC, Lozovoy MA, Bahls LD, Morimoto HK, Simão TN, Matsuo T, et al. Blood pressure decrease with ingestion of a soy product (kinako) or fish oil in women with metabolic syndrome: role of adiponectin and nitric oxide. Br J Nutr. 2012;108:1435-42.

24. Stern MP. Diabetes and cardiovascular disease. The "common soil" hypothesis. Diabetes. 1995;44:369-74.

25. Kip KE, Marroquin OC, Kelley DE, Johnson BD, Kelsey SF, Shaw LJ, et al. Clinical importance of obesity versus the metabolic syndrome in cardiovascular risk in women. A report from the Women's Ischemia Syndrome evaluation (WISE) Study. Circulation. 2004;109:706-13.

26. Furukawa S, Fujita T, Shimabukuro M, Iwaki M, Yamada Y, Nakajima Y, et al. Increased oxidative stress in obesity and its impact on metabolic syndrome. J Clin Invest. 2004;114:1752-61.

27. Keaney JF Jr, Larson MG, Vasan RS, Wilson PW, Lipinska I, Corey D, et al. Obesity and systemic oxidative stress: clinical correlates

of oxidative stress in the Framingham Study. Arterioscler Thromb Vasc Biol. 2003;23:434-9.

28. Simão ANC, Lozovoy MA, Dichi I. Metabolic syndrome: new targets for an old problem. Expert Opin Ther Targets. 2012;16:147-50.

29. Zurawska-Płaksej E, Grzebyk E, Marciniak D, Szymańska-Chabowska A, Piwowar A. Oxidatively modified forms of albumin in patients with risk factors of metabolic syndrome. J Endocrinol Invest. 2014;37:819-27.

30. Venturini D, Simão ANC, Dichi I. Advanced oxidation protein products are more related to metabolic syndrome components than biomarkers of lipid peroxidation. Nutr Res. 2015;35:759-65.

31. Zahedi Asl S, Ghasemi A, Azizi F. Serum nitric oxide metabolites in subjects with metabolic syndrome. Clin Biochem. 2008;41:1342-7.

32. Bahadoran Z, Mirmiran P, Ghasemi A, Azizi F. Serum nitric oxide metabolites are associated with the risk of hypertriglyceridemic-waist phenotype in women: Tehran lipid and glucose study. Nitric Oxide. 2015;50:52-7.

33. Elizalde M, Rydén M, van Harmelen V, Eneroth P, Gyllenhammar H, Holm C, et al. Expression of nitric oxide synthases in subcutaneous adipose tissue of nonobese and obese humans. J Lip Res. 2000;41:1244-51.

34. Esposito K, Ciotola M, Schisano B, Misso L, Giannetti G, Ceriello A, et al. Oxidative stress in the metabolic syndrome. J Endocrinol Invest. 2006;29:791-5.

35. Mineo C, Deguchi H, Griffin JH, Shaul PW. Endothelial and antithrombotic actions of HDL. Circ Res. 2006;98:1352-64.

36. Wilson PW, D'Agostino RB, Sullivan L, Parise H, Kannel WB. Overweight and obesity as determinants of cardiovascular risk: the Framingham experience. Arch Intern Med. 2002;162:1867-72.

37. Hermann M, Flammer A, Lüscher TF. Nitric oxide in hypertension. J Clin Hypertens (Greenwich). 2006;8:17-29.

38. Besler C, Heinrich K, Rohrer L, Doerries C, Riwanto M, Shih DM, et al. Mechanisms underlying adverse effects of HDL on eNOS-activating pathways in patients with coronary artery disease. J Clin Invest. 2011;121:2693-708.

15

Androgen insensitivity syndrome

Rafael Loch Batista[1], Elaine M. Frade Costa[1], Andresa de Santi Rodrigues[1,2],
Nathalia Lisboa Gomes[1], José Antonio Faria Jr.[1], Mirian Y. Nishi[1,2],
Ivo Jorge Prado Arnhold[1], Sorahia Domenice[1],
Berenice Bilharinho de Mendonca[1,2]

ABSTRACT

Androgenic insensitivity syndrome is the most common cause of disorders of sexual differentiation in 46,XY individuals. It results from alterations in the androgen receptor gene, leading to a frame of hormonal resistance, which may present clinically under 3 phenotypes: complete (CAIS), partial (PAIS) or mild (MAIS). The androgen receptor gene has 8 exons and 3 domains, and allelic variants in this gene occur in all domains and exons, regardless of phenotype, providing a poor genotype – phenotype correlation in this syndrome. Typically, laboratory diagnosis is made through elevated levels of LH and testosterone, with little or no virilization. Treatment depends on the phenotype and social sex of the individual. Open issues in the management of androgen insensitivity syndromes includes decisions on sex assignment, timing of gonadectomy, fertility, physcological outcomes and genetic counseling. Arch Endocrinol Metab. 2018;62(2):227-35

Keywords
Androgen insensitivity syndrome; androgen receptor; disorders of sex development; 46,XY DSD

[1] Unidade de Endocrinologia do Desenvolvimento, Laboratório de Hormônios e Genética Molecular/ LIM42, Hospital das Clínicas, Disciplina de Endocrinologia, Faculdade de Medicina da Universidade de São Paulo (FMUSP), São Paulo, SP, Brasil
[2] Laboratório de Sequenciamento em Larga Escala (SELA), Faculdade de Medicina da Universidade de São Paulo (FMUSP), São Paulo, SP, Brasil

Correspondence to:
Berenice Bilharinho de Mendonca
Hospital das Clínicas,
Laboratório de Hormônios
e Genética Molecular
Av. Dr. Enéas de Carvalho Aguiar, 155,
2° andar, Bloco 6
05403-900 – São Paulo, SP, Brasil
beremen@usp.br

INTRODUCTION

Androgen Insensitivity Syndrome (AIS) is an X-linked genetic disease and it is the most common cause of disorders of sex development (DSD) in 46,XY individuals (1). The phenotype ranges from normal female external genitalia in the complete form (CAIS) to normal male external genitalia associated with infertility and/or gynecomastia in the mild form (MAIS). A large spectrum of undervirilized male external genitalia is observed in the partial form (PAIS) (2). Mutations in the androgen receptor gene (*AR*) are found in most individuals with CAIS but in less individuals with PAIS (3).

AIS was first described by Morris, in 1953, with the clinical description of 82 female patients with testes but female phenotype and for this reason Morris named the syndrome as testicular feminization (4). Later, this syndrome was characterized for being a condition resulting from a complete or partial resistance to androgens in 46,XY individuals with normal male gonad development (5).

PAIS should be considered in all individuals with atypical genitalia at birth regardless of the degree of external genitalia virilization and MAIS is a possible diagnosis in males with persistent gynecomastia and or infertility (6).

Role of Androgens in Male Fetal Development: androgens are key elements for appropriate internal and external male sex differentiation. After normal testes development, the Leydig cells produce testosterone, which promotes Wolffian duct differentiation into epididymes, vasa deferentia and seminal vesicles (7). The conversion of testosterone to dihydrotestosterone by the 5α-reductase type 2 enzyme promotes male external genitalia differentiation (8). In humans, the critical period for genitalia virilization occurs between 8 and 14 weeks of gestation and depends on the presence of androgens and of a functioning androgen receptor (9). Impairment of androgen secretion and defects in the androgen receptor will compromise the virilization process.

THE HUMAN ANDROGEN RECEPTOR

The *AR* gene is located at chromosome Xq11-12, is encoded by eight exons and codifies a 919 aminoacids protein (Figure 1). The *AR* is a ligand-dependent transcription factor composed by three functional domains as the other nuclear receptors: a large N-terminal domain (NTD) (residues 1-555), a DNA-binding domain (DBD) (556-623 residues), a hinge domain (624-665 residues) and a C-terminal ligand-binding domain (LBD) (666–919 residues) (10). The NTD is encoded by exon 1 and contains a ligand-independent transactivation function 1 (AF1), which contains two distinct transcription activation units: Tau-1 (aminoacids 100-370) and Tau-5 (aminoacids 360-485), that are essential for full *AR* activity. The DBD is composed by two zinc fingers and connects the *AR* to promoter and enhancer regions of *AR* regulated genes by direct nuclear DNA binding allowing the activate functions of NTD and LBD (11). The LBD is encoded by exons 4-8 and contains 11 α-helices associated with two anti-parallel β-sheets in a sandwich-like conformation with a central ligand binding pocket, in which the ligand can bind (12).

CLINICAL PRESENTATION

CAIS prevalence in 46,XY males is estimated from 1 in 20.400 to 1 in 99.100 (13). Except in cases of familial inheritance, CAIS is diagnosed in three scenarios: in fetal life when prenatal sex determination disclosed a 46,XY karyotype in a fetus with female external genitalia; in childhood in a girl with inguinal hernia or at puberty in females with primary amenorrhea (14). The presence of inguinal hernia in a female child is rare and could indicate a CAIS diagnosis (13). Patients with AIS developed breasts with estradiol levels in normal male range suggesting that the lack of androgen action is the main driver of breast development in these patients, rather than an increased estrogen secretion. Menstrual cycles do not appear since normal production of anti-mullerian hormone (AMH) by the testis impeded uterus, cervix and proximal vagina to development. A shortened blind-ending vagina is observed in almost all patients and the vaginal measurement varied from 2.5 to 8 cm in CAIS and 1.5 – 4 cm in PAIS. Pubic and axillary hair are sparse or absent (1,14).

Final height in CAIS is above normal mean female height, probably due to the action of the growth-controlling gene (GCY) located at the Y chromosome (15). Interestingly, newborns with CAIS have the same size of male newborns, suggesting that postnatal factors are involved in the final height in these individuals (16). In our cohort, the final height of CAIS individuals (165.7 ± 8.9 cm) was taller than described for Brazilian females, but lower than expected for Brazilian males (15).

Differential diagnosis of CAIS includes complete gonadal dysgenesis, Mayer-Rokitanski-Kuster-Hauser syndrome and Mullerian ducts anomalies (1). Biosynthetic enzyme deficiencies are rarely a differential diagnosis for CAIS (8,17).

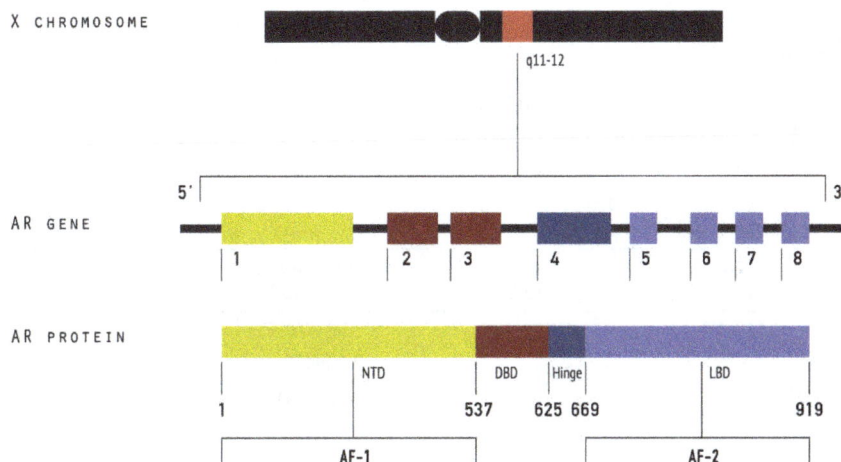

Figure 1. A schematic representation of androgen receptor gene and androgen receptor protein.

The PAIS clinical phenotype varies according to the degree of *AR* residual function and ranges from proximal hypospadias to micropenis (18). Hypospadias are a common finding with an estimated prevalence of 1:8000 male births and *AR* sequencing is necessary to exclude PAIS diagnosis (19). Gynecomastia observed at puberty time in patients with atypical genitalia can be indicative of PAIS (2,20). Differential diagnosis of PAIS includes all causes resulting in a undervirilized male external genitalia such as chromosomal defects (Klinefelter syndrome), genetic diseases (Smith-Lemli-Opitz syndrome, Denys-Drash syndrome, Frasier syndrome), partial gonadal dysgenesis, LH receptor defects, biosynthetic enzyme deficiencies (17,20-lyase deficiency, P450 oxidoreductase deficiency, 17β-hydroxysteroid dehydrogenase deficiency type 3, 5α-reductase 2 deficiency and hypospadias in small for gestation age boys (8,17).

MAIS is associated with *AR* mutations but without external genitalia abnormalities (6). This diagnosis could be suspected in the investigation of male infertility or in pubertal gynecomastia (14,18). There are few *AR* mutations associated exclusively with MAIS, but this condition is probably underdiagnosed (3,6).

MAIS can also manifest in a patient with neurological disorder characterized by bulbar and muscular atrophy (Kennedy's disease). This condition is due to the hyperexpansion of the CAG repeats (> 38), present in *AR* exon 1 (21). These patients present with normal male external genitalia, but testosterone resistance will develop with disease progression. For MAIS, the differential diagnosis includes other causes of male infertility.

ENDOCRINE FEATURES

In AIS the endocrine profile is consistent with androgen resistance characterized by elevated or normal basal serum testosterone levels associated with high serum LH levels (22). Elevated serum AMH and testosterone levels in a newborn suggest the diagnosis of androgen insensitivity and also exclude the diagnosis of complete gonadal dysgenesis (23). In postpuberal patients estradiol levels are normal or slightly elevated for a male individual (22). This pattern is seen at mini-puberty or after puberty. During childhood when gonadotropin axis is not activated, a hCG stimulation is necessary to evaluate testosterone secretion by Leydig cells (24). In MAIS, hormone concentrations are usually normal, but elevated serum LH and testosterone levels could be found in these patients (19).

Typically in AIS, basal testosterone and LH levels are elevated demonstrating the impairment of androgen negative feedback on the anterior pituitary (22). In contrast, FSH levels are usually normal in AIS. This is explained by the fact that FSH is mainly regulated by gonadal inhibin (25). Although there are differences in the *AR* residual function among the mutated receptors between CAIS and PAIS phenotypes, no difference are observed in hormonal levels (20,22). Serum LH, FSH estradiol, DHT were not different in subjects with CAIS and PAIS (Table 1).

MOLECULAR DEFECTS IN THE ANDROGEN RECEPTOR GENE

The AIS diagnosis is confirmed by the presence of allelic variants in the *AR* gene (1,26). About 30% of *AR* mutations in AIS are *de novo* and sequencing of the entire *AR* gene is recommended for all 46,XY DSD newborns, regardless of a familial history of DSD or AIS (26). In the absence of allelic variants in *AR* a multiplex ligation-dependent probe amplification (MLPA) can be helpful in order to detect deletions, insertions and duplications in the *AR* gene (26). There are more than 1000 *AR* mutations described in a website database

Table 1. Basal hormone levels in patients with AIS

Phenotype	LH (U/L)	FSH (U/L)	Testosterone ng/dL	Estradiol pg/mL	Reference
CAIS	14 – 43*	3.5 – 16*	186 – 1033*	10 – 40*	(22)
n = 11	26**	7.4**	342**	27**	
PAIS	9 – 32*	– 34*	157 – 1592*	20 – 109*	(22)
n = 14	26**	5.0**	1032	49	
CAIS	5.5 – 51	0.4 – 16**	173 – 1497*	4.8 – 70*	(60)
n = 42	18.5	3.5*	576**	30.7**	

* Range; ** Median.

associated with AIS and prostate cancer (http://www. mcgill.ca/androgendb) and around 600 of them were described in AIS (3). Mutations are found along the *AR* gene, being more frequent in exon 1 (the largest *AR* exon, which encodes the NTD). Defects in the NTD domain are more frequent in CAIS's patients and variants in exons 5 and 6 (that encode LBD) are more frequent in PAIS's patients (3). Almost all *AR* mutations in MAIS were found in the NTD, but there is a low number of *AR* mutations related to this phenotype.

The most common *AR* allelic variants in all AIS phenotypes are non-synonymous point mutations. Insertions and deletions causing a frameshift leading to a premature stop codon downstream are more frequently reported in CAIS's patients. Allelic variants affecting mRNA splicing are reported in CAIS and PAIS phenotypes. Rarely, synonymous allelic variants affecting splicing sites has been described in PAIS (27) and in CAIS individuals (28).

Large structural mutations (exon 1 deletion, exon 2 duplication, exon 3 deletion, exon 4-8 (LBD domain) deletion and deletion of entire *AR* gene) have been described but are very rare in AIS (3). Interesting, a deletion of an entire exon (exon 4) was previously described in a phenotypic male with azoospermia (29).

Postzygotic *AR* allelic variants resulting in somatic mosaicism are rarely described in AIS (30). In this situation the variant appears in heterozygote instead of hemizygote state. *AR* allelic variants in heterozygosis was also identified in some individuals with 47,XXY karyotype causing AIS (31).

There is not a perfect correlation between genotype and phenotype in AIS. In the *AR* mutation database, there are some *AR* allelic variants that can cause different phenotypes (Table 2). The explanation for this is not completely understood. It is hypothesized that *AR* co-regulators (activators and repressors) are implicated with this phenomenon. Other possibilities are variations in the level of 5α-reductase type 2 activity resulting in different DHT availability, and the presence

of germ-line *AR* allelic variants at a post zygote stage conferring somatic mosaicism (31).

CLINICAL MANAGEMENT OF AIS

AIS patients have complex issues including functional, sexual and psychosocial aspects. Sex assignment, external genitalia adequacy for social sex, hormonal replacement, psychosexual outcome, ideal time for gonadectomy, infertility and genetic counseling are issues that need attention in AIS care. All of them demand flexible, sensible and individualized procedures to achieve good results.

CLINICAL MANAGEMENT OF CAIS

After diagnosis, the first aspect to be considered is the time for bilateral gonadectomy. In a girl, maintenance of the gonads will allow spontaneous breast development, though breast development is similar with estrogen replacement in gonadectomized females. So far, gonadectomy is performed at early age, in order to avoid the risk of malignancies and the psychosocial difficulties in submitting an adolescent female to gonadectomy (24). When gonadectomy is performed before puberty, estrogen replacement is necessary to induce puberty. In general, hormonal replacement is started at the age of 11-12 years with oral or transdermal estrogen. Both ways are adequate and the patient and family can choose the route in which the compliance will be better (18). Due to the absence of uterus, progesterone replacement is not necessary.

Genitoplasty is not necessary in CAIS and vaginal dilation promotes an adequate vaginal length vaginal dilation should occur after puberty or when the patient refers to desire to initiate sexual activity (32). Most of the individuals (80%) who were submitted to vaginal dilation referred satisfactory and some of them reported dyspareunia (33). There are many vaginoplasty techniques (34), but non-surgical dilation is effective, safe, non expensive and normalizes vaginal length and

Table 2. *AR* allelic variants identified in more than one AIS phenotype (3)

Allelic variants	Phenotype
p.Leu174, p.Arg616Pro, p.Asn693del, p.Asn706Ser,p.Gly744Val, p.Met746Phe, p.Met750Val, p.Trp752*, p.Ala766Thr, p.Pro767Ser, p.Arg775His, p.Arg841His, p.Ile843Thr, p.Val867Met, p.Val890Met, p.Ser704Gly	CAIS, PAIS
p.Pro392Ser, p.Leu548Phe, p.Arg616His, p.Asp696Asn, p.Met781Ile, p.Arg856His, p.Ala646Asp	CAIS, PAIS, MAIS
p.Tyr572His, p.Arg608Gly, p.Asn757Ser, p.Arg789Ser, p.Gln799Glu, p.Thr801Ile, p.Ser815Asn, p.Leu822Val, p.Ala871Gly, p.Gly216Arg, p.Arg608Gly	PAIS, MAIS

sex intercourse (32). Because of that, surgical creation of a vagina should be avoid regardless of the surgical technique (32).

CLINICAL MANAGEMENT OF PAIS

PAIS diagnosis is usually suspected in a newborn with atypical genitalia and palpable gonads. Most of the patients are raised as male. The degree of external genitalia virilization is related to the residual AR function and can be predictive of androgen response at puberty. In male patients, correction of cryptorchidism and hypospadias are recommended as soon as possible, preferably before two years of age (35).

PAIS males frequently develop gynecomastia at puberty and surgical correction is generally necessary (22). High testosterone or DHT trials (intramuscular or topic testosterone esters or topic DHT) can be use to increase penile length and to improve other virilization signs (18,30). The results are unpredictable but are usually limited. Maximum virilization effect is observed after 6 months of high androgen usage treatment, subsequently, androgen therapy can be withdrawn in the patients with normal testes and preserved testosterone secretion.

For individuals raised as females, bilateral gonadectomy is recommended in childhood to avoid virilization and to eliminate the risk of testicular tumors (36). Genitoplasty is usually necessary in PAIS females and estrogen replacement is mandatory at pubertal time, with similar recommendation as describe for CAIS patients (15).

For MAIS, there is little information about clinical outcomes. Gynecomastia and infertility are the usual clinical presentation of this phenotype (6) and mastectomy is recommended for gynecomastia correction. This phenotype is observed in individuals with Kennedy's disease, which is more commonly known as spinal and bulbar muscular atrophy (SBMA). This syndrome is caused by an excessive number of CAG

Table 3. Types of androgen receptor allelic variants related to AIS reported in the androgen receptor mutations database

Type of defect	CAIS	PAIS	MAIS
Non-synonymous	155	125	41
Stop codon	57	2	0
Indel	41	4	2
Duplication	6	0	0
Total	259	131	43

repeats in the *AR* exon 1 and a number of patients also have testicular atrophy, gynecomastia, oligospermia and erectile dysfunction (37).

HORMONAL REPLACEMENT IN AIS

Hormonal replacement is mandatory for all gonadectomized individuals. In females, the purpose is the development of secondary sexual characteristics and an adequate and bone mass (2). Estrogen can be introduced in low doses (one quarter of the adult dose), at 9 – 11 years of age, with titration of this dosage every 6 months (20). The time for complete feminization is expected to be about 2 years. Oral or transdermic estrogen are alternative ways for estrogen replacement. The initial dose is 0.25 mg/day of 17β-estradiol increasing the dose each 6 months considering the progression of breast development. After complete breast development, a regular dose can be introduced (1-2 mg/day of 17β-estradiol continuously) (9).

In male individuals, the testes are able to produce testosterone. In male AIS, at pubertal age, high testosterone doses (200–500 mg twice a week) can be used, in order to increase the penile size and to promote virilization (1). Maximum penile length is obtained after six months of treatment with high testosterone doses. After this period, the dose of testosterone when necessary should return to the maintenance dose. The use of DHT in male PAIS has been tested (0.3 mg/kg of androstanolone gel 2.5% for 4 months) and mixed results were obtained following DHT therapy (38).

GONADAL TUMOR RISK IN AIS

Disorders of sex development are recognized as a risk factor for type II germ cell tumors (GCTs). These tumors are classified as seminomatous and non-seminomatous types (39). The seminomatous tumors referred to seminoma (testis) and to dysgerminoma (ovary and dysgenetic gonads). In the non-seminomatous group, many differentiated variants can be identified according to the cellular origin, being the teratomas from somatic differentiation, yolk sac tumor and choriocarcinoma from extra-embryonic differentiation, and embryonal carcinoma from stem cells (27). These tumors derivate from a non-invasive precursor named carcinoma *in situ* – CIS – or Intrabular germ cell neoplasia unclassified – IGCNU). In 2016, the World Health Organization suggested to change the nomenclature of this initial germinative neoplastic lesion from CIS or IGCNU to germ cell neoplasia *in situ* (GCNIS) (40). GCNIS are always non-invasive, but 50% of GCNIS progress to invasive GCTs within 5 years. The risk of GCTs development is related to the presence of a Y chromosome, but is not the same for the different etiologies of 46,XY DSD. So far, some factors, as chronological age and gonadal location can influence GCTs development (41).

In CAIS, the risk of GCTs is considered low and related to age (36). The estimated risk of gonadal tumors in CAIS gonads was about 0.8% - 22% (42). However, most old series included patients without confirmed AR mutation or without description of age at gonadectomy. The reports of malignant GCTs before puberty in CAIS are very rare (43). There is only one documented report of an invasive yolk-sac tumor in a CAIS individual before puberty. This occurred in a 17-months-old CAIS girl with abdominal gonads (44). After puberty, the risk is low, but not negligible. In a study, including 133 patients with CAIS, the gonads' histological and immunohistochemical findings showed a prevalence of 1.5% (2/133) for malignancies (45). The low incidence of GCTs in CAIS individuals can be explain by the rapid decline of germ cells after the first year of life (46).

PAIS individuals may maintain their germ cells because of the presence of residual androgen receptor responsiveness, differently of CAIS (46). Therefore, the incidence of GCTs in PAIS (15%) is higher than in CAIS (42). In cases of PAIS with untreated undescended testes the GCTs risk may be as high as 50% (47). Therefore, laparoscopic bilateral gonadectomy is indicated in all PAIS females and orquidopexy in scrotum in the male patients (48).

In patients who maintained the gonads, a careful monitoring including ultrasonography (US) or MRI has been suggested (43). Due to easy access and low cost, US remain the first choice for monitoring retained gonads. MRI has demonstrated adequate sensitivity to detect benign gonadal lesions, such as cysts or Sertoli cell adenomas, but failed to detect GCNIS (49). Annual US follow-up of labioscrotal and/or inguinal gonads is recommended. For abdominal gonads monitoring MRI is more helpful (50).

FERTILITY IN AIS

A normal androgen receptor is necessary for normal male reproduction, because testosterone and FSH, are essential factors for male spermatogenesis. Therefore, mutations in the androgen receptor gene have been searched in order to identify possible causes for male infertility. As previously described, infertility may be the only clinical manifestation of undervirilization in MAIS phenotype (6,51).

The strategy to obtain fertility in AIS individuals has not been defined yet (52). In CAIS, there is absence of uterus and testes histology reveals incomplete spermatogenesis, increased fibrosis, Leydig cell hyperplasia and low frequency of spermatogonia conferring a very low potential to fertility. In addition, the viability of male germ cells in CAIS is restricted to the first two years of life and for fertility in adult life germ cells should be preserved before this age (46). In PAIS individuals, some residual androgen receptor function is preserved, but not usually enough to promote fertility (46). Indeed, infertility is the rule in AIS (22).

Probably, fertility is the most sensitive outcome which depends of an intact androgen receptor. For it, MAIS individuals can present only infertility (6,51). However, the p.G824K and p.R840C *AR* variant allelics, were found in male individuals with preserved fertility (51,53).

A successful fertility was recently described in a PAIS individual harboring the p.V686A *AR* variant, after prolonged high-dose testosterone therapy (250 mg of testosterone enanthate weekly by four years) causing improvement in sperm count. The gonadotropin concentrations remained unaffected and intracytoplasmic sperm injection with a single sperm directly into an egg resulted in proved fertility (54).

In general, infertility in AIS is the rule. The evidence of sperm count improvement after high doses of testosterone (as described above) can be an indicative of fertility success, but should be tested in further studies as well as the use of aromatase inhibitors and clomiphene citrate to obtain fertility in these patients

PSYCHOLOGICAL OUTCOMES

Psychological support is essential for AIS individuals and their parents, in general (55). Dialogue about fertility, sexuality and karyotype are delicated issues to be approached with AIS individuals.

The gender identity, gender role and sexual orientation show a female pattern in CAIS individuals. In PAIS patients, in general, gender identity aligned with both sex of rearing male or female (56).

Gender change is very rarely described in CAIS and there are just four cases of gender change in individuals with CAIS (57). Therefore, gender dysphoria in CAIS is considered truly transgenderism. However, sexual functioning and sexual quality of life demonstrated less-positive outcome in CAIS patients in comparison with normal woman (58).

Although there is no inconsistency in gender identity, male PAIS individuals show disappointment with undervirilization signs. The absence or paucity of facial and body hair, the high-pitched voice compromised their self-perception of manhood (59). In female individuals, low scores in feminility scales have been reported (58). An impairment of sexual functioning is reported in male and female PAIS individuals (58).

CONCLUSION

AIS is the most common molecular diagnosis in newborns with 46,XY DSD and results of an *AR* defect. It has an X-linked inheritance and affects 50% of the male offspring. In CAIS, the diagnosis can be done intrauterus, at birth, childhood or after puberty. In PAIS, the diagnosis is usually at birth due to the atypical external genitalia. In MAIS, the diagnosis should be considered in cases of pubertal gynecomastia and male infertility. *AR* defects are found along *AR* gene in all AIS phenotypes. Non-synonymous point mutations are the commonest *AR* defects reported in AIS. Molecular diagnosis is achieved in almost all patients with CAIS and in a lower frequency in PAIS individuals. AIS is characterized by elevated serum LH and testosterone. In CAIS, there is a low risk of GCTs before puberty and postponing surgery to after puberty may allow the development of spontaneous puberty. In PAIS there is a risk of GCTs in 15% of the patients, and bilateral gonadectomy is recommended at childhood in all individuals raised in the female social sex. For males with PAIS, the testis should be placed in the scrotum and regularly monitored. Fertility was described in one PAIS individuals, and therapeutic strategy for successful fertility could be experienced in PAIS and MAIS individuals. In AIS, gender identity usually follows the sex of rearing, but quality of sexual life, sexual functioning and quality of life can be slightly compromised and are important issues for keeping patients in psychological care.

Funding: this work was supported by: *Fundação de Amparo à Pesquisa do Estado de São Paulo* Grant 2013/02162-8, *Núcleo de Estudos e Terapia Celular e Molecular* (NETCEM) and *Conselho Nacional de Desenvolvimento Científico e Tecnológico* Grant 303002/2016-6 (to B.B.M.); *Fundação de Amparo à Pesquisa do Estado de São Paulo* 2014/50137-5 (to SELA).

REFERENCES

1. Melo KFS, Mendonça BB, Billerbeck AEC, Costa EMF, Latronico AC, Arnhold IJP. [Androgen insensitivity syndrome: clinical, hormonal and molecular analysis of 33 cases]. Arq Bras Endocrinol Metab. 2005;49(1):87-97.

2. Mendonca BB, Costa EM, Belgorosky A, Rivarola MA, Domenice S. 46,XY DSD due to impaired androgen production. Best Pract Res Clin Endocrinol Metab. 2010;24(2):243-62.

3. Gottlieb B, Beitel LK, Nadarajah A, Paliouras M, Trifiro M. The androgen receptor gene mutations database: 2012 update. Hum Mutat. 2012;33(5):887-94.

4. Morris JM. The syndrome of testicular feminization in male pseudohermaphrodites. Am J Obstet Gynecol. 1953;65(6):1192-211.

5. McPhaul MJ, Marcelli M, Zoppi S, Griffin JE, Wilson JD. Genetic basis of endocrine disease. 4. The spectrum of mutations in the androgen receptor gene that causes androgen resistance. J Clin Endocrinol Metab. 1993;76(1):17-23.

6. Carmina E. Mild androgen phenotypes. Best Pract Res Clin Endocrinol Metab. 2006;20(2):207-20.

7. Imperato-McGinley J, Zhu YS. Androgens and male physiology the syndrome of 5alpha-reductase-2 deficiency. Mol Cell Endocrinol. 2002;198(1-2):51-9.

8. Mendonca BB, Batista RL, Domenice S, Costa EM, Arnhold IJ, Russell DW, et al. Steroid 5α-reductase 2 deficiency. J Steroid Biochem Mol Biol. 2016;163:206-11.

9. Mendonca BB, Domenice S, Arnhold IJ, Costa EM. 46,XY disorders of sex development (DSD). Clin Endocrinol (Oxf) 2009;70:173-87.

10. Tan MH, Li J, Xu HE, Melcher K, Yong EL. Androgen receptor: structure, role in prostate cancer and drug discovery. Acta Pharmacol Sin. 2015;36(1):3-23.

11. Clinckemalie L, Vanderschueren D, Boonen S, Claessens F. The hinge region in androgen receptor control. Mol Cell Endocrinol. 2012;358(1):1-8.

12. Nadal M, Prekovic S, Gallastegui N, Helsen C, Abella M, Zielinska K, et al. Structure of the homodimeric androgen receptor ligand-binding domain. Nat Commun. 2017;8:14388.

13. Oakes MB, Eyvazzadeh AD, Quint E, Smith YR. Complete androgen insensitivity syndrome – a review. J Pediatr Adolesc Gynecol. 2008;21(6):305-10.

14. Hughes IA, Werner R, Bunch T, Hiort O. Androgen insensitivity syndrome. Semin Reprod Med. 2012;30(5):432-42.

15. Danilovic DL, Correa PH, Costa EM, Melo KF, Mendonca BB, Arnhold IJ. Height and bone mineral density in androgen insensitivity syndrome with mutations in the androgen receptor gene. Osteoporos Int. 2007;18(3):369-74.

16. Miles HL, Gidlöf S, Nordenström A, Ong KK, Hughes IA. The role of androgens in fetal growth: observational study in two genetic models of disordered androgen signalling. Arch Dis Child Fetal Neonatal Ed. 2010;95(6):F435-8.

17. Mendonca BB, Gomes NL, Costa EM, Inacio M, Martin RM, Nishi MY, et al. 46,XY disorder of sex development (DSD) due to 17β-hydroxysteroid dehydrogenase type 3 deficiency. J Steroid Biochem Mol Biol. 2017;165(Pt A):79-85.

18. Mongan NP, Tadokoro-Cuccaro R, Bunch T, Hughes IA. Androgen insensitivity syndrome. Best Pract Res Clin Endocrinol Metab. 2015;29(4):569-80.

19. Qiao L, Tasian GE, Zhang H, Cunha GR, Baskin L. ZEB1 is estrogen responsive in vitro in human foreskin cells and is over expressed in penile skin in patients with severe hypospadias. J Urol. 2011;185(5):1888-93.

20. Arnhold IJ, Melo K, Costa EM, Danilovic D, Inacio M, Domenice S, et al. 46,XY disorders of sex development (46,XY DSD) due to androgen receptor defects: androgen insensitivity syndrome. Adv Exp Med Biol. 2011;707:59-61.

21. Madeira JLO, Souza ABC, Cunha FS, Batista RL, Gomes NL, Rodrigues AS, et al. A severe phenotype of Kennedy disease associated with a very large CAG repeat expansion. Muscle Nerve 2018;57(1):E95-7.

22. Melo KF, Mendonca BB, Billerbeck AE, Costa EM, Inácio M, Silva FA, et al. Clinical, hormonal, behavioral, and genetic characteristics of androgen insensitivity syndrome in a Brazilian cohort: five novel mutations in the androgen receptor gene. J Clin Endocrinol Metab. 2003;88(7):3241-50.

23. Edelsztein NY, Grinspon RP, Schteingart HF, Rey RA. Anti-Müllerian hormone as a marker of steroid and gonadotropin action in the testis of children and adolescents with disorders of the gonadal axis. Int J Pediatr Endocrinol. 2016;2016:20.

24. Ahmed SF, Cheng A, Hughes IA. Assessment of the gonadotrophin-gonadal axis in androgen insensitivity syndrome. Arch Dis Child. 1999;80(4):324-9.

25. Lahlou N, Bouvattier C, Linglart A, Rodrigue D, Teinturier C. [The role of gonadal peptides in clinical investigation]. Ann Biol Clin (Paris). 2009;67(3):283-92.

26. Achermann JC, Domenice S, Bachega TA, Nishi MY, Mendonca BB. Disorders of sex development: effect of molecular diagnostics. Nat Rev Endocrinol. 2015;11(8):478-88.

27. Hellwinkel OJ, Holterhus PM, Struve D, Marschke C, Homburg N, Hiort O. A unique exonic splicing mutation in the human androgen receptor gene indicates a physiologic relevance of regular androgen receptor transcript variants. J Clin Endocrinol Metab. 2001;86(6):2569-75.

28. Batista RL, Rodrigues ADS, Nishi MY, Gomes NL, Faria JAD Junior, Moraes DR, et al. A recurrent synonymous mutation in the human androgen receptor gene causing complete androgen insensitivity syndrome. J Steroid Biochem Mol Biol. 2017;174:14-16.

29. Akin JW, Behzadian A, Tho SP, McDonough PG. Evidence for a partial deletion in the androgen receptor gene in a phenotypic male with azoospermia. Am J Obstet Gynecol. 1991;165(6 Pt 1):1891-4.

30. Köhler B, Lumbroso S, Leger J, Audran F, Grau ES, Kurtz F, et al. Androgen insensitivity syndrome: somatic mosaicism of the androgen receptor in seven families and consequences for sex assignment and genetic counseling. J Clin Endocrinol Metab. 2005;90(1):106-11.

31. Batista RL, Rodrigues AS, Nishi MY, Feitosa ACR, Gomes NLRA, Junior JAF, et al. Heterozygous nonsense mutation in the androgen receptor gene associated with partial androgen insensitivity syndrome in an individual with 47,XXY karyotype. Sex Dev. 2017;11(2):78-81.

32. Ismail-Pratt IS, Bikoo M, Liao LM, Conway GS, Creighton SM. Normalization of the vagina by dilator treatment alone in Complete Androgen Insensitivity Syndrome and Mayer-Rokitansky-Kuster-Hauser Syndrome. Hum Reprod. 2007;22(7):2020-4.

33. Costa EM, Mendonca BB, Inácio M, Arnhold IJ, Silva FA, Lodovici O. Management of ambiguous genitalia in pseudohermaphrodites: new perspectives on vaginal dilation. Fertil Steril. 1997;67(2):229-32.

34. Hayashida SA, Soares JM Jr, Costa EM, da Fonseca AM, Maciel GA, Mendonça BB, et al. The clinical, structural, and biological features of neovaginas: a comparison of the Frank and the McIndoe techniques. Eur J Obstet Gynecol Reprod Biol. 2015;186:12-6.

35. Sircili MH, e Silva FA, Costa EM, Brito VN, Arnhold IJ, Dénes FT, et al. Long-term surgical outcome of masculinizing genitoplasty in large cohort of patients with disorders of sex development. J Urol. 2010;184(3):1122-7.

36. Cools M, Looijenga LH, Wolffenbuttel KP, T'Sjoen G. Managing the risk of germ cell tumourigenesis in disorders of sex development patients. Endocr Dev. 2014;27:185-96.

37. Fischbeck KH. A role for androgen reduction treatment in Kennedy disease? Muscle Nerve. 2013;47(6):789.

38. Becker D, Wain LM, Chong YH, Gosai SJ, Henderson NK, Milburn J, et al. Topical dihydrotestosterone to treat micropenis secondary to partial androgen insensitivity syndrome (PAIS) before, during, and after puberty – a case series. J Pediatr Endocrinol Metab. 2016;29(2):173-7.

39. Wünsch L, Holterhus PM, Wessel L, Hiort O. Patients with disorders of sex development (DSD) at risk of gonadal tumour development: management based on laparoscopic biopsy and molecular diagnosis. BJU Int. 2012;110(11 Pt C):E958-65.

40. Moch H, Cubilla AL, Humphrey PA, Reuter VE, Ulbright TM. The 2016 WHO Classification of Tumours of the Urinary System and Male Genital Organs-Part A: Renal, Penile, and Testicular Tumours. Eur Urol. 2016;70(1):93-105.

41. van der Zwan YG, Cools M, Looijenga LH. Advances in molecular markers of germ cell cancer in patients with disorders of sex development. Endocr Dev. 2014;27:172-84.

42. Looijenga LH, Hersmus R, Oosterhuis JW, Cools M, Drop SL, Wolffenbuttel KP. Tumor risk in disorders of sex development (DSD). Best Pract Res Clin Endocrinol Metab. 2007;21(3):480-95.

43. Döhnert U, Wünsch L, Hiort O. Gonadectomy in Complete Androgen Insensitivity Syndrome: Why and When? Sex Dev. 2017;11(4):171-4.

44. Handa N, Nagasaki A, Tsunoda M, Ohgami H, Kawanami T, Sueishi K, et al. Yolk sac tumor in a case of testicular feminization syndrome. J Pediatr Surg. 1995;30(9):1366-7.

45. Chaudhry S, Tadokoro-Cuccaro R, Hannema SE, Acerini CL, Hughes IA. Frequency of gonadal tumours in complete androgen insensitivity syndrome (CAIS): A retrospective case-series analysis. J Pediatr Urol. 2017;13(5):498.e1-498.e6.

46. Kaprova-Pleskacova J, Stoop H, Brüggenwirth H, Cools M, Wolffenbuttel KP, Drop SL. Complete androgen insensitivity syndrome: factors influencing gonadal histology including germ cell pathology. Mod Pathol. 2014;27(5):721-30.

47. Kathrins M, Kolon TF. Malignancy in disorders of sex development. Transl Androl Urol. 2016;5(5):794-8.

48. Hiort O, Birnbaum W, Marshall L, Wünsch L, Werner R, Schröder T, et al. Management of disorders of sex development. Nat Rev Endocrinol. 2014;10(9):520-9.

49. Nakhal RS, Hall-Craggs M, Freeman A, Kirkham A, Conway GS, Arora R, et al. Evaluation of retained testes in adolescent girls and women with complete androgen insensitivity syndrome. Radiology. 2013;268(1):153-60.

50. Cools M, Looijenga L. Update on the pathophysiology and risk factors for the development of malignant testicular germ cell tumors in complete androgen insensitivity syndrome. Sex Dev. 2017;11(4):175-81.

51. Hiort O, Holterhus PM. Androgen insensitivity and male infertility. Int J Androl. 2003;26(1):16-20.

52. Finlayson C, Fritsch MK, Johnson EK, Rosoklija I, Gosiengfiao Y, Yerkes E, et al. Presence of germ cells in disorders of sex

development: implications for fertility potential and preservation. J Urol. 2017;197(3 Pt 2):937-43.

53. Chu J, Zhang R, Zhao Z, Zou W, Han Y, Qi Q, et al. Male fertility is compatible with an Arg(840)Cys substitution in the AR in a large Chinese family affected with divergent phenotypes of AR insensitivity syndrome. J Clin Endocrinol Metab. 2002;87(1):347-51.

54. Tordjman KM, Yaron M, Berkovitz A, Botchan A, Sultan C, Lumbroso S. Fertility after high-dose testosterone and intracytoplasmic sperm injection in a patient with androgen insensitivity syndrome with a previously unreported androgen receptor mutation. Andrologia. 2014;46(6):703-6.

55. Cohen-Kettenis PT. Psychosocial and psychosexual aspects of disorders of sex development. Best Pract Res Clin Endocrinol Metab. 2010;24(2):325-34.

56. Mendonca BB. Gender assignment in patients with disorder of sex development. Curr Opin Endocrinol Diabetes Obes. 2014;21(6):511-4.

57. Bermúdez de la Vega JA, Fernández-Cancio M, Bernal S, Audí L. Complete androgen insensitivity syndrome associated with male gender identity or female precocious puberty in the same family. Sex Dev. 2015;9(2):75-9.

58. de Vries AL, Doreleijers TA, Cohen-Kettenis PT. Disorders of sex development and gender identity outcome in adolescence and adulthood: understanding gender identity development and its clinical implications. Pediatr Endocrinol Rev. 2007;4(4):343-51.

59. Callens N, Van Kuyk M, van Kuppenveld JH, Drop SLS, Cohen-Kettenis PT, Dessens AB, et al. Recalled and current gender role behavior, gender identity and sexual orientation in adults with Disorders/Differences of Sex Development. Horm Behav. 2016;86:8-20.

60. Doehnert U, Bertelloni S, Werner R, Dati E, Hiort O. Characteristic features of reproductive hormone profiles in late adolescent and adult females with complete androgen insensitivity syndrome. Sex Dev. 2015;9(2):69-74.

16

Impact of free thyroxine levels and other clinical factors on bare metal stent restenosis

Uğur Canpolat[1], Osman Turak[1], Fırat Özcan[1], Fatih Öksüz[1], Mehmet Ali Mendi[1], Çağrı Yayla[1], Sinan Aydoğdu[1]

ABSTRACT

Objective: Thyroid hormones have both direct and indirect effects on thermogenesis such as modulating vascular smooth muscle cell proliferation. However, the influence of more subtle changes in thyroid hormones on coronary atherosclerosis remains a matter of speculation. Smooth muscle cells play a crucial role in the pathogenesis of in-stent restenosis (ISR). However, the relationship between free thyroxine (fT4) and ISR has not been studied. In the present study, we aimed to assess the role of preprocedural serum fT4 level on the development of ISR in patients undergoing coronary bare metal stent (BMS) implantation. **Materials and methods:** We enrolled and analyzed clinical, biochemical, and angiographic data from 705 consecutive patients without a history of primary thyroid disease [mean age 60.3 ± 9.3 years, 505 (72%) male]; all patients had undergone BMS implantation and further control coronary angiography owing to stable or unstable angina pectoris. Patients were divided into 3 tertiles based on preprocedural serum fT4 levels. **Results:** ISR was observed in 53 (23%) patients in the lowest tertile, 82 (35%) patients in the second tertile, and 107 (46%) patients in the highest fT4 tertile (p < 0.001). Using multiple logistic regression analysis, five characteristics emerged as independent predictors of ISR: diabetes mellitus, smoking, HDL-cholesterol, stent length, and preprocedural serum fT4 level. In receiver operating characteristics curve analysis, fT4 level > 1.23 mg/dL had 70% sensitivity and 73% specificity (AUC: 0.75, p < 0.001) in predicting ISR. **Conclusion:** Higher preprocedural serum fT4 is a powerful and independent predictor of BMS restenosis in patients with stable and unstable angina pectoris. Arch Endocrinol Metab. 2017;61(2):130-6.

Keywords
Serum free thyroxine; bare metal stent; restenosis

[1] Türkiye Yüksek Ihtisas Training and Research Hospital, Cardiology Clinic, Ankara, Turkey

Correspondence to:
Uğur Canpolat
Türkiye Yüksek İhtisas
Training and Research Hospital,
Cardiology Clinic, Sıhhiye
06100 – Ankara, Turkey
dru_canpolat@yahoo.com

INTRODUCTION

Thyroid hormones (TH) falling within and outside of the normal range have both direct and indirect effects on atherogenesis (1). While TH indirectly modifies atherosclerotic risk factors such as lipid profile (2,3) and blood pressure (4), direct effects act via vascular smooth muscle cells, altering vascular tone (5), angiotensin-II type 1 receptor modulating the proliferation of vascular smooth muscle cells (6), upregulation of basic fibroblast growth factor causing enhanced angiogenesis (7), modulating the maturation and functioning of macrophages (8), and acting on the renin-angiotensin system (9,10). However, clinical studies yield conflicting results and mechanistic explanations remain elusive (11-13).

In-stent restenosis (ISR) continues to be a major pitfall for interventional cardiologists, and numerous efforts have been made to predict or resolve this important problem

(14,15). Various reactions following percutaneous coronary intervention (PCI) mediated vascular damage occur in sequence including inflammation, granulation, extracellular matrix remodeling, and vascular smooth muscle cell proliferation and migration, which result in neointimal hyperplasia and restenosis (16,17). Besides procedural factors, we hypothesize that patient-related factors such as preprocedural TH status may also be important in the development of ISR. Although previous evidence has shown several roles for THs in angiogenesis, macrophage functioning, and vascular smooth muscle cell function and proliferation, to the best of our knowledge, there has been no study investigating any possible association between pre-procedural TH levels and ISR. Here, we aimed to evaluate the association of TH levels before successful bare metal stent (BMS) implantation in predicting ISR in patients with stable and unstable angina pectoris.

MATERIALS AND METHODS

We retrieved clinical, laboratory, and angiographic data of consecutive patients who had undergone successful BMS implantation between January 2008 and August 2010 at our tertiary center hospital. The inclusion criteria were as follows: (a) patients with stable or unstable angina, (b) coronary angiography showing *de-novo* lesions without a history of the previous PCI, and (c) patients who received coronary BMS implantation. Patient data was accessed retrospectively with the time of interest being the point at which the patients underwent BMS implantation after control coronary angiography was performed because of clinical indications that included anginal symptoms and abnormal non-invasive test results (either treadmill exercise test or myocardial perfusion scintigraphy), thus recalling clinical, angiographic, and laboratory characteristics at that time. As such, we were able to collect the data from 772 patients. Patients with unstable angina pectoris were identified according to the definition of Braunwald (18). As part of our preprocedural protocol, thyroid hormone levels were obtained prior to coronary angiography for all patients. Patients were excluded from analysis if they had been using thyroid replacement therapy or anti-thyroid drugs (n = 8), showed clinical evidence of neoplastic diseases (n = 2), heart failure [left ventricular ejection fraction (LVEF) of < 50%] (n = 18), renal dysfunction [estimated glomerular filtration rate (eGFR) of < 90 mL/min/1.73 m²] (n = 20), hepatic and hemolytic disorders (n = 1), chronic inflammatory disease (n = 3), used therapy with amiodarone (n = 7), or had any active infectious disease (n = 2) or sepsis (n = 1), alcohol consumption (n = 3), and patients having major adverse event during follow-up (n = 2), leaving 705 patients to be included in the study for analysis.

Clinical and demographic characteristics of patients encompassing age, gender, history of arterial hypertension, diabetes mellitus, smoking, family history of coronary artery disease, LVEF, and medications used were noted. In addition, serum levels of fasting blood glucose, serum creatinine, and lipid panel including total cholesterol, low-density lipoprotein cholesterol, high-density lipoprotein cholesterol, and triglyceride levels were recorded. Our study was in compliance with the principles outlined in the Declaration of Helsinki and approved by Institutional Ethics Committee.

All laboratory data were obtained from venous blood samples up to 6 h before stent implantation. Complete blood count and serum lipid/biochemistry panel were measured according to standard methods. Measurement of thyroid-stimulating hormone (TSH) (reference range, 0.34–5.6 µIU/mL), free triiodothyronine (fT3) (reference range, 2.5–3.9 pg/mL), and free thyroxine (fT4) (reference range, 0.54–1.24 ng/dL) levels was performed with a Beckman Coulter DXI 800 auto analyzer (Beckman Coulter, Brea, CA, USA) using the chemiluminescence method. Intra assay coefficients of variations were as follows: 4.1% for fT3, 3.4% for fT4, and 5.3% for TSH.

Coronary interventions were performed according to the current practice guidelines and were recorded in digital storage for further analysis. The degree of coronary stenosis was visually estimated by experienced interventional cardiologists. A luminal narrowing > 50% in a major subepicardial vessel (left anterior descending, left circumflex, or right coronary artery) was defined as significant stenosis. Each patient received aspirin plus clopidogrel (loading dose 300 or 600 mg) before or during coronary intervention. Unfractionated heparin 100 U/kg was administered at the beginning of the procedure to keep the activated clotting time > 200 s. The access site for PCI was at the physician's preference (femoral or radial). The usage of glycoprotein IIb/IIIa (GpIIbIIIa) inhibitors and pre- or post-dilatation after stent implantation of the lesion was at the operator's discretion. Successful PCI was defined as a < 20% decrease in diameter stenosis and residual stenosis < 5% in diameter with final thrombolysis in myocardial infarction (TIMI) grade 3 flow without any major complications. After stent placement, clopidogrel was administered for 1 month and aspirin was used indefinitely. During routine clinical follow-up, coronary angiography was performed on clinical indications secondarily in patients with stable or unstable angina pectoris. Control coronary angiograms were recorded with Judkins technique and interpreted by two, independent cardiologists who were blinded to the patients' data. The evaluation of stenosis was conducted using the conventional visual assessment technique. ISR was accepted as narrowing of > 50% in an otherwise normal diameter, including 5 mm proximal and distal to the stent edge, according to the results of control coronary angiographies (19). Intra- and inter-observer variabilities of stent restenosis analysis were minimal in a representative subset of 100 patients. The interpretations of the two investigators on the presence or absence of ISR was 95% and 97%, respectively.

Intra-observer variability was assessed by the same investigator. The two readings were concordant for the presence or absence ISR in 98% and 97%, respectively.

Analyses were performed using SPSS 20.0 (SPSS, Inc., Chicago, Illinois). Continuous data were presented as median (minimum-maximum range) or mean ± standard deviation. To test the distribution pattern, the Kolmogorov–Smirnov test was used. The study population was assigned to tertiles based on the preprocedural fT4 level. Comparisons of multiple mean values were conducted by using the Kruskal–Wallis tests or analysis of variance as appropriate. Categorical variables were summarized as percentages and compared with the chi-square test. The effects of different variables on ISR were calculated by univariate analysis for each variable. Variables for which the unadjusted p-value was < 0.10 in the logistic regression analysis were identified as potential risk markers and were included in the full model. We reduced the model using stepwise, multivariate logistic regression analyses and eliminated potential risk markers using likelihood ratio tests. An exploratory evaluation of additional cut points was performed using receiver operating characteristics (ROC) curve analysis. A p-value of < 0.05 was considered statistically significant.

RESULTS

A total 705 patients [mean age 60.3 ± 9.3 years, 505 (72%) male] were grouped into tertiles according to the preprocedural fT4 levels. The baseline clinical, laboratory, and angiographic data of the study groups are summarized in Table 1. All diabetic patients included in the study had a diagnosis of type 2 diabetes mellitus. The mean period between the two coronary angiograms for the entire study population was 20.2 ± 4.5 months. While the TSH [median 1.34 (0.95–1.95) vs 1.22 (1.03–1.54), p = 0.48] and fT3 [median 2.96 (2.75–3.18) vs 2.85 (2.60–3.10), p = 0.11] levels were similar between patients with and without ISR, the fT4 levels were significantly higher in patients with ISR [median 1.45 (1.25–1.67) vs 1.20 (1.02–1.38), p < 0.001] (Figure 1). No difference was found in GpIIbIIIa inhibitor use, pre-dilatation rate, or post-dilatation rates among fT4 tertile groups (Table 1) and among the without/with ISR groups [GpIIbIIIa inhibitor use: 36 (7.7%) for without ISR vs 14 (5.9%) for with ISR, p = 0.232; pre-dilatation rate: 27 (8.8%) for without ISR vs 11 (4.6%) for with ISR, p = 0.325;

post-dilatation rate: 17 (3.6%) for without ISR vs 7 (2.9%) for with ISR, p = 0.404].

The rate of ISR showed an incremental trend from tertile 1 to 3 (23%, 35%, and 46%, p < 0.001, respectively) (Figure 2). Similarly, higher fT4 levels before stent implantation were associated with an increased risk for ISR by logistic regression analysis. Assuming fT4 level as a continuous variable in multiple logistic regression analysis, diabetes mellitus, smoking, HDL-C, stent length, and fT4 levels emerged as independent predictors of ISR (Table 2). When fT4 tertiles were analyzed as a categorical (tertile 1 reference) variable in multiple logistic regression analysis, the relative risk of ISR in the highest tertile was 5.31 (95% CI: 3.44–8.19, p < 0.001) and 2.98 for tertile 2 (95% CI: 1.92–4.63, p < 0.001) as compared to the lowest tertile of the fT4 levels.

The ROC curve explored the relation between preprocedural fT4 and ISR. Area under the curve was 0.75 (95% confidence interval 0.72–0.79; p < 0.001). Preprocedural fT4 with a cut-off level of > 1.23 ng/dL well predicted ISR with a sensitivity of 70% and specificity of 73% (Figure 3).

In subgroup analyses, patients with subclinical hyperthyroidism (12/18 patients) displayed a higher rate of ISR during follow-up compared to subclinical hypothyroidism (3/10 patients) and euthyroidism (227/677 patients) (66.7% vs 30% and 33.5%, p < 0.001). In another subgroup analysis that included only diabetic and/or smoking patients, the impact of fT4 on ISR was analyzed. We found that among diabetic patients who did not smoke, the rate of ISR was higher in Tertile 3 [39 (36.4%)] of fT4 compared to Tertile 1 [22 (14.4%)] and Tertile 2 [46 (34.3%)] (p < 0.001). Serum fT4 level was still significantly associated with ISR in patients with diabetes who did not smoke (OR: 3.6, p < 0.001). Among smokers who did not have diabetes, the rate of ISR was higher in Tertile 3 [66 (50.8%)] for fT4 compared to Tertile 1 [22 (11.6%)] and Tertile 2 [52 (31.3%)] (p < 0.001). The serum fT4 level was significantly associated with ISR in non-diabetic smokers (OR: 6.08, p < 0.001). When these same two populations were excluded from the analysis, the rate of ISR was higher in Tertile 3 [18 (35.3%)] for fT4 compared to Tertile 1 [13 (10.9%)] and Tertile 2 [24 (29.6%)] (p < 0.001). However, the serum fT4 level did not reach a high enough statistical significance to show an association with ISR when diabetic and smoking patients were excluded from the analysis.

Table 1. Baseline characteristics of study sample according to preprocedural free thyroxine tertiles

Variables	Tertile 1 n = 235 1.02 (0.91-1.15)	Tertile 2 n = 235 1.23 (1.13-1.37)	Tertile 3 n = 235 1.49 (1.37-1.68)	p value
	Free Thyroxine (ng/dL)			
Age (years)	60.4 ± 9.1	59.7 ± 9.2	61.1 ± 9.5	0.52
Male gender	178 (77%)	160 (68%)	167 (71%)	0.18
Type 2 DM	53 (23%)	70 (30%)	84 (35%)	0.002
Current smoker	80 (34%)	94 (40%)	115 (49%)	< 0.001
Hypertension	131 (56%)	124 (53%)	135 (57%)	0.58
Cause of stent implantation				
Stable angina pectoris	150 (64%)	146 (68%)	140 (60%)	0.34
Unstable angina pectoris	85 (36%)	89 (38%)	95 (40%)	0.34
No of coronary arteries narrowed				
1 vessel	43 (18%)	56 (24%)	53 (23%)	0.31
2 vessel	192 (82%)	179 (76%)	182 (77%)	0.31
Target coronary artery				
Left anterior descending artery	124 (53%)	100 (43%)	103 (44%)	0.01
Right coronary artery	50 (21%)	83 (35%)	76 (32%)	0.01
Left circumflex artery	61 (26%)	52 (21%)	56 (24%)	0.01
Stent diameter (mm)	3 (2.75-3)	3 (2.5-3)	3 (2.75-3)	0.67
Stent length (mm)	15 (12-18)	15 (13-18)	16 (13-18)	0.31
Periprocedural GpIIbIIIa inhibitor adminisitration	18 (7.7%)	15 (6.4%)	17 (7.2%)	0.86
Pre-dilatation rate	13 (5.5%)	11 (4.7%)	14 (6.0%)	0.82
Post-dilatation rate	8 (3.4%)	7 (3.0%)	9 (3.8%)	0.88
In-hospital medications				
Beta blocker	81%	82%	79%	0.78
ACEi	71%	73%	70%	0.81
CCB	4%	4%	3%	0.84
ARB	5%	6%	5%	0.74
Statins	86%	89%	87%	0.68
LVEF (%)	60.1 ± 3.7	61.0 ± 3.9	59.5 ± 3.4	0.53
Fasting glucose (mg/dL)	104 (92-131)	104 (92-137)	113 (95-144)	0.04
HDL-C (mg/dL)	43 (35-47)	40 (34-46)	35 (30-42)	0.02
LDL-C (mg/dL)	105 (81-134)	107 (83-137)	104 (82-130)	0.73
Triglycerides (mg/dL)	143 (100-207)	140 (100-183)	135 (94-180)	0.18
TSH (µIU/mL)	1.28 (0.12-6.0)	1.40 (0.05-5.90)	1.30 (0.02-5.50)	0.596
Free triiodothyronine (pg/mL)	2.8 (2.6-3.1)	2.9 (2.6-3.2)	2.9 (2.7-3.2)	0.28
Hemoglobin (g/dL)	14.2 ± 2.0	14.0 ± 1.7	13.7 ± 1.6	0.03
Platelet count (×10^9/L)	251.9 ± 32.2	248.7 ± 34.5	255.6 ± 32.3	0.41
Period between the two CAG (months)	20.9 ± 4.4	20.3 ± 5.2	19.3 ± 4.1	0.17
In-stent restenosis	53 (23%)	82 (35%)	107 (46%)	< 0.001

Data are median (minimum-maximum range), means ± S.D. or n (%).
ACEi: angiotensin converting enzyme inhibitors; ARB: angiotensin receptor blockers; CAG: coronary angiography; CCB: calcium channel blocker; DM: diabetes mellitus; HDL-C: high density lipoprotein cholesterol; LDL-C: low density lipoprotein cholesterol; LVEF: left ventricular ejection fraction.

Table 2. Predictors of in-stent restenosis in univariable and multivariable logistic regression analyses

Variables	Univariable		Multivariable	
	OR (95% CI)	p value	OR (95% CI)	p value
Age (years)	1.02 (0.90-1.13)	0.52	-	-
Diabetes mellitus	1.35 (1.12-1.55)	< 0.001	1.21 (1.08-1.33)	< 0.001
Smoking	1.47 (1.08-1.87)	< 0.001	1.87 (1.19-2.55)	0.001
HDL-C (mg/dL)	0.91 (0.86-0.96)	0.001	0.94 (0.89-0.98)	0.02
LDL-C (mg/dL)	1.05 (0.94-1.15)	0.27	-	-
Triglycerides (mg/dL)	1.02 (0.85-1.20)	0.46	-	-
Hemoglobin (g/dL)	1.12 (0.95-1.31)	0.19	-	-
Stent length (mm)	1.33 (1.15-1.51)	0.001	1.30 (1.11-1.48)	0.001
Stent diameter (mm)	1.05 (0.96-1.14)	0.31	-	-
LVEF (%)	1.07 (0.94-1.19)	0.14	-	-
Free thyroxine (ng/dL)	1.17 (1.09-1.25)	0.001	1.05 (1.02-1.08)	0.02
Free triiodothyronine (pg/mL)	1.02 (0.94-1.11)	0.51		
Period between the two CAG (months)	0.93 (0.88-0.97)	0.01	0.97 (0.92-1.03)	0.10

CAG: coronary angiography; CI: confidence interval; HDL-C: high density lipoprotein cholesterol; LDL-C: low density lipoprotein cholesterol; LVEF: left ventricular ejection fraction; OR: odds ratio.

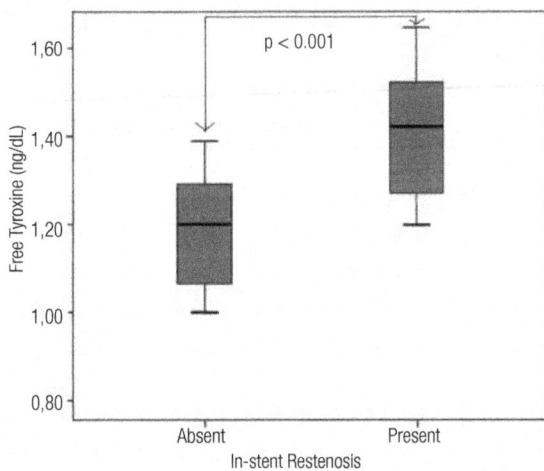

Figure 1. Comparison of serum fT4 levels among patients with and without in-stent restenosis.

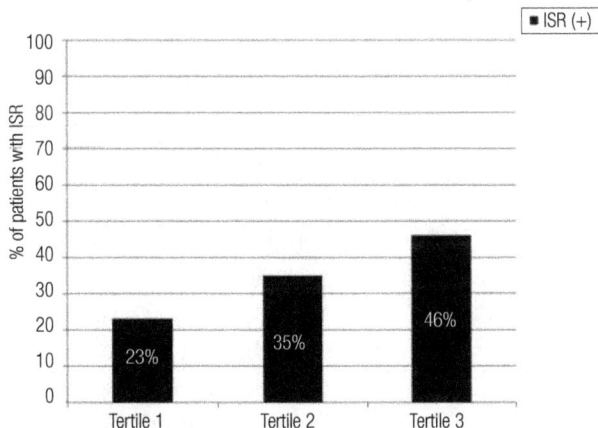

Figure 2. Percentages of the patients developing in-stent restenosis stratified by tertile of preprocedural serum fT4 levels.

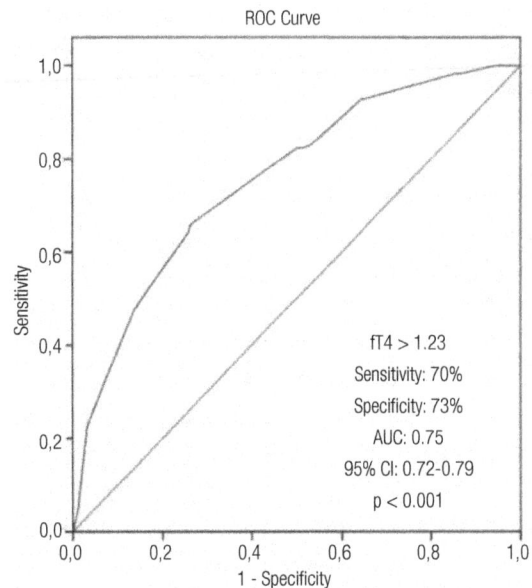

Figure 3. Receiver operating characteristic curve of pre-procedural serum fT4 levels for predicting in-stent restenosis after bare metal stent implantation. AUC: Area under curve; CI: confidence interval.

DISCUSSION

Three major findings arose from our study: (i) preprocedural serum fT4 is a significant, independent predictor of further ISR in patients with stable or unstable angina pectoris undergoing successful BMS implantation, (ii) patients in the highest tertile of serum fT4 are at greater risk, and preprocedural fT4 > 1.23 ng/dl have a 70% sensitivity and 73% specificity in predicting ISR, and (iii) other well-known predictors of ISR including diabetes mellitus, smoking, lower HDL-C, and increased stent length were also important.

PCI for ischemic coronary heart disease is well-known as a pioneering innovation for interventional cardiologists. However, ISR represents a major nightmare for interventionalists and efforts are ongoing to circumvent this serious problem (15,20). Along with technical issues, several cellular and molecular pathways play a role in coronary wall injury after PCI (14,21). Cellular response to mechanical vascular damage initiated immediately after PCI includes an early phase, consisting of platelet activation and inflammation, followed by an intermediate phase of granulation tissue corresponding to vascular smooth muscle cell migration and proliferation, and a late phase of neointima formation and finally progression to ISR (21). Although the exact etiopathogenesis remains to be fully elucidated, various pre-, peri-, and post-procedural risk factors represent possible actors in the development of ISR (14). The clinical parameter that most consistently increases the risk of ISR is diabetes mellitus (22). The common hypothesis for this effect is that hyperglycemia induces endothelial dysfunction and a proinflammatory state with increased cytokine production (23,24). These pathways enhance neointima formation, which promotes the development of ISR. Although smoking is established as a conventional risk factor for atherosclerosis, there is a possible protective effect associated with smoking that might result in the development of ISR after PCI. The data regarding the impact of smoking on ISR have been contradictory (25-27). Hong and cols. (28) evaluated 840 patients with drug-eluting stent implantation and showed that current smoking was a predictor of ISR in diabetic patients (OR: 1.923, 95% CI: 1.055–4.725). In another study, Ma and cols. (29) also showed that current smoking increases the risk of ISR in ST-segment elevation MI patients undergoing drug-eluting stent implantation. Furthermore, among the lesion-related factors, lesion length and thereby stent length are the most consistent factors that were associated ISR (30). Consistent with previous studies, we have also found that diabetes mellitus, smoking, and stent length are significantly associated with ISR.

The role of THs, particularly fT4, in the pathogenesis of atherosclerosis is unclear and controversial. It has been suggested that THs act both directly and indirectly on atherogenesis by altering vascular tone, modulating macrophage functions, enhancing angiogenesis, and

regulating vascular smooth muscle cell proliferation (5-10). Jung and cols. (11) reported that higher serum fT4 levels even within the normal reference range were significantly associated with both the presence and severity of coronary artery disease in 192 patients with stable angina pectoris. In contrast, Auer and cols. (12) showed that higher serum fT4 levels were inversely correlated with the severity of coronary atherosclerosis and higher thyrotropin levels correlated positively. The reasons proposed to underlie the differences in the study results are as follows: i) study populations that are too small to detect an association between subtle changes in fT4 level and coronary atherosclerosis because of the narrow reference range for serum fT4 level; ii) inclusion of heterogeneous patient groups having either stable angina pectoris or acute coronary syndrome. Therefore, to clarify the exact association of THs with coronary atherosclerosis, more specific studies should be designed. The findings of experimental and clinical studies investigating the fT4-atherosclerosis relationship and ISR mechanisms have been coupled, and we have found that high pre-procedural serum fT4 is a powerful and independent predictor of BMS restenosis in patients with stable or unstable angina pectoris. We hypothesize that serum fT4 increases the risk of ISR through enhanced activity of the renin–angiotensin system and proliferation of vascular smooth muscle cells. To the best of our knowledge, this is the first study demonstrating such an association.

Our results raise some clinical implications. The pre-procedural fT4 level may identify patients with a higher risk for ISR with high relevance for clinical routine practice, and close follow-up in those patients is warranted. Furthermore, it is unclear in such a population, at what level or range the serum fT4 should be kept to prevent ISR. Prospective, large-scale studies evaluating the impact of thyroxin replacement or anti-thyroid therapy on ISR should be designed to confirm our study findings and to decide which interval of TH levels are safe for patients undergoing PCI.

Our study should be interpreted within several limitations. First, the study was designed in a retrospective manner representing a single-center experience with only BMS restenosis. Thus, a causal relationship cannot be established between THs and ISR. Second, the definition of ISR was based on visual assessment rather than on a more quantitative and informative intravascular ultrasound or optical coherence tomography. Third, the serum fT4 level was only measured before stent implantation. The levels of serum fT4 have the potential to change over time in an individual patient.

In summary, higher preprocedural serum fT4 is a powerful and independent predictor of BMS restenosis in patients with stable and unstable angina pectoris.

Acknowledgement: none.

Funding: this study was not funded by any institution.

REFERENCES

1. Ichiki T. Thyroid hormone and atherosclerosis. Vascul Pharmacol. 2010;52:151-6.

2. Morris MS, Bostom AG, Jacques PF, Selhub J, Rosenberg IH. Hyperhomocysteinemia and hypercholesterolemia associated with hypothyroidism in the third US National Health and Nutrition Examination Survey. Atherosclerosis. 2001;155:195-200.

3. Danese MD, Ladenson PW, Meinert CL, Powe NR. Clinical review 115: effect of thyroxine therapy on serum lipoproteins in patients with mild thyroid failure: a quantitative review of the literature. J Clin Endocrinol Metab. 2000;85:2993-3001.

4. Fommei E, Iervasi G. The role of thyroid hormone in blood pressure homeostasis: evidence from short-term hypothyroidism in humans. J Clin Endocrinol Metab. 2002;87:1996-2000.

5. Ojamaa K, Klemperer JD, Klein I. Acute effects of thyroid hormone on vascular smooth muscle. Thyroid. 1996;6:505-12.

6. Fukuyama K, Ichiki T, Takeda K, Tokunou T, Iino N, Masuda S, et al. Downregulation of vascular angiotensin II type 1 receptor by thyroid hormone. Hypertension. 2003;41:598-603.

7. Tomanek RJ, Doty MK, Sandra A. Early coronary angiogenesis in response to thyroxine: growth characteristics and upregulation of basic fibroblast growth factor. Circ Res. 1998;82:587-93.

8. Perrotta C, Buldorini M, Assi E, Cazzato D, De Palma C, Clementi E, et al. The thyroid hormone triiodothyronine controls macrophage maturation and functions: protective role during inflammation. Am J Pathol. 2014;184:230-47.

9. Marchant C, Brown L, Sernia C. Renin-angiotensin system in thyroid dysfunction in rats. J Cardiovasc Pharmacol. 1993;22:449-55.

10. Sernia C, Marchant C, Brown L, Hoey A. Cardiac angiotensin receptors in experimental hyperthyroidism in dogs. Cardiovasc Res. 1993;27:423-8.

11. Jung CH, Rhee EJ, Shin HS, Jo SK, Won JC, Park CY, et al. Higher serum free thyroxine levels are associated with coronary artery disease. Endocrine J. 2008;55:819-26.

12. Auer J, Berent R, Weber T, Lassnig E, Eber B. Thyroid function is associated with presence and severity of coronary atherosclerosis. Clin Cardiol. 2003;26:569-73.

13. Singh S, Duggal J, Molnar J, Maldonado F, Barsano CP, Arora R. Impact of subclinical thyroid disorders on coronary heart disease, cardiovascular and all-cause mortality: a meta-analysis. Int J Cardiol. 2008;125:41-8.

14. Jukema JW, Verschuren JJ, Ahmed TA, Quax PH. Restenosis after PCI. Part 1: pathophysiology and risk factors. Nat Rev Cardiol. 2012;9:53-62.

15. Jukema JW, Ahmed TA, Verschuren JJ, Quax PH. Restenosis after PCI. Part 2: prevention and therapy. Nat Rev Cardiol. 2012;9:79-90.

16. Liu MW, Roubin GS, King SB, 3rd. Restenosis after coronary angioplasty. Potential biologic determinants and role of intimal hyperplasia. Circulation. 1989;79:1374-87.

17. Welt FG, Rogers C. Inflammation and restenosis in the stent era. Arterioscler Thromb Vasc Biol. 2002;22:1769-76.

18. Braunwald E. Unstable angina: an etiologic approach to management. Circulation. 1998;98:2219-22.

19. Gaspardone A, Crea F, Versaci F, Tomai F, Pellegrino A, Chiariello L, et al. Predictive value of C-reactive protein after successful coronary-artery stenting in patients with stable angina. Am J Cardiol. 1998;82:515-8.

20. Stettler C, Wandel S, Allemann S, Kastrati A, Morice MC, Schömig A, et al. Outcomes associated with drug-eluting and bare-metal stents: a collaborative network meta-analysis. Lancet. 2007;370:937-48.

21. Inoue T, Croce K, Morooka T, Sakuma M, Node K, Simon DI. Vascular inflammation and repair: implications for re-endothelialization, restenosis, and stent thrombosis. JACC Cardiovasc Interv. 2011;4:1057-66.

22. Gilbert J, Raboud J, Zinman B. Meta-analysis of the effect of diabetes on restenosis rates among patients receiving coronary angioplasty stenting. Diabetes Care. 2004;27:990-4.

23. Lee MS, David EM, Makkar RR, Wilentz JR. Molecular and cellular basis of restenosis after percutaneous coronary intervention: the intertwining roles of platelets, leukocytes, and the coagulation-fibrinolysis system. J Pathol. 2004;203:861-70.

24. Aronson D, Edelman ER. Revascularization for coronary artery disease in diabetes mellitus: angioplasty, stents and coronary artery bypass grafting. Rev Endocr Metab Disord. 2010;11:75-86.

25. Cohen DJ, Doucet M, Cutlip DE, Ho KK, Popma JJ, Kuntz RE. Impact of smoking on clinical and angiographic restenosis after percutaneous coronary intervention: another smoker's paradox? Circulation. 2001;104:773-8.

26. Park CB, Park HK. Identification of independent risk factors for restenosis following bare-metal stent implantation: Role of bare-metal stents in the era of drug-eluting stents. Exp Ther Med. 2013;6:840-6.

27. Hu RT, Liu J, Zhou Y, Hu BL. Association of smoking with restenosis and major adverse cardiac events after coronary stenting: A meta-analysis. Pak J Med Sci. 2015;31:1002-8.

28. Hong SJ, Kim MH, Ahn TH, Ahn YK, Bae JH, Shim WJ, et al. Multiple predictors of coronary restenosis after drug-eluting stent implantation in patients with diabetes. Heart. 2006;92:1119-24.

29. Ma S, Yang D, Zhang X, Tang B, Li D, Sun M, et al. Comparison of restenosis rate with sirolimus-eluting stent in STEMI patients with and without diabetes at 6-month angiographic follow-up. Acta Cardiol. 2011;66:603-6.

30. Singh M, Gersh BJ, McClelland RL, Ho KK, Willerson JT, Penny WF, et al. Clinical and angiographic predictors of restenosis after percutaneous coronary intervention: insights from the Prevention of Restenosis With Tranilast and Its Outcomes (PRESTO) trial. Circulation. 2004;109:2727-31.

17

Radiation exposure and thyroid cancer

Maria Laura Iglesias[1], Angelica Schmidt[2], Abir Al Ghuzlan[1], Ludovic Lacroix[1], Florent de Vathaire[1,3], Sylvie Chevillard[4], Martin Schlumberger[1]

ABSTRACT

The association between radiation exposure and the occurrence of thyroid cancer has been well documented, and the two main risk factors for the development of a thyroid cancer are the radiation dose delivered to the thyroid gland and the age at exposure. The risk increases after exposure to a mean dose of more than 0.05-0.1 Gy (50-100mGy). The risk is more important during childhood and decreases with increased age at exposure, being low in adults. After exposure, the minimum latency period before the appearance of thyroid cancers is 5 to 10 years. Papillary carcinoma (PTC) is the most frequent form of thyroid carcinoma diagnosed after radiation exposure, with a higher prevalence of the solid subtype in young children with a short latency period and of the classical subtype in cases with a longer latency period after exposure. Molecular alterations, including intra-chromosomal rearrangements, are frequently found. Among them, *RET/PTC* rearrangements are the most frequent. Current research is directed on the mechanism of genetic alterations induced by radiation and on a molecular signature that can identify the origin of thyroid carcinoma after a known or suspected exposure to radiation. Arch Endocrinol Metab. 2017;61(2):180-7.

Keywords

Differentiated thyroid carcinoma; radiation-induced thyroid cancer; radiation exposure; chernobyl accident

[1] Institut Gustave Roussy, Université Paris-Sud, Villejuif, France
[2] Division of Endocrinology, Hospital de Clínicas, University of Buenos Aires Buenos Aires, Argentina
[3] Cancer and Radiation Team, INSERM Unit 1018, Villejuif, France
[4] CEA, Institute of Cellular and Molecular Radiobiology, Laboratory of Experimental Cancerology, CEA, Fontenay-aux-Roses, France

Correspondence to:
Maria Laura Iglesias
Institut Gustave Roussy,
114 Rue Edouard Vaillant
94800 – Villejuif, France
maria.iglesias@gustaveroussy.fr

INTRODUCTION

The thyroid gland is highly sensitive to the carcinogenic effects of exposure to ionizing radiation during childhood and adolescence. The first relationship between radiation exposure and thyroid carcinoma was reported in 1950 after irradiation of the thymus soon after birth (1). Thyroid carcinoma was the first solid malignant tumor found with an increased incidence among Japanese atomic bomb survivors (2). Later, an increased risk of thyroid carcinoma was observed as a consequence of fallout from thermonuclear explosion in the Marshall Islands (3) and from the nuclear plant accident in Chernobyl (4). The risk is significantly increased for radiation doses to the thyroid of 50-100 mGy, and for higher doses, the risk increases with increasing radiation doses to the thyroid gland (5). The risk is maximal for radiation exposure during the first years of life and decreases with increasing age at exposure, and is low in exposed adults.

One third of thyroid tumors occurring after radiation exposure are malignant, and most radiation-induced thyroid cancers are papillary thyroid carcinoma (PTC). PTC occurs at least 5 to 10 years after radiation exposure and may occur years or decades after the exposure (6). These cancers have a clinical behavior similar to that of PTC that occurs at the same age in non-irradiated individuals and that are usually not aggressive (7).

As demonstrated for sporadic thyroid carcinomas (8), the apparent incidence of radiation-induced thyroid cancer is closely related to the modalities and intensity of screening. In South Korea where screening procedures were introduced in 2000, the apparent incidence increased by 15 folds in the subsequent years; in 2014, the "Physician Coalition for Prevention of Overdiagnosis of Thyroid Cancer" discouraged screening with ultrasound (US), resulting in a decrease in thyroid cancer incidence by 40% within 3 months (9). Similarly, the prevalence of thyroid cancer in Belarus after the Chernobyl accident or in Japan after the Fukushima accident is much higher at ultrasonography screening that at clinical examination in both exposed and non-exposed populations (10). Although most studies showed an increased incidence of thyroid cancer in patients who were exposed to radiation during childhood and adolescence, it is important to take into account that the extent of this increase could be determined by the screening procedures used to detect thyroid abnormalities.

We reviewed the current perspectives of this pathology and its clinical management.

EPIDEMIOLOGICAL DATA

External radiation

From 1920 until the 50s, external radiation was used for the treatment of children with benign conditions such as the enlargement of the thymus, skin angiomas, adenoids or neck lymph nodes, acnea, otitis, or tinea capitis. External radiation therapy to the neck for malignant diseases, such as Hodgkin's disease, may deliver high radiation doses to the thyroid gland (11), but even external radiation therapy for a thoracic or abdominal tumor in young children may deliver significant radiation doses to the thyroid gland, because of their small body size (12).

Nuclear exposure

On August 6, 1945, the U.S. Army Air Forces detonated a fission bomb over the Japanese city of Hiroshima and another bomb three days later over the city of Nagasaki. Since 1950, the Radiation Effects Research Foundation has been investigating the late health effects of the radiation exposure in atomic bomb survivors. In the cohort of 105,401 subjects, 371 thyroid cancers were identified from 1958 through 2005. The excess relative risk of thyroid cancer at age 60 after exposure at 1Gy at age 10 was estimated as 1.28 (95% confidence interval: 0.59–2.70). The risk decreased with increasing age at exposure and was minimal for those exposed after age 20. About 36% of the thyroid cancer cases among subjects exposed before age 20 were attributable to radiation exposure (13).

In March 1954, after the Bravo nuclear test on the Bikini atoll, 245 individuals were exposed to external beta and gamma radiation and to internally deposited radionuclides. Nearly 80% of the thyroid radiation dose was due to short-lived radioactive isotopes of iodine. Treatment of exposed subjects with levothyroxine was initiated in 1965, when cases of hypothyroidism and thyroid nodules were discovered. Thirty-four years after the test explosion, 55 (22%) thyroid nodules, including 16 (7%) thyroid carcinomas, were diagnosed in the 245 exposed subjects. Twenty-two (1.5%) nodules,

including 7 (0.5%) carcinomas, were found in 1,495 unexposed subjects from the same geographical region (3,14). The prevalence of hypothyroidism, thyroid nodules, and thyroid carcinoma in exposed subjects increased with the radiation dose to the thyroid gland. Females were at a higher risk (3.7 fold) of developing a thyroid nodule than males, and the risk decreased with increasing age at exposure. In 1987, the study was expanded to subjects living on atolls away from Bikini Island and showed that the frequency of thyroid nodules increased with shorter distances from Bikini Island. A more recent study was unable to confirm or refute these conclusions (15). The risk of radiation-induced thyroid tumors in fact decreases with longer follow-up, whereas the risk of spontaneous thyroid tumors increases with older age.

In 1986, after the accident at the nuclear power plant at Chernobyl in Ukraine, huge amounts of radioactivity were released in the atmosphere (over 10^{19} Bq), including large amounts of radioactive iodines (16). The radiation dose to the thyroid gland was high in Belarus, Ukraine, and South Russia because of the high level of contamination (no food restriction, no shielding, late evacuation of only some contaminated populations) and because the uptake of radioiodines in the thyroid gland was high (iodine deficiency and no iodine prophylaxis). Because of wind during the days after the accident, the radiation cloud spread over large territories in northern and western Europe. The first cases of thyroid cancers were observed in contaminated young children in 1990, only 4 years after the accident in Minsk and Kiev centers (16). The incidence of childhood thyroid carcinoma then increased, and in 1995, the incidence rate of childhood thyroid carcinoma in Belarus reached 40 per million. It is estimated that 7,000 thyroid cancer cases occurred among the 2 million highly contaminated subjects who were younger than 18 years at the time of the accident. In children, a strong relationship was found between the dose of radiation delivered to the thyroid gland and the risk of developing a thyroid cancer (17).

Important differences exist between the nuclear bombing in Japan and the accident at Chernobyl; during the atomic bombing, the irradiation was instantaneous due to gamma rays and neutrons that were released by the atomic explosion, and the entire body was irradiated. In Chernobyl, the emitted radiation involved beta and gamma rays from radioactive iodines (mainly[131] I), which were concentrated into the thyroid gland, and the exposure lasted for days, resulting in radiation doses to the thyroid gland that were 1,000 to 10,000 folds higher than the doses to other organs (16).

On March 11, 2011, during the Fukushima nuclear plant accident in Japan, large amounts of radioactive isotopes, including ^{131}I, were released. However, the radiation dose to the thyroid gland was low because the authorities ordered shielding, evacuation from the most contaminated territories, and food restriction. Furthermore, the thyroid uptake of iodine was low in relation to the high iodine alimentary intake. The average thyroid dose of residents was < 1 mSv, with a maximal dose to the thyroid gland of 33mSv., and during the 5 years following the accident, there was no increased incidence of clinical thyroid cancers (1 to 5 per million children) (10). The 300,000 people aged 18 years or younger who were living in Fukushima prefecture at the time of the accident are being submitted to ultrasonography screening. During the first screening assessment, 100 cases of thyroid cancer were found in the screened population, and a similar incidence was found in a Japanese control population of non-exposed children and adolescents. These cases were discovered soon after the accident, and in those who developed a thyroid cancer, the radiation dose to the thyroid was low (< 10 mSv.), and there is no evidence that thyroid cancer incidence is increasing with time. Therefore, there is no obvious relationship with the nuclear meltdown; furthermore, the age distribution at occurrence of thyroid cancer is similar to that observed in France and Italy in non-exposed children and was different from the age distribution observed at Chernobyl (18). The detection of these cases is related to the sensitivity of screening procedures.

FACTORS MODIFYING THE SENSITIVITY TO DEVELOPING RADIATION-RELATED THYROID CARCINOMA

Dose

The main risk factor for the development of a thyroid cancer after radiation exposure is the radiation dose delivered to the thyroid gland. In the pooled analysis of seven studies (5), which was recently extended to 12 studies (18), the risk of thyroid cancer significantly increased after a mean dose to the thyroid during childhood as low as 0.05 to 0.1 Gy (50 to 100mGy). Nevertheless, there is no dose limit below which the risk

can be totally excluded (19). For this reason, irradiating procedures such as CT scan that may deliver up to 10 mSv should be avoided in young children whenever possible, and when performed, it should deliver a minimal radiation dose.

At doses above 0.05 - 0.1 Gy, the risk increases linearly with the dose up to 20–29 Gy (OR: 9.8, 3.2–34.8), and at doses higher than 30 Gy, there is a reduction in dose response (20). This is consistent with the cell-killing hypothesis, but the risk remains significant (19,21).

In children exposed to a dose of 1 Gy to the thyroid, the relative risk of thyroid carcinoma ranges among series from 5.1 to 8.5 (17,19). It was estimated that 88% of the thyroid cancers in this group of patients are attributable to radiation exposure (5,19). A similar relative risk was observed after external radiation exposure and in contaminated children who lived in Belarus and Ukraine at the time of the Chernobyl accident (17).

In the past, it was thought that the dose rate (Gy/time unit) was an important parameter because radiation-induced thyroid tumors were observed after exposure to external radiation at high dose rates, but the study of subjects exposed to ^{131}I for medical conditions in Sweden did not reveal any increased risk of thyroid cancer (22). Also, the occurrence of thyroid tumors in the Marshall Islands was attributed to the exposure to short-lived radioisotopes of iodine. In fact, Swedish subjects were adults at the time of exposure and at an age when people are poorly sensitive to the carcinogenetic effects of radioiodine (see below). The consequences of the Chernobyl accident clearly showed that low-dose-rate exposure due to radioactive iodine contamination, including with ^{131}I, may induce thyroid tumors at a young age with similar risk factors compared to external radiation exposure at a high dose rate.

Age and latency

In the pooled analysis of 12 studies, the patients exposed to external radiation before the age of 4 years showed a fivefold greater risk per Gy of developing a thyroid cancer relative to those aged 10–14 years (19). Likewise, a study of thyroid cancer after external radiation therapy for childhood cancer found a 10-fold higher excess relative risk per Gy (ERR/Gy) for those treated with radiation at age 0–1 year relative to those aged 15–20 years (19,23). Similar data were observed in Japanese survivors of atomic bombings and after the Chernobyl accident, for whom the risk was maximal when exposed at a young age and decreased with increasing age at exposure (17,24).

The risk of thyroid cancer after exposure to external radiation was believed to be 2-3 fold higher in females than in males, but this gender effect was not confirmed in the pooled analysis of 12 studies (19) and was not found in contaminated children after the Chernobyl accident (24).

After exposure to radiation, the minimum latency period for the development of thyroid cancer was 5 to 10 years (5,6,25,26). However, a shorter interval was observed after the Chernobyl accident that may be related to the large number of contaminated children among whom few cases of thyroid cancer occurred earlier, representing a significant increased incidence due to the rarity of the disease in the general population at that young age (4). The risk increases and peaks at 20-35 years, declining thereafter; but in survivors of the Nagasaki and Hiroshima bombings, an excess risk is still present at 60 years after exposure (5,13).

Iodine status and other conditions

In the case of iodine deficiency, the thyroid uptake of radioactive iodine is high, resulting in high radiation doses to the thyroid gland. Iodine deficiency may also increase the proliferation rate of thyroid cells that may facilitate the occurrence of thyroid cancers, and this may have occurred in contaminated children in Belarus, Ukraine, and Russia (17,26,27).

In a cohort of 4,338 5-year survivors of solid childhood cancer, the thyroid cancer risk increased after splenectomy and decreased after high radiation doses to the pituitary gland. The authors hypothesized that after splenectomy, the immunological alterations could be involved in the development of thyroid carcinoma and that, after pituitary irradiation, low serum TSH levels will result in lower thyroid stimulation (12).

Until recently, chemotherapy administration was not considered to be a risk factor for thyroid carcinoma after radiation therapy for a childhood cancer or as a potential radiation dose response-modifier (5). However, it is currently considered that chemotherapy during childhood increases the risk of subsequent thyroid carcinoma by 4 folds if given alone and that the risk of chemotherapy is additive to the risk of radiation therapy when both are given (19).

The risk of thyroid carcinoma per unit of radiation dose to the thyroid was higher in subjects with a body mass index (BMI) higher than 25 or a larger BSA (body surface area) (12).

These data show that the risk for any radiation dose to the thyroid gland may be modified by many factors, but as already stated, screening biases should always be kept in mind.

Other thyroid pathologies

Several other thyroid abnormalities may be caused by radiation exposure (28). The risk of hypothyroidism, probably as a consequence of cellular death, increases with the radiation dose.

In a study of 4,091 Hiroshima and Nagasaki survivors, autoimmune thyroid diseases were not associated with radiation exposure (29). In a study of patients irradiated for Hodgkin's disease, the risk of Graves' disease was significantly increased (11). Finally, several studies have indicated that low-doses of radiation to the thyroid could be associated with an increased prevalence of anti-thyroid antibodies (30), but these associations remain controversial.

Personal and familial susceptibility

A familial susceptibility to radiation-induced thyroid cancer has been suggested by the pedigree of some families in which several irradiated individuals have developed a thyroid tumor more often that would be expected by chance. Also, the association of thyroid, parathyroid, salivary gland, or neural tumors in a subject exposed to radiation to the neck suggests a predisposition to develop tumors after radiation exposure. However, the natural history of the thyroid cancer was not altered by any familial concordance (31).

PATHOLOGY AND MOLECULAR BIOLOGY

PTC is the most frequent form of thyroid carcinoma diagnosed after radiation exposure. After the Chernobyl accident, most young children had a solid or follicular PTC subtype with an aggressive behavior and a short latency period, whereas older children had more frequently classical PTC that was less aggressive and was discovered after a longer latency period. Solid subtype was also frequently observed in the rare PTC that occurred in young children in the absence of any radiation exposure, demonstrating that this subtype is associated with a younger age at occurrence of the tumor (16,32).

Ionizing radiations induce DNA damage either directly or by generating reactive oxygen species (ROS) (16). The thyroid tissue contains a high quantity of NADPH oxidases, which are specialized ROS-generating enzymes that are known as NOX/DUOX. Radiation exposure increases DUOX1 expression, leading to an important production of ROS in the thyroid gland after radiation exposure, and this may explain its high sensitivity to radiation (33). This DNA damage includes single- or double-strand breaks that will result in deletions and chromosomal rearrangements.

Normal thyrocytes multiply during body growth, especially before the age of 5 years, and this will favor the accumulation of genetic defects after radiation exposure. Mitotic rate decreases with age and becomes very low in adults. This may explain the high sensitivity of the thyroid gland to the carcinogenic effects of radiation at birth, which decreases with increasing age, becoming low or not significant after the age of 15-20 years (5,16,26,27).

In PTC occurring after radiation exposure, intra-chromosomal rearrangements are frequently observed. RET/PTC rearrangements consist in the fusion of the tyrosine kinase domain of RET with the NH2 terminal domain of another gene that is ubiquitously expressed, resulting in the constitutive expression of the transcript. RET/PTC3 rearrangement was the most frequently observed rearrangement in aggressive PTC that occurred in young children soon after the Chernobyl accident, and RET/PTC1 rearrangement was more frequently observed in classical PTC that occurred later after the accident. Other RET/PTC rearrangements have been found in Chernobyl thyroid cancers that may differ either by the partner gene or by the breakpoint site (34-40). In a series of 26 papillary thyroid cancers that occurred in highly contaminated children in Ukraine, kinase fusion oncogenes resulting from intra-chromosomal rearrangements that activate the mitogen-activated kinase pathway (MAP kinase pathway) were found in 23 (including RET/PTC, BRAF, and TRK rearrangements), and BRAF (n = 2) and TSHR (n = 1) gene point mutations were found in only 3 tumors (36). In contrast, in 27 sporadic papillary thyroid cancers that occurred in non-contaminated children from Ukraine, gene rearrangements were found in 9, and BRAF (n = 7) or NRAS (n = 2) gene

point mutations were found in 9 tumors, and no driver mutation was found in 9 tumors. In conclusion, in radiation-induced PTC, gene rearrangements are frequently found and point mutations are infrequent; in rare PTCs occurring in children in the absence of previous radiation exposure, RET/PTC gene rearrangements are more frequent than in adults but less frequent than in radiation-induced PTC (41).

A transcriptomic signature that includes genes that are differently expressed in sporadic tumors relative to tumors occurring after external radiation exposure during childhood permits the distinction of these two groups of tumors with a sensitivity of 0.92 and a specificity of 0.85 (42). Furthermore, this signature allows for classifying tumors from Belarus and Ukraine as either sporadic or occurring in highly contaminated subjects during the Chernobyl accident (43). These data confirm previous studies (44-47) and suggest that radiation-induced tumors may have some specific molecular characteristics, but this should be confirmed on a larger series of tumors.

MANAGEMENT

The risk of developing a thyroid cancer and its temporal pattern of occurrence is of clinical importance for the long-term surveillance of late effects of radiation to the neck. In daily practice, the clinician could be in front of patients who have been exposed to external radiation or patients with thyroid abnormalities that require the search for a history of radiation exposure (28).

In the case of external radiation exposure, the risk of radiation-induced thyroid tumor can be estimated according to the age at exposure and the dose delivered to the thyroid gland; additionally, it is important to search for other effects of radiation and a personal or family history of head and neck tumors.

An exhaustive physical examination and ultrasonography of the thyroid gland and of lymph node areas are performed. Also abnormalities that may be induced by radiation exposure to the neck such as tumors of the salivary glands, hyperparathyroidism, and neural tumors should be screened.

Laboratory tests include screening for hypothyroidism (TSH) and hyperparathyroidism (calcium). Radiation exposure during childhood increases the risk of hyperparathyroidism, and this risk increases with radiation doses (48,49). Subjects exposed to radiation with high Tg levels and with a normal clinical examination have an increased risk of developing thyroid nodules (50).

Patients with a history of radiation exposure during childhood (Figure 1) should be submitted to follow-up for life. Patients without abnormalities can be evaluated every 1 to 5 years, according to risk factors.

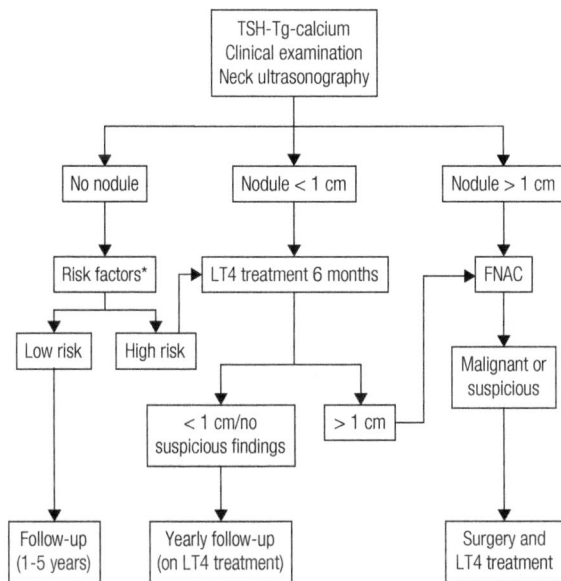

Figure 1. Work-up of subjects with a history of external radiation during childhood.

* Risk factors include young age at radiation exposure, high radiation dose to the neck, personal and familial susceptibility, and elevated serum Tg concentrations. Levothyroxine therapy is considered if needed to maintain a TSH in the low-to-normal reference range.

Solid thyroid nodules larger than 1 cm in diameter are submitted to fine needle biopsy for cytology. If multiple nodules are found, the fine needle biopsy is indicated in nodules that are suspicious at ultrasound. Patients with sub-centimeter nodules are controlled every 1-2 years with ultrasonography.

Hypothyroidism is treated with levothyroxine. In addition, levothyroxine treatment is considered in euthyroid patients with high risk factors and in patients with small nodules in order to maintain the serum TSH levels in the low normal range.

If the cytology suggests the presence of a papillary carcinoma, a total thyroidectomy is recommended. Total thyroidectomy is also performed when surgery has been decided for an apparently benign nodule, with the aim of reducing the risk of nodule recurrence.

PREVENTION

Evaluation of the consequences of the Chernobyl accident has clearly demonstrated that contamination with radioactive isotopes of iodine during childhood increases the risk of developing a thyroid cancer. It is therefore warranted to avoid any thyroid irradiation in case of atmospheric contamination by means of shielding, food restrictions, and evacuation if necessary and with the administration of large amounts of stable iodine.

Stable iodine, administered as potassium iodide (KI), inhibits the thyroid uptake of radioactive iodine by more than 98% if it is administered several hours before contamination, by 90% at the time of the contamination, and by 50% if it is given 6 hours after the accident. Uptake will be low during 48-72 hours and then will re-increase.

KI prophylaxis should be administered in priority to children and pregnant women. It is not recommended for people over 60 years or those with cardio-vascular disease. KI can induce thyrotoxicosis in subjects with nodular goiter or thyroid autonomy. In Poland, after the Chernobyl accident, KI doses were distributed to over 18 million subjects, and no case of thyrotoxicosis has been reported, and only a few subjects had symptoms (51). The newborns of mothers who took KI at the end of their pregnancies had increased serum TSH at birth, but this was transient, and no neurological sequelae were observed.

In France, KI was distributed to the population that lives within 10 kilometers of one of the 19 French nuclear power plants (52). In case of atmospheric contamination, the public authorities will establish the need for and timing of iodine prophylaxis.

In France, each tablet contains 65 mg of KI (equivalent to 50 mg of iodine) with a chemical stability of at least 5 years. The tablets can be dissolved in water, milk, or fruit juice and can be divided in 4 pieces. It is not recommended to ingest these tablets with an empty stomach. The recommended doses are: 100 mg of iodine (130 mg KI, two tablets) for adult subjects (including pregnant women); 50 mg of iodine (65 mg KI, one tablet) for children below 13 years of age; 25 mg of iodine (32.5 mg KI, half tablet) for children below 3 years of age; 12.5 mg of iodine (16 mg KI, quarter tablet) for newborns.

For the International Atomic Energy Agency, the intervention level for the administration of stable iodine is when the thyroid gland of children may receive an estimated dose of 50 mSv or more (53,54). Western nuclear reactors are fitted with filters that will decrease the magnitude of atmospheric contamination and with an isolating barrier (not present at the Chernobyl plant), which should ensure a delay of several hours between a serious accident and the release of radioactive material into the atmosphere. Public authorities must capitalize on this time interval to organize iodine prophylaxis.

CONCLUSION

The consequences of radiation exposure of the thyroid gland are well known. The risk of thyroid carcinoma after exposure to doses higher than 0.05 - 0.1 Gy is higher in younger children at the time of exposure. All efforts should be performed to avoid any radiation exposure during childhood.

Acknowledgements: Université Paris Sud – Faculté de Médecine Paris Sud (Kremlin-Bicêtre). Diplôme Universitaire Européen de Recherche Translationnelle Et Clinique en Cancérologie – DUERTECC.

REFERENCES

1. Duffy BJ, Fitzgerald PJ. Thyroid cancer in childhood and adolescence. A report on twenty-eight cases. Cancer. 1950;3(6):1018-32.

2. Socolow EL, Hashizume A, Neriishi S, Niitani R. Thyroid carcinoma in man after exposure to ionizing radiation. A summary of the findings in Hiroshima and Nagasaki. N Engl J Med. 1963;268: 406-10.

3. Conard RA, Dobyns BM, Sutow WW. Thyroid neoplasia as late effect of exposure to radioactive iodine in fallout. JAMA. 1970;214(2):316-24.

4. Kazakov VS, Demidchik EP, Astakhova LN. Thyroid cancer after Chernobyl. Nature. 1992;359(6390):21.

5. Ron E, Lubin JH, Shore RE, Mabuchi K, Modan B, Pottern LM, et al. Thyroid cancer after exposure to external radiation: a pooled analysis of seven studies. 1995. Radiat Res. 2012;178(2):AV43-60.

6. Schneider AB, Ron E, Lubin J, Stovall M, Gierlowski TC. Dose-response relationships for radiation-induced thyroid cancer and thyroid nodules: evidence for the prolonged effects of radiation on the thyroid. J Clin Endocrinol Metab. 1993;77(2):362-9.

7. Naing S, Collins BJ, Schneider AB. Clinical behavior of radiation-induced thyroid cancer: factors related to recurrence. Thyroid. 2009;19(5):479-85.

8. Vaccarella S, Franceschi S, Bray F, Wild CP, Plummer M, Dal Maso L. Worldwide thyroid-cancer epidemic? The increasing impact of overdiagnosis. N Engl J Med. 2016;375(7):614-7.

9. Ahn HS, Welch HG. South Korea's thyroid-cancer "epidemic" -- Turning the tide. N Engl J Med. 2015;373(24):2389-90.

10. Suzuki S, Suzuki S, Fukushima T, Midorikawa S, Shimura H, Matsuzuka T, et al. Comprehensive survey results of childhood thyroid ultrasound examinations in Fukushima in the first four years after the Fukushima Daiichi Nuclear Power Plant accident. Thyroid. 2016;26(6):843-51.

11. Hancock SL, Cox RS, McDougall IR. Thyroid diseases after treatment of Hodgkin's disease. N Engl J Med. 1991;325(9):599-605.

12. de Vathaire F, Haddy N, Allodji RS, Hawkins M, Guibout C, El-Fayech C, et al. Thyroid radiation dose and other risk factors of thyroid carcinoma following childhood cancer. J Clin Endocrinol Metab. 2015;100(11):4282-90.

13. Furukawa K, Preston D, Funamoto S, Yonehara S, Ito M, Tokuoka S, et al. Long-term trend of thyroid cancer risk among Japanese atomic-bomb survivors: 60 years after exposure. Int J Cancer. 2013;132(5):1222-6.

14. Dobyns BM, Hyrmer BA. The surgical management of benign and malignant thyroid neoplasms in Marshall Islanders exposed to hydrogen bomb fallout. World J Surg. 1992;16(1):126-39.

15. Takahashi T, Schoemaker MJ, Trott KR, Simon SL, Fujimori K, Nakashima N, et al. The relationship of thyroid cancer with radiation exposure from nuclear weapon testing in the Marshall Islands. J Epidemiol. 2003;13(2):99-107.

16. Williams D. Radiation carcinogenesis: Lessons from Chernobyl. Oncogene. 2008;27(Suppl. 2):S9-18.

17. Cardis E, Kesminiene A, Ivanov V, Malakhova I, Shibata Y, Khrouch V, et al. Risk of thyroid cancer after exposure to 131I in childhood. J Natl Cancer Inst. 2005;97(10):724-32.

18. Pacini F, Vorontsova T, Demidchik EP, Molinaro E, Agate L, Romei C, et al. Post-Chernobyl thyroid carcinoma in Belarus children and adolescents: comparison with naturally occurring thyroid carcinoma in Italy and France. J Clin Endocrinol Metab. 1997;82(11):3563-9.

19. Veiga LHS, Holmberg E, Anderson H, Pottern L, Sadetzki S, Adams MJ, et al. Thyroid cancer after childhood exposure to external radiation: an updated pooled analysis of 12 studies. Radiat Res. 2016;185(5):473-84.

20. Sigurdson AJ, Ronckers CM, Mertens AC, Stovall M, Smith SA, Liu Y, et al. Primary thyroid cancer after a first tumour in childhood (the Childhood Cancer Survivor Study): a nested case-control study. Lancet. 2005;365(9476):2014-23.

21. Gray LH. Radiation biology and cancer. In: Cellular radiation biology: a collection of works presented at the 18th Annual Symposium on Experimental Cancer Research 1964. Baltimore: Williams and Wilkins; 1965; 7-25.

22. Holm LE, Wiklund KE, Lundell GE, Bergman NA, Bjelkengren G, Ericsson UB, et al. Cancer risk in population examined with diagnostic doses of 131I. J Natl Cancer Inst. 1989;81(4):302-6.

23. Veiga LHS, Lubin JH, Anderson H, de Vathaire F, Tucker M, Bhatti P, et al. A pooled analysis of thyroid cancer incidence following radiotherapy for childhood cancer. Radiat Res. 2012;178(4):365-76.

24. Boice JD. Thyroid disease 60 years after Hiroshima and 20 years after Chernobyl. JAMA. 2006;295(9):1060-2.

25. de Vathaire F, Hardiman C, Shamsaldin A, Campbell S, Grimaud E, Hawkins M, et al. Thyroid carcinomas after irradiation for a first cancer during childhood. Arch Intern Med. 1999;159(22):2713-9.

26. Saad AG, Kumar S, Ron E, Lubin JH, Stanek J, Bove KE, et al. Proliferative activity of human thyroid cells in various age groups and its correlation with the risk of thyroid cancer after radiation exposure. J Clin Endocrinol Metab. 2006;91(7):2672-7.

27. Williams ED, Abrosimov A, Bogdanova T, Demidchik EP, Ito M, LiVolsi V, et al. Morphologic characteristics of Chernobyl-related childhood papillary thyroid carcinomas are independent of radiation exposure but vary with iodine intake. Thyroid. 2008;18(8):847-52.

28. Sinnott B, Ron E, Schneider AB. Exposing the thyroid to radiation: a review of its current extent, risks, and implications. Endocr Rev. 2010;31(5):756-73.

29. Imaizumi M, Usa T, Tominaga T, Neriishi K, Akahoshi M, Nakashima E, et al. Radiation dose-response relationships for thyroid nodules and autoimmune thyroid diseases in Hiroshima and Nagasaki atomic bomb survivors 55-58 years after radiation exposure. JAMA. 2006;295(9):1011-22.

30. Eheman CR, Garbe P, Tuttle RM. Autoimmune thyroid disease associated with environmental thyroidal irradiation. Thyroid. 2003;13(5):453-64.

31. Momani MS, Shore-Freedman E, Collins BJ, Lubin J, Ron E, Schneider AB. Familial concordance of thyroid and other head and neck tumors in an irradiated cohort: analysis of contributing factors. J Clin Endocrinol Metab. 2004;89(5):2185-91.

32. Schlumberger M, De Vathaire F, Travagli JP, Vassal G, Lemerle J, Parmentier C, et al. Differentiated thyroid carcinoma in childhood: long term follow-up of 72 patients. J Clin Endocrinol Metab. 1987;65(6):1088-94.

33. Ameziane-El-Hassani R, Talbot M, de Souza Dos Santos MC, Al Ghuzlan A, Hartl D, Bidart J-M, et al. NADPH oxidase DUOX1 promotes long-term persistence of oxidative stress after an exposure to irradiation. Proc Natl Acad Sci U S A. 2015;112(16):5051-6.

34. Leeman-Neill RJ, Brenner AV, Little MP, Bogdanova TI, Hatch M, Zurnadzy LY, et al. RET/PTC and PAX8/PPARγ chromosomal rearrangements in post-Chernobyl thyroid cancer and their association with iodine-131 radiation dose and other characteristics. Cancer. 2013;119(10):1792-9.

35. Challeton C, Bounacer A, Du Villard JA, Caillou B, De Vathaire F, Monier R, et al. Pattern of ras and gsp oncogene mutations in radiation-associated human thyroid tumors. Oncogene. 1995;11(3):601-3.

36. Ricarte-Filho JC, Li S, Garcia-Rendueles MER, Montero-Conde C, Voza F, Knauf JA, et al. Identification of kinase fusion oncogenes in post-Chernobyl radiation-induced thyroid cancers. J Clin Invest. 2013;123(11):4935-44.

37. Rabes HM, Demidchik EP, Sidorow JD, Lengfelder E, Beimfohr C, Hoelzel D, et al. Pattern of radiation-induced RET and NTRK1 rearrangements in 191 post-Chernobyl papillary thyroid carcinomas: biological, phenotypic, and clinical implications. Clin Cancer Res. 2000;6(3):1093-103.

38. Fugazzola L, Pilotti S, Pinchera A, Vorontsova TV, Mondellini P, Bongarzone I, et al. Oncogenic rearrangements of the RET proto-oncogene in papillary thyroid carcinomas from children exposed to the Chernobyl nuclear accident. Cancer Res. 1995;55(23):5617-20.

39. Ito T, Seyama T, Iwamoto KS, Mizuno T, Tronko ND, Komissarenko IV, et al. Activated RET oncogene in thyroid cancers of children from areas contaminated by Chernobyl accident. Lancet. 1994;344(8917):259.

40. Klugbauer S, Lengfelder E, Demidchik EP, Rabes HM. High prevalence of RET rearrangement in thyroid tumors of children from Belarus after the Chernobyl reactor accident. Oncogene. 1995;11(12):2459-67.

41. Sassolas G, Hafdi-Nejjari Z, Ferraro A, Decaussin-Petrucci M, Rousset B, Borson-Chazot F, et al. Oncogenic alterations in papillary thyroid cancers of young patients. Thyroid. 2012;22(1):17-26.

42. Ory C, Ugolin N, Levalois C, Lacroix L, Caillou B, Bidart JM, et al. Gene expression signature discriminates sporadic from post-radiotherapy-induced thyroid tumors. Endocr Relat Cancer. 2011;18(1):193-206.

43. Ory C, Ugolin N, Schlumberger M, Hofman P, Chevillard S. Discriminating gene expression signature of radiation-induced thyroid tumors after either external exposure or internal contamination. Genes. 2011;3(1):19-34.

44. Port M, Boltze C, Wang Y, Röper B, Meineke V, Abend M. A radiation-induced gene signature distinguishes post-Chernobyl from sporadic papillary thyroid cancers. Radiat Res. 2007;168(6):639-49.

45. Stein L, Rothschild J, Luce J, Cowell JK, Thomas G, Bogdanova TI, et al. Copy number and gene expression alterations in radiation-induced papillary thyroid carcinoma from Chernobyl pediatric patients. Thyroid. 2010;20(5):475-87.

46. Suzuki K, Mitsutake N, Saenko V, Yamashita S. Radiation signatures in childhood thyroid cancers after the Chernobyl accident: possible roles of radiation in carcinogenesis. Cancer Sci. 2015;106(2):127-33.

47. Ugolin N, Ory C, Lefevre E, Benhabiles N, Hofman P, Schlumberger M, et al. Strategy to find molecular signatures in a small series of rare cancers: validation for radiation-induced breast and thyroid tumors. PloS One. 2011;6(8):e23581.

48. Fujiwara S, Sposto R, Shiraki M, Yokoyama N, Sasaki H, Kodama K, et al. Levels of parathyroid hormone and calcitonin in serum among atomic bomb survivors. Radiat Res. 1994;137(1):96-103.

49. Colaço SM, Si M, Reiff E, Clark OH. Hyperparathyroidism after radioactive iodine therapy. Am J Surg. 2007;194(3):323-7.

50. Schneider AB, Bekerman C, Leland J, Rosengarten J, Hyun H, Collins B, et al. Thyroid nodules in the follow-up of irradiated individuals: comparison of thyroid ultrasound with scanning and palpation. J Clin Endocrinol Metab. 1997;82(12):4020-7.

51. Nauman J, Wolff J. Iodide prophylaxis in Poland after the Chernobyl reactor accident: benefits and risks. Am J Med. 1993;94(5):524-32.

52. Le Guen B, Stricker L, Schlumberger M. Distributing KI pills to minimize thyroid radiation exposure in case of a nuclear accident in France. Nat Clin Pract Endocrinol Metab. 2007;3(9):611.

53. International Agency for Energy Atomic (IAEA). Intervention Criteria in a Nuclear or Radiation Emergency. 1994.

54. International Commission on Radiological Protection (IRCP). Principles for Intervention for Protection of the Public in a Radiological Emergency. 1991.

18

Evaluation of salivary oxidative parameters in overweight and obese young adults

Eduardo Ottobelli Chielle[1], Jeferson Noslen Casarin[1]

ABSTRACT

Background: Obesity is characterized by a deposition of abnormal or excessive fat in adipose tissue, and is linked with a risk of damage to several metabolic and pathological processes associated with oxidative stress. To date, salivary oxidative biomarkers have been minimally explored in obese individuals. Thus, the aim of this study was to assess the concentrations of salivary oxidative biomarkers (ferric-reducing antioxidant power, uric acid, sulfhydryl groups) and lipid peroxidation in obese and overweight young subjects. **Materials and methods:** Levels of lipid peroxidation, ferric-reducing antioxidant power, uric acid, and SH groups were determined in the saliva and serum of 149 young adults, including 54 normal weight, 27 overweight, and 68 obese individuals. Anthropometric measurements were also evaluated. **Results:** Salivary levels of ferric-reducing antioxidant power, sulfhydryl groups, and lipid peroxidation, as well as serum levels of ferric-reducing antioxidant power, uric acid, and lipid peroxidation were higher in obese patients when compared with individuals with normal weight. There were correlations between salivary and serum ferric-reducing antioxidant power and salivary and serum uric acid in the obese and normal-weight groups. **Conclusions:** Our results indicate that the increase in salivary levels of ferric-reducing antioxidant power, sulfhydryl groups, and lipid peroxidation, and serum levels of ferric-reducing antioxidant power, uric acid, and lipid peroxidation could be related to the regulation of various processes in the adipose tissue. These findings may hold promise in identifying new oxidative markers to assist in diagnosing and monitoring overweight and obese patients. Arch Endocrinol Metab. 2017;61(2):152-9.

Keywords
Obesity; biomarkers; oxidative stress; saliva; antioxidants

[1] Departamento de Ciências da Saúde, Laboratório de Bioquímica Clínica, Universidade do Oeste de Santa Catarina (Unoesc), São Miguel do Oeste, SC, Brasil

Correspondence to:
Eduardo Ottobelli Chielle
Rua Oiapoc, 211
89900-000 – São Miguel do Oeste, SC, Brasil
eduardochielle@yahoo.com.br

INTRODUCTION

Reactive oxygen species (ROS) and reactive nitrogen species (RNS) play an important role in cell signaling and metabolic pathways in physiological conditions. On the other hand, decreased antioxidant levels and/or increased production of reactive metabolites may disrupt homeostatic processes and lead to oxidative damage (1,2). Oxidative/nitrosative stress may have a serious impact on cell viability and induce cellular responses leading to cell death (3). Many studies have shown a connection between oxidative molecular damage and pathophysiological mechanisms associated with severe diseases such as atherosclerosis (4), neurodegenerative disorders (5), and diabetes, and an important role in the etiopathogenesis of inflammatory diseases (6). There is also a relationship between oxidative stress and aging processes (7).

Obesity is associated with an increase in oxidative stress, defined as an increased load of free radicals comprised of ROS and RNS generated during cellular metabolism (8). These free radicals are chemically reactive molecules that may damage cellular proteins, membranes, and DNA. The increase in oxidative stress is considered to be involved in the pathogenesis of insulin resistance and type 2 diabetes (T2DM) associated with obesity (9,10). Data from studies with cell culture systems have shown that products of oxidative stress impair insulin-mediated translocation of GLUT4 in myotubes and adipocytes and suppress the transcription of the insulin gene in β cells and adiponectin in adipocytes (11,12).

On the other hand, most cells have an adequate protective system to circumvent harmful oxidative events. This system is composed of antioxidant enzymes (superoxide dismutase, catalase, and many other peroxidases) and nonenzymatic antioxidants, including the glutathione (SH groups), uric acid, ascorbate, and ferric-reducing antioxidant power (FRAP) (13). Was observed a progressive increase TBARS levels in accordance with the increase in body weight and progressive decrease in SH groups and FRAP according to body weight gain (14). The increased oxidative stress in vascular walls is involved in the pathogenesis of atherosclerosis, hypertension and induces damage to cell structures, including membranes, proteins, and ADN and this contributes to disorders cardiometabolic (15).

The major antioxidant capacity toward named oxidants is represented by numerous thiol groups (SH groups) in intracellular and extracellular compartments. At the same time, thiols are also the major targets for ROS and RNS. It is well known that the serum SH groups levels are modified in many diseases, including obesity, indicating that SH groups content is a useful biochemical marker of "in vivo" oxido-reduction reactions (16). Membrane SH groups are liable to be modified by different oxidants or alkylating agents, increasing their membrane permeability to different ions, such as Ca^{++}, which can promote excitotoxicity, by RNS and ROS that lead to lipid peroxidation, increasing the levels of TBARS and decreased concentration of SH groups in membrane proteins (17). Thiol-containing molecules with SH bonds such as glutathione (GSH) suppress oxidative damage and involve the maintenance of the cell redox status. In healthy tissues, these antioxidants work in cooperative to maintain the pro oxidant antioxidant balance and prevent tissue damage and disease (18).

The saliva also has antioxidant properties attributed to its composition of enzymatic (mostly peroxidase system) and nonenzymatic compounds (uric acid, glutathione, sialic acid), which may be determined in salivary samples (19,20). Sampling of human saliva is an attractive means to diagnose and monitor diseases since the saliva may be collected easily and noninvasively. Analysis of the saliva may also be beneficial to predict the progression of future diseases (14,21,22). As a clinical tool, saliva has many advantages over serum, including ease of collection, storing, and shipping. Saliva is composed of organic and inorganic elements and represents an important fluid in the oral cavity that has been used as a sample to diagnose and control the treatment of systemic diseases and disorders (23). Measurement of oxidative biomarkers in the saliva to examine numerous clinical conditions has increased over the last decade (24).

Thus, considering the fact that obesity is a chronic state that involves diverse pathways such as oxidative stress, inflammation, and endothelial dysfunction, the aim of this study was to assess the salivary and serum levels of oxidative biomarkers in obese and overweight subjects and analyze the correlation between salivary and serum parameters.

MATERIALS AND METHODS

Study population

Participants were recruited from January to August 2014 in São Miguel do Oeste located in south of Brazil. The protocol of the study was approved by the Ethics Committee of the University of West Santa Catarina (UNOESC, N° 219.091) and all participants provided writ- ten informed consent. Experiments were performed in 149 subjects. A total of 54 normal weight subjects with gender-matched healthy volunteers served as a control group (32 females and 22 males). The subjects with increased weight were divided in two subgroups, matching for sex, age, and body mass index, and were enrolled as follows: 1) 27 overweight subjects (17 females and 10 males); 2) 68 obese young subjects (41 females and 27 males). The participants were non-smokers and were not using any medications, as shown in Table 1.

Anthropometric measurements

All measures were taken in the Anthropometry Laboratory at the University of West Santa Catarina, São Miguel do Oeste, SC (Table 1). Standing height (H, cm) was measured to the nearest 0.1 cm using a wall-mounted stadiometer (Charder model HM-210D). Weight (W, kg) was measured to the nearest 0.1 kg using a calibrated electronic scale (Toledo model 2124). BMI was calculated as W/H^2 (kg/m^2). Waist circumference (WC), neck circumference (NC) and hip circumference (HC) was measured in centimeters with a flexible tape to the nearest 0.1 cm. For AC the tape was applied above the iliac crest with the subject standing with the abdomen relaxed, arms at sides and feet together. NC for the participant remained in the same position and tape was placed on half of the neck on the hyoid bone. The percentages of fat and fat weight were determined by bioimpedance (Biodynamics Model 450). Systolic and diastolic pressure (SBP, DBP) was measured in the individual after being seated and resting for 10 minutes, with a digital apparatus and were expressed in mmHg. All measurements were taken on the left side of the body, according to standardized procedures by Weiner and Lourie (11). During the anthropometric measurements, all participants were barefoot and clothed appropriately.

Indices and classifications

According to the World Health Organization, underweight was defined as BMI < 18.5 kg/m^2, normal weight as BMI 18.5–24.9 kg/m^2, overweight as BMI 25–29.9 kg/m^2, and obesity as a BMI > 30 kg/m^2 (12), all without comorbidities. According to Gallagher and cols. (13) % fat $\geq$ 20% (males) and % fat $\geq$ 33% (females) are the cut-points adopted to define over fatness, corresponding to overweight classification using BMI in a population of young adults. According to the National Institute for Health and Clinical Excellence guidelines, WC $\geq$ 102 cm for men and $\geq$ 88 cm for women are prerequisite risk factors for the diagnosis of the metabolic syndrome, as Waist-Hip Ratio (WHR) $\geq$ 0.9 for males and $\geq$ 0.8 females (25).

Saliva sampling

A well defined and standardized protocol was used for collection, storage, and processing of all the samples under the exactly same conditions. Unstimulated saliva samples were collected in the morning after fasting for at least 8 h. Brushing teeth, smoking, eating or drinking anything but water for at least 60 min prior to sampling were prohibited. For the collection of salivary samples, patients were asked to put and keep the cotton swab under tongue for Laboratory analyzes 3 min and then to place it back directly into the plastic container according to the manufacture's instruction (Salivette tubes, Sarstedt, Nümbrecht, Germany). The collections were made in the laboratory under the guidance and supervision of researchers. Immediately after collecting the saliva samples were centrifuged for 10 min at 1100g, fractionated in eppendorf and were stored at –20°C until analysis (19). Approximately 200 µL of thawed saliva samples was processed for enzymatic and biochemical tests. To avoid the effects of protein degradation, the samples that had been thawed were not reused.

Laboratory methods

Determination of Ferric-Reducing Antioxidant Power (FRAP): salivary and serun FRAP levels were measured according to Singh and cols., (20). Two hundred µL of prewarmed 37°C FRAP reagent (1 volume of 3 mol/L acetate buffer, pH 3.6 + 1 vol of 10 mmol/L 2,4,6-tripyridyl-S-triazine in 40 mmol/L HCl + 1 vol of 20 mmol/L FeCl$_3$) was mixed with 20 µL of saliva. Absorbance was read at 593 nm. Ferrous sulphate was used as standard and the concentration of FRAP was expressed in µmol/L. All other chemicals were obtained from Sigma Chemical Co. (St. Louis, MO, USA).

Determination of Thiobarbituric Acid Reactive Substances (TBARS): lipid peroxidation was estimated in plasma and salivary by measurement of thiobarbituric acid reactive substances (TBARS) according to the method of Lapenna and cols. (23), using 1% phosphoric acid and 0.6% thiobarbituric acid (TBA). The reaction product was measured spectrophotometrically at 532 nm and the results were expressed in nmol TBARS/mL.

Determination of Protein thiol groups (SH groups): protein thiol groups were assayed in salivary and plasma by the method of Boyne and Ellman (24) which consist of the reduction of 5.5'-dithio(bis-nithrobenzoic) acid (DTNB) in pH 7.0, measured at 412 nm. The results were expressed in nmol P-SH/mL.

Statistical analysis

The data were analyzed using Statistica 6.0 software (StatSoft, Tulsa, OK, USA). Data are expressed as means $\pm$ SD or median (interquartile ranges). The Kolmogorov-Smirnov test was used to examine the distribution of variables. Comparisons of baseline data among the groups were performed using One-way ANOVA followed by Tukey's test or Kruskal Wallis test followed by Dunn's Multiple Comparison Test. Spearman or Pearson correlation coefficients were calculated to describe crude associations between variables (bivariate correlation) and the effect of potential confounding factors was tested in multivariate linear regression models. A p-value of < 0.05 was considered statistically significant.

RESULTS

The baseline characteristics of the study participants are described in Table 1. As expected, systolic blood pressure (SBP) and diastolic blood pressure (DBP), weight, body mass index (BMI), neck, hip and waist circumferences, body fat percentage, and body fat mass were higher in obese when compared with normal-weight subjects ($p < 0.0001$).

Levels of salivary FRAP and SH groups were significantly elevated in the obese group when compared with the normal-weight group ($p < 0.05$ and $p < 0.0001$, respectively). There were no significant differences in levels of salivary uric acid among the groups. The degree of lipid peroxidation, measured by levels of salivary TBARS, were significantly higher in the obese group compared with the normal-weight group ($p < 0.0001$), as shown in Table 2.

Serum levels of FRAP, uric acid, and TBARS were significantly elevated in the obese group when compared with the normal-weight group ($p < 0.05$, $p < 0.0001$, and $p < 0.05$, respectively). In contrast, levels of SH groups were significantly decreased in the obese group when compared with the normal-weight group ($p < 0.0001$), as shown in Table 3.

Correlation analyses were performed between antioxidant parameters and salivary and serum lipid peroxidation levels among the study groups. As shown in Table 4, there were significant correlations between salivary and serum levels of uric acid ($r = 0.5162$, $p < 0.0001$) and FRAP ($r = 0.4361$, $p = 0.001$) in the normal-weight group. This positive correlation was also observed in the obese group ($r = 0.4205$ and $p = 0.0004$ for uric acid, and $r = 0.4482$ and $p = 0.0001$ for FRAP), as shown in Table 5. No other positive correlations were observed in the other groups and parameters.

Table 1. Baseline characteristics of study participants

	Groups		
	Normal weight	Overweight	Obese
N	54	27	68
Male/Female	22/32	10/17	27/41
Age (years)	21.0 (19.8-24.0)	24.0 (21.0-26.0)	25.0 (22.0-27.0)
Weight (kg)	60.1 ± 9.4	77.2 ± 7.0[a]	97.7 ± 16.0[ab]
Height (cm)	167.8 ± 7.3	167.0 ± 8.3	166.8 ± 10.5
BMI (kg/m²)	20.9 (19.3 – 22.6)	28.1 (26.5 – 28.7)[a]	34.1 (32.4 – 37.5)[ab]
NC (cm)	36.0 ± 4.3	36.0 ± 3.3	38.8 ± 3.5[ab]
WC (cm)	72.3 ± 6.8	87.7 ± 6.3[a]	104.2 ± 13.7[ab]
HC (cm)	95.7 ± 6.2	107.1 ± 5.5[a]	117.8 ± 8.9[ab]
SBP (mmHg)	120.9 ± 11.7	126.3 ± 11.2	136.7 ± 14.2[ab]
DBP (mmHg)	72.0 (67.8 – 80.0)	81.0 (73.0 – 89.0)[a]	86.0 (77.0 – 93.0)[a]
Body fat (%)	25.3 (18.9 – 28.9)	33.3 (27.4 – 36.8)[a]	38.7 (34.8 – 41.6)[ab]
Fat body mass (kg)	14.9 (12.7 – 17.9)	24.2 (21.0 – 28.3)[a]	36.1 (31.1 – 40.7)[ab]

Data are expressed as means ± SD or median (interquartile ranges). Data were processed for analysis for One-way ANOVA followed by Tukey's test or Kruskal Wallis test followed by Dunn's Multiple Comparison Test. BMI: body mass index; NC: neck circumference; WC: waist circumference; HC: hip circumference; SBP: systolic blood pressure; DBP: diastolic blood pressure.
[a] $p < 0.0001$ compared to normal weight group.
[b] $p < 0.0001$ compared to overweight group.

Table 2. Concentration of salivary antioxidants and lipid peroxidation in the groups studied

	Groups		
	Normal weight	Overweight	Obese
N	54	27	68
Uric acid (mg/dL)	1.7 (1.4 – 2.4)	1.8 (1.4 – 2.6)	1.9 (1.4 – 2.3)
FRAP (mmol/L)	0.37 (0.29 – 0.46)	0.38 (0.35 – 0.48)	0.45 (0.35 – 0.59)[a]
SH groups (nmol P-SH/mL)	15.1 ± 8.9	20.9 ± 8.7[b]	22.22 ± 8.8[b]
TBARS (mmol/L)	20.7 ± 7.2	23.4 ± 7.9	28.2 ± 11.6[b]

Data are expressed as means ± SD or median (interquartile ranges). Normality was assessed by Kolmogorov-Smirnov test. Data were processed for analysis, where One-way ANOVA followed by Tukey's test, and Kruskal-Wallis test followed by Dunn's Multiple Comparison Test.
[a] $p < 0.05$, [b] $p < 0.0001$ compared to normal weight group.

Table 3. Concentration of serum antioxidants and lipid peroxidation in the groups studied

	Groups		
	Normal weight	Overweight	Obese
N	54	27	68
Uric acid (mg/dL)	3.8 ± 1.0	4.2 ± 1.0	4.7 ± 1.7[b]
FRAP (mmol/L)	0.89 ± 0.20	0.98 ± 0.25	1.05 ± 0.22[a]
SH groups (nmol P-SH/mL)	143.6 ± 21.7	123.2 ± 25.1	105.4 ± 24.2[bc]
TBARS (mmol/L)	5.1 (4.6 – 6.5)	6.0 (5.0 – 7.4)	6.6 (5.4 – 8.3)[a]

Data are expressed as means ± SD or median (interquartile ranges). Normality was assessed by Kolmogorov-Smirnov test. Data were processed for analysis, where One-way ANOVA followed by Tukey's test, and Kruskal-Wallis test followed by Dunn's Multiple Comparison Test.
[a] $p < 0.05$, [b] $p < 0.0001$ compared to Normal Weight Group, [c] $p < 0.0001$ compared to Overweight Group.

Table 4. Correlation between antioxidants salivary and serum in normal weight group

	Saliva	Serum	p and r value
Uric Acid (mg/dL)	1.7 (1.4 – 2.4)	3.8 ± 1.0	r = 0.5162
			p < 0.0001
FRAP (mmol/L)	0.37 (0.29 – 0.46)	0.89 ± 0.20	r = 0.4361
			p = 0.001

Data are expressed as means ± SD or median (interquartile ranges). Normality was assessed by Kolmogorov-Smirnov test. Data were processed for analysis by Pearson or Spearman correlation.

Table 5. Correlation between antioxidants salivary and serum in group obese

	Saliva	Serum	p and r value
Uric Acid (mg/dL)	1.9 (1.4 – 2.3)	4.7 ± 1.7	r = 0.4205
			p = 0.0004
FRAP (mmol/L)	0.45 (0.35 – 0.59)	1.05 ± 0.22	r = 0.4482
			p = 0.0001

Data are expressed as means ± SD or median (interquartile ranges). Normality was assessed by Kolmogorov-Smirnov test. Data were processed for analysis by Pearson or Spearman correlation.

DISCUSSION

Sampling of human saliva is an attractive means to diagnose and monitor diseases since the saliva may be collected easily and noninvasively. Saliva has been widely used to study a variety of molecules and biochemical substances. Salivary analysis may also be helpful in predicting the development of future diseases (26,27). In the present study, we investigated antioxidant parameters and markers of lipoperoxidation in the saliva of healthy young adults with obesity and overweight to verify if the excessive body fat would influence these parameters. We then correlated the results in the saliva with those in the serum.

The nonenzymatic parameters evaluated in this study were selected based on their specific antioxidant properties (28): (i) the FRAP test quantifies the general capacity of the saliva to chelate and inactivate metal ions (mainly $Fe^{2+/3+}$) involved in the formation of highly reactive ROS/RNS, such as hydroxyl radicals (using the Fenton reaction); (ii) uric acid is both a preventive (chelating) antioxidant and a scavenger of free radicals that have already been produced; and (iii) SH groups are considered the nonenzymatic antioxidant frontline in most body fluids, and their measurement accurately identifies the redox (pro/antioxidant) balance in the saliva.

TBARS are products of lipid peroxidation often used to determine the balance between oxidation and antioxidation (29). The present data demonstrated an increase in TBARS concentration ($p = 0.0002$) in the saliva and serum ($p < 0.05$) in obese patients compared with non-obese individuals. These results suggest an increased generation of reactive species with potential to cause damage to cell membranes. Physiologically, an increase in O_2 and H_2O_2 production can increase the levels of TBARS. Obesity associated with a dyslipidemic profile, characterized by high levels of triglycerides and low-density lipoprotein (LDL) and low levels of high-density lipoprotein (HDL), promotes lipid peroxidation through formation of free radicals and ROS. Lipid oxidation generates some products, including TBARS, F_2-isoprostanes, and MDA, which are used as markers of oxidative stress (30).

SH groups (mixed disulfides of proteins and low-molecular-weight thiols) are very early products of protein oxidation generated during oxidative stress, formed a few seconds after oxygen radicals are generated. As a result, the assessment of the extent and specificity of this process during oxidative stress is one of the best measurements of the primary effects of oxygen radicals. S-thiolation has been correlated in many cases with changes in protein function. Hence, the estimation of salivary levels of protein thiol indicates the status of the oxidative stress (31,32). Many studies have observed changes in protein thiols, including alterations in glutathione levels in various diseases in which oxidative stress occurs (33,34). Oxidative stress is considered to be involved in the pathogenesis of insulin resistance associated with obesity (35).

In this study, salivary protein thiols were significantly increased ($p < 0.0001$) in obese patients when compared with normal-weight individuals. Similar results have been reported in studies measuring salivary and serum levels of antioxidants (peroxidase, superoxide dismutase, salivary total antioxidant status) in patients with type 1 diabetes mellitus. Increased antioxidant levels have been observed in these patients, indicating a compensation of the antioxidant systems against oxidative stress (36).

Corroborating with the above, FRAP levels were significantly higher ($p < 0.05$) in the saliva of patients in the obese group. This may reflect a compensation of the obese body against oxidative stress to neutralize reactive species since several paths generating oxidative stress are activated in obesity (37). Studies in obese diabetic subjects, compared with normal men and women matched for weight, have shown higher oxidative stress in obese individuals (12), as evidenced in this study by the increased production of TBARS.

In the acute phase of obesity, levels of antioxidants appear to be increased, but as the obesity becomes chronic, the antioxidant reserve depletes over time (9). In addition to a deficiency in antioxidants in individuals with obesity and excessive fat tissue, other mechanisms may contribute to the increased oxidative stress: hyperglycemia, increased muscle activity to bear the excessive weight, hypertension, chronic inflammation, endothelial production of EROS, and hyperleptinemia (37).

We observed no significant differences in uric acid levels in the saliva among the studied groups, although this compound has been noted to increase with increases in BMI. However, we observed that the serum of patients in the obese group had a greater concentration of uric acid. Uric acid, one of the largest hydrophilic antioxidants in the body, inhibits the action of free radicals on organic molecules, such as those that make up the cell membrane and the genetic material (26). However, the sharp increase in the concentration of uric acid appears to be a protective factor against oxidative stress, whereas its chronic increase is associated with a risk of chronic diseases (38).

Data from a series of studies have shown a strong and independent correlation between serum uric acid and insulin resistance in subjects with metabolic syndrome. Evidence has also shown that serum uric acid is a strong predictor of future development of diabetes (39,40). In this context, an important result of the present study was to detect higher concentrations of uric acid in obese individuals.

Oxidative stress occurring in obesity contributes to the oxidation of proteins in the plasma; these proteins may then undergo functional changes, in particular, loss of metabolic, enzymatic, and immunological properties (8). Protein thiol groups are the most susceptible to oxidation. Among proteins with antioxidant properties, powerful nonenzymatic antioxidants stand out such as glutathione, which has an important antioxidant action (7). Plasma thiol groups serve as antioxidants capable of removing oxidants responsible for initiating peroxidation, the main responsible for oxidative damage to proteins (40).

Our results demonstrate a significant plasma reduction in SH groups in the obese group compared with the normal-weight group. Since the serum levels of TBARS were significantly higher in the obese group, this effect was probably due to a requirement for neutralization of ROS, which are produced in greater amounts in this group. Plasma SH groups are antioxidants that scavenge

oxidants that initiate peroxidation and are quantitatively the major manifestation of oxidative protein damage (18). In obesity, the increase in carbonyl protein and a concomitant reduction in plasma thiol groups may be a possible mechanism contributing to atherosclerosis, insulin resistance, and hypertension (41). These data demonstrate a consumption of thiol groups to combat overproduction of free radicals and ROS produced during oxidative stress.

The results showed a progressive increase in serum FRAP levels in relation to BMI, in addition to significantly higher levels in obese volunteers. This reinforces our line of thought in which we consider this compound to be produced in greater amounts to offset the increased oxidative stress in the obese group since FRAP levels indicate the total plasma antioxidant capacity.

The second objective of this study was to correlate the salivary and serum parameters. We found a significant positive correlation between salivary and serum levels of uric acid and FRAP in the obese and normal-weight group, suggesting that measurement of salivary antioxidants could be used in the future to assess the antioxidant status of obese patients.

In conclusion, the results of this study showed that obese young patients presented significant changes in salivary biomarkers when compared normal-weight volunteers. Changes in salivary and serum levels of FRAP, SH groups, uric acid, and TBARS in obese subjects suggest major changes in oxidative status in these individuals. These findings are particularly important since they show an oxidative and inflammatory imbalance frequently observed in obesity. These results could help determine the pathways involved in obesity-related oxidative stress that are relevant to the development of obesity in young individuals. The results demonstrated a good correlation between salivary and serum biomarkers. There was a good replication in the results and maybe in the future, salivary can be used instead of blood to measure these oxidative biomarkers. Hence, we conclude that in addition to physical characteristics, levels of salivary FRAP and SH groups are indicators of oxidative stress in young obese individuals. Salivary analysis may prove to be a noninvasive, patient-friendly technique to assess the antioxidant status in these cases.

Acknowledgments: the work had the financial support of the Brazilian National Research Council (CNPq), FAPE – UNOESC (Research Support Fund). The authors wish to thank the University of West of Santa Catarina (UNOESC), SC, Brazil, for support in this study.

REFERENCES

1. Arana C, Cutando A, Ferrera MJ, Gómez-Moreno G, Worf CV, Bolaños MJ, et al. Parameters of oxidative stress in saliva from diabetic and parenteral drug addict patients. J Oral Pathol Med. 2006;35(9):554-9.

2. Haidari M, Ali M, Gangehei L, Chen M, Zhang W, Cybulsky MI. Increased oxidative stress in atherosclerosis-predisposed regions of the mouse aorta. Life Sci. 2010;87(3-4):100-10.

3. Pazdro R, Burgess JR. The role of vitamin E and oxidative stress in diabetes complications. Mech Ageing Dev. 2010;131(4):276-86.

4. Sohal RS, Mockett RJ, Orr WC. Mechanisms of aging: an appraisal of the oxidative stress hypothesis. Free Radic Biol Med. 2002;33(5):575-86.

5. Al-Aubaidy HA, Jelinek HF. Oxidative DNA damage and obesity in type 2 diabetes mellitus. Eur J Endocrinol. 2011;164(6):899-904.

6. Maddux BA, See W, Lawrence JC Jr, Goldfine AL, Goldfine ID, Evans JL. Protection against oxidative stress-induced insulin resistance in rat L6 muscle cells by mircomolar concentrations of alpha-lipoic acid. Diabetes. 2001;50(2):404-10.

7. Furukawa S, Fujita T, Shimabukuro M, Iwaki M, Yamada Y, Nakajima Y, et al. Increased oxidative stress in obesity and its impact on metabolic syndrome. J Clin Invest. 2004;114(12):1752-61.

8. Rudich A, Tirosh A, Potashnik R, Hemi R, Kanety H, Bashan N. Prolonged oxidative stress impairs insulin-induced GLUT4 translocation in 3T3-L1 adipocytes. Diabetes. 1998;47(10):1562-9.

9. Rodriguez de Sotillo D, Velly AM, Hadley M, Fricton JR. Evidence of oxidative stress in temporomandibular disorders: a pilot study. J Oral Rehabil. 2011;38(10):722-8.

10. Lee YH, Wong DT. Saliva: an emerging biofluid for early detection of diseases. Am J Dent. 2009;22(4):241-8.

11. Weiner JS, Lourie JA. Practical human biology. London: Academic Press, 1981.

12. James PT, Leach R, Kalamara E, Shayeghi M. The worldwide obesity epidemic. Obes Res. 2001;9 Suppl 4:228S-33S.

13. Gallagher D, Heymsfield SB, Heo M, Jebb SA, Murgatroyd PR, Sakamoto Y. Healthy percentage body fat ranges: an approach for developing guidelines based on body mass index. Am J Clin Nutr. 2000;72(3):694-701.

14. Chielle EO, Bonfanti G, De Bona KS, Moresco RN, Moretto MB. Adenosine deaminase, dipeptidyl peptidase-IV activities and lipid peroxidation are increased in the saliva of obese young adult. Clin Chem Lab Med. 2015;53(7):1041-7.

15. Grundy SM, Brewer HB Jr, Cleeman JI, Smith SC Jr, Lenfant C; National Heart, Lung, and Blood Institute; American Heart Association. Definition of metabolic syndrome: report of the National Heart, Lung, and Blood Institute/American Heart Association conference on scientific issues related to definition. Arterioscler Thromb Vasc Biol. 2004;24(2):e13-8.

16. Calabrese V, Bella R, Testa D, Spadaro F, Scrofani A, Rizza V, et al. Increased cerebrospinal fluid and plasma levels of ultraweak chemiluminescence are associated with changes in the thiol pool and lipid-soluble fluorescence in multiple sclerosis: the pathogenic role of oxidative stress. Drugs Exp Clin Res. 1998;24(3):125-31.

17. Staroń A, Mąkosa G, Koter-Michalak M. Oxidative stress in erythrocytes from patients with rheumatoid arthritis. Rheumatol Int. 2012;32(2):331-4.

18. Ramprasath T, Senthil Murugan P, Prabakaran AD, Gomathi P, Rathinavel A, Selvam GS. Potential risk modifications of GSTT1, GSTM1 and GSTP1 (glutathione-S-transferases) variants and their association to CAD in patients with type-2 diabetes. Biochem Biophys Res Commun. 2011;407(1):49-53.

19. Sereg M, Toke J, Patócs A, Varga I, Igaz P, Szücs N, et al. Diagnostic performance of salivary cortisol and serum osteocalcin measurements in patients with overt and subclinical Cushing's syndrome. Steroids. 2011;76(1-2):38-42.

20. Singh N, Bhardwaj P, Pandey RM, Saraya A. Oxidative stress and antioxidant capacity in patients with chronic pancreatitis with and without diabetes mellitus. Indian J Gastroenterol. 2012;31(5):226-31.

21. Rahim MA, Rahim ZH, Ahmad WA, Hashim OH. Can saliva proteins be used to predict the onset of acute myocardial infarction among high-risk patients? Int J Med Sci. 2015;12(4):329-35.

22. Zhou L, Wang K, Li Q, Nice EC, Zhang H, Huang C. Clinical proteomics-driven precision medicine for targeted cancer therapy: current overview and future perspectives. Expert Rev Proteomics. 2016;13(4):367-81.

23. Lapenna D, Ciofani G, Pierdomenico SD, Giamberardino MA, Cuccurullo F. Reaction conditions affecting the relationship between thiobarbituric acid reactivity and lipid peroxides in human plasma. Free Radic Biol Med. 2001;31(3):331-5.

24. Boyne AF, Ellman GL. A methodology for analysis of tissue sulfhydryl components. Anal Biochem. 1972;46(2):639-53.

25. Ashwell M, Hsieh SD. Six reasons why the waist-to-height ratio is a rapid and effective global indicator for health risks of obesity and how its use could simplify the international public health message on obesity. Int J Food Sci Nutr. 2005;56(5):303-7.

26. Vincent HK, Taylor AG. Biomarkers and potential mechanisms of obesity-induced oxidant stress in humans. Int J Obes (Lond). 2006;30(3):400-18.

27. Skrha J, Sindelka G, Kvasnicka J, Hilgertová J. Insulin action and fibrinolysis influenced by vitamin E in obese Type 2 diabetes mellitus. Diabetes Res Clin Pract. 1999;44(1):27-33.

28. Erdeve O, Siklar Z, Kocaturk PA, Dallar Y, Kavas GO. Antioxidant superoxide dismutase activity in obese children. Biol Trace Elem Res. 2004;98(3):219-28.

29. Sautin YY, Johnson RJ. Uric acid: the oxidant-antioxidant paradox. Nucleosides Nucleotides Nucleic Acids. 2008;27(6):608-19.

30. Tsouli SG, Liberopoulos EN, Mikhailidis DP, Athyros VG, Elisaf MS. Elevated serum uric acid levels in metabolic syndrome: an active component or an innocent bystander? Metabolism. 2006;55(10):1293-301.

31. Yoo TW, Sung KC, Shin HS, Kim BJ, Kim BS, Kang JH, et al. Relationship between serum uric acid concentration and insulin resistance and metabolic syndrome. Circ J. 2005;69(8):928-33.

32. Rho YH, Woo JH, Choi SJ, Lee YH, Ji JD, Song GG. Association between serum uric acid and the Adult Treatment Panel III-defined metabolic syndrome: results from a single hospital database. Metabolism. 2008;57(1):71-6.

33. Himmelfarb J, McMonagle E. Albumin is the major plasma protein target of oxidant stress in uremia. Kidney Int. 2001;60(1):358-63.

34. Himmelfarb J, McMonagle E, McMenamin E. Plasma protein thiol oxidation and carbonyl formation in chronic renal failure. Kidney Int. 2000;58(6):2571-8.

35. Uzun H, Konukoglu D, Gelisgen R, Zengin K, Taskin M. Plasma protein carbonyl and thiol stress before and after laparoscopic gastric banding in morbidly obese patients. Obes Surg. 2007;17(10):1367-73.

36. Lubrano V, Balzan S. Enzymatic antioxidant system in vascular inflammation and coronary artery disease. World J Exp Med. 2015;5(4):218-24.

37. Cejvanovic V, Asferg C, Kjær LK, Andersen UB, Linneberg A, Frystyk J, et al. Markers of oxidative stress in obese men with and without hypertension. Scand J Clin Lab Invest. 2016 Sep 26:1-6.

38. Shani M, Vinker S, Dinour D, Leiba M, Twig G, Holtzman EJ, et al. High normal uric acid levels are associated with an increased risk of diabetes in lean, normoglycemic healthy women. J Clin Endocrinol Metab. 2016;101(10):3772-8.

39. Wang ZN, Li P, Jiang RH, Li L, Li X, Li L, et al. The association between serum uric acid and metabolic syndrome among adolescents in northeast China. Int J Clin Exp Med. 2015;8(11):21122-9.

40. Xue B, Tan JB, Ning F, Sun JP, Zhang KY, Liu L, et al. Association between serum uric acid and prevalence of type 2 diabetes diagnosed using HbA1c criteria among Chinese Adults in Qingdao, China. Biomed Environ Sci. 2015;28(12):884-93.

41. Mori T, Ogawa S, Cowely AW Jr, Ito S. Role of renal medullary oxidative and/or carbonyl stress in salt-sensitive hypertension and diabetes. Clin Exp Pharmacol Physiol. 2012;39(1):125-31.

19

Radioactive iodine-refractory differentiated thyroid cancer: an uncommon but challenging situation

Angelica Schmidt[1,2], Laura Iglesias[2], Michele Klain[3],
Fabián Pitoia[1], Martin J. Schlumberger[2]

ABSTRACT

Radioiodine (RAI)-refractory thyroid cancer is an uncommon entity, occurring with an estimated incidence of 4-5 cases/year/million people. RAI refractoriness is more frequent in older patients, in those with large metastases, in poorly differentiated thyroid cancer, and in those tumors with high 18-fluordeoxyglucose uptake on PET/CT. These patients have a 10-year survival rate of less than 10%. In recent years, new therapeutic agents with molecular targets have become available, with multikinase inhibitors (MKIs) being the most investigated drugs. Two of these compounds, sorafenib and lenvatinib, have shown significant objective response rates and have significantly improved the progression-free survival in the two largest published prospective trials on MKI use. However, no overall survival benefit has been achieved yet. This is probably related to the crossover that occurs in most patients who progress on placebo treatment to the open treatment of these studies. In consequence, the challenge is to correctly identify which patients will benefit from these treatments. It is also crucial to understand the appropriate timing to initiate MKI treatment and when to stop it. The purpose of this article is to define RAI refractoriness, to summarize which therapies are available for this condition, and to review how to select patients who are suitable for them. Arch Endocrinol Metab. 2017;61(1):81-9

Keywords

Differentiated thyroid cancer; radioactive iodine refractory thyroid cancer; tyrosine kinase inhibitors

[1] Division of Endocrinology,
Hospital de Clínicas,
University of Buenos Aires
Buenos Aires, Argentina
[2] Institut Gustave Roussy, Université
Paris-Saclay, Villejuif, France
[3] Università Federico II di
Napoli, Napoli, Italia

Correspondence to:
Angelica Schmidt
Division of Endocrinology,
Hospital de Clínicas,
University of Buenos Aires
Córdoba 2351, 5th Floor,
Buenos Aires 1424, Argentina
angelica.schm@gmail.com

INTRODUCTION

Despite the high and increasing incidence of differentiated thyroid carcinomas (DTCs), only a few patients (less than 10% of patients with clinical disease) will develop distant metastases. Two thirds of these patients will become refractory to the treatment with radioactive iodine (RAI), and they represent 4-5 new cases/year/million. After the discovery of advanced RAI-refractory disease, the 10-year survival rate is usually less than 10% and the mean life expectancy is 3-5 years (1). Systemic chemotherapy has limited efficacy with a high toxicity rate (2). Multikinase inhibitors (MKIs) are the most investigated drugs. Two of these compounds, sorafenib and lenvatinib, have shown objective response rates and have significantly improved the progression-free survival rates in the two largest published prospective randomized trials performed with an MKI in patients with advanced refractory DTC. However, no overall survival benefit has been demonstrated yet. This is probably related to the crossover that occurs in most patients who progress on placebo treatment to the open treatment (3,4).

The aim of this review is to define RAI refractoriness and summarize the therapies currently available. We also aim to analyze the most appropriate timings to initiate and to stop MKI treatment.

Defining RAI refractoriness

RAI treatment is the first-line systemic treatment in patients with advanced disease (5). Achieving a cure with RAI treatments is frequent in young patients with small metastases from well-differentiated thyroid cancer who have high uptake of RAI in neoplastic foci. These patients represent about one third of all patients with an advanced form of the disease. Partial response and long-term stabilization may be obtained, but cure is rarely achieved in the other two thirds of patients with an advanced form of the disease, who will be classified as refractory at some point during their life (1,6).

It is important to recognize at which point RAI treatment is no longer beneficial for DTC patients in order to avoid unnecessary treatments that may lead to severe adverse events (AEs) and to consider alternative local or systemic therapies (5,7). Indeed, the practitioner should ascertain that decreased RAI uptake is not due to iodine contamination or to insufficient TSH (thyrotropin) stimulation (8). When this has been excluded, there are different possible scenarios (5,6):

Metastatic disease that does not take up radioactive iodine at the time of the first I¹³¹ treatment

For these patients, treatment with I^{131} does not provide any benefit. This group includes patients with structurally evident disease with no RAI uptake on a diagnostic, whole-body scan. In some of these patients, RAI uptake may be observed on post therapy scans but usually will not be high enough to induce any therapeutic benefit (9).

Ability to take up RAI lost after previous evidence of uptake

This is frequently observed in patients with multiple large metastases, and it is generally due to the eradication of differentiated tumor cells with RAI uptake, with persistence of those poorly differentiated clones that will continue growing (6).

RAI uptake retained in some lesions but not in others

This situation is also frequently seen in patients with multiple large metastases, and progression is likely to occur in metastases without RAI uptake, in particular when high 18-fluorodeoxyglucose (¹⁸FDG) uptake is present (10,11).

Metastatic disease that progresses despite substantial uptake of RAI

When structural progression occurs within 12 to 16 months after the course of an adequate RAI treatment, subsequent RAI treatment, even with higher activities, will be ineffective (12).

Absence of complete response to treatment after > 600 mCi of cumulative activity of RAI

The situation is less clear in patients who still have visible RAI uptake in all lesions and who are not cured, despite several treatment courses, but in whom disease does not progress according to Response Evaluation Criteria In Solid Tumors (RECIST) 1.1 criteria (13). The probability of obtaining a cure with further RAI treatment is low, and the risk of AEs increases with further treatments (1,5,7). The decision to continue RAI treatment is generally based on the magnitude of tumor response to previous treatment courses, the persistence of a significant RAI

uptake, a low ¹⁸FDG uptake in tumor foci, and the absence of detectable side effects (6).

High uptake of ¹⁸FDG on PET/CT scan

The likelihood of obtaining a complete response is reduced when ¹⁸FDG uptake on PET/CT scanning is high in the tumor foci. However, the decision to abandon RAI therapy should not be based only on the presence or intensity of ¹⁸FDG uptake (14-17).

Advanced disease and unfeasible thyroidectomy

When the thyroid gland has not been removed, RAI treatment is usually not administered and RAI uptake status cannot be assessed. These patients are usually managed as iodine-refractory patients (6).

Rationale for the use of MKIs

Genetic alterations inducing the activation of the *RAS-RAF-MEK-ERK* and *PI3K/Akt/mTOR* signaling pathways are found in the majority of DTCs (18). Angiogenic factors are also involved in the cellular control of differentiation, proliferation, and survival. Vascular endothelial growth factor (VEGF) stimulates endothelial cell proliferation and is a key to tumor angiogenesis. VEGF has an important role in thyroid cancer development, and its expression level correlates with advanced disease (19,20). As a consequence, MKIs targeting angiogenesis have recently been used with encouraging results in clinical trials involving patients with progressive and unresectable RAI-refractory disease (3,4,21).

When to initiate an MKI?

One main challenge is properly selecting patients for systemic therapy. As all these medications can cause a decrease in quality of life (QoL) and life-threatening, adverse effects, it is important to identify which patients may benefit from and should be placed on therapy. Patients with distant metastases may have a disease that does not progress for years. In these patients, it is recommended to keep TSH suppression therapy with levothyroxine and imaging every 3-12 months (CT scan, ¹⁸FDG-PET/CT scan, or MRI) based on the disease burden and location of lesions (5,22). Although serum thyroglobulin (Tg) levels are measured as a biomarker of the disease extent, patients should not be identified as having progressive disease only on the basis of rising levels of serum Tg. Rapidly increasing serum

Tg levels should, however, lead to more frequent and comprehensive imaging in efforts to identify structural correlates (23).

In general, the appropriate indications to initiate a MKI treatment are (5,24,25) as follow:

Rapidly progressive disease and large tumor burden

Large, multiple tumors greater than 1-2 cm in size that are rapidly progressing (within < 12 months) should be considered for treatment; in these patients, treatment should preferably be initiated before the occurrence of symptoms (6,26).

In contrast, patients with smaller tumors (< 1 cm) or with only a few lesions and with no documented progression rarely require immediate, systemic treatment with an MKI (6).

For patients with smaller tumors that are rapidly progressing (< 6-12 months) or for those who have large tumors that progress slowly (> 12 months), the decision to treat or not (or to postpone treatment) is less clear and should be considered on a case-by-case basis (6,26,27).

Symptomatic disease and the risk of local complications

Dyspnea or painful bone lesions should first be submitted to focal therapy. Also, symptomatic treatment modalities are always warranted, as well as bisphosphonates or an anti-RANK ligand antibody in patients with bone metastases. Cases of ineffectiveness or with the presence of tumor foci near the respiratory–digestive axis or large vessels may be an indication to initiate treatment, even in patients with no demonstrated progression before the occurrence of tumor involvement of the trachea or esophagus and before encasement of great vessels that may contraindicate the use of an MKI with respect to the risk of bleeding (28).

Good overall performance status and acceptable life expectancy

Before initiation, a comprehensive review is necessary to ascertain the patient's suitability for therapy. An initial evaluation includes assessment of the patient's performance status. Little is known about the tolerability of MKIs in patients with a poor performance status (*e.g.*, ECOG 2 or more) because all trials with MKIs have excluded these patients (29).

Absence of comorbidities or contraindications

Cardiovascular history, poor blood pressure control, and hematological, renal, and hepatic abnormalities may contraindicate any MKI treatment or may indicate treatment initiation at a lower dosage (Table 1) (5,28).

Table 1. Contraindications or factors discouraging MKI treatment

Intestinal or liver disease	Active or recent diverticulitis, inflammatory bowel disease, or recent bowel resection
	Laboratory: AST-ALT > 5 times the upper limit of normal range; increased bilirubin level
High risk of bleeding	Recent gastrointestinal hemorrhage or hemoptysis, coagulopathy, or anticoagulant treatment
	Tumor involvement of the larynx, trachea–bronchus axis or the pharyngo-esophagus axis Encasement of great vessels
High cardiovascular risk	Unstable angina, myocardial infarction, or stroke within 6 months prior to MKI initiation
Poorly controlled hypertension	Uncontrolled hypertension; start antihypertensive treatment first if blood pressure is > 140/90 mmHg
Prolonged QTc interval	≥ 450 msec
	History of ventricular arrhythmias and bradyarrhythmias
Renal impairment	CrCl < 60 ml/min
	Proteinuria ≥ 1g/24h
Recent tracheal radiation therapy	Within 6 months prior to MKI initiation Increased risk of bleeding/fistula
Cachexia, poor nutrition, sarcopenia	Care should improve performance status
Untreated brain metastases	Controversial
Recent suicidal ideation	Suicide has been reported in depressed patients receiving MKIs
Concomitant medication that induces or inhibits CYP3A4	Avoid or substitute for another drug. If a CYP3A4-inhibiting drug cannot be eliminated, consider a dose reduction in the MKI
Life expectancy	If it is too brief systemic therapy will not be justified

ALT: alanine aminotransferase; AST: aspartate aminotransferase; CrCl: creatinine clearance.

Good compliance to treatment

Due to the duration of treatment, the potential for toxicities, and the need for regular monitoring, patients must be aware that the follow-up will be close and may be prolonged for years.

Which agents are available?

Multikinase inhibitors

Sorafenib

Sorafenib targets *BRAF, RET, VEGFR 1–3, PDGFR,* and *c-KIT* and was the first agent approved (in 2013) for the treatment of refractory DTC, based on the DECISION trial, a randomized, placebo-controlled, phase III trial (30,31). A total of 417 adult patients with progressive advanced RAI-refractory DTC were randomized 1 to 1 to sorafenib (800 mg daily) or a placebo. The median progression-free survival (PFS) of patients treated with sorafenib was significantly improved compared to the placebo (10.8 vs. 5.8 months; p < 0.0001). Disease control rate, including partial responses (PRs in 12% of patients) and stable disease (SD > 23 weeks), was achieved in 54% of patients treated with sorafenib. There was no difference in overall survival (OS), even after correction of the potential benefits of the crossover in patients from the placebo group who crossed over to the sorafenib treatment upon disease progression. AEs occurred in almost all patients, but most were grade 1 or 2. The most frequent AEs were dermatological – hand–foot syndrome (76%), alopecia (67%), and rash or desquamation (50%) – but also included diarrhea (68%), fatigue (49%), weight loss (46%), and hypertension (40%). Serious AEs occurred in more than 30% of patients, the most frequent being secondary malignancy (4.3%), dyspnea (3.4%), and pleural effusion (2.9%). The dose was decreased in 64% of cases, and the drug was discontinued due to AEs in 19% of patients (32).

Lenvatinib

Lenvatinib targets *VEGFR1-3, FGFR1-4, PDGFR-b, RET,* and *c-KIT* and was labeled in 2014 based on the SELECT trial (33). SELECT, a phase III trial, enrolled a total of 392 patients with progressive, advanced RAI-refractory DTC who were randomized 2 to 1 to lenvatinib (24 mg/day) (n = 261) or a placebo (n = 131). The median PFS was significantly improved compared to the placebo (18.3 months vs. 3.6 months; p < 0.001). The PFS benefit was found among all subgroups, including patients previously treated with another MKI (25% of patients), distinct histology subtypes (i.e., papillary, poorly differentiated, follicular, and oncocytic), and site of metastases, and was independent of the *BRAF* and *RAS* mutational status of the tumor. In addition, a significant objective response rate of 64.8% was documented among

patients treated with lenvatinib, including complete responses in 4 patients; furthermore, a prolonged stable disease (longer than 23 weeks) was observed in 15% of patients. Responses occurred rapidly after initiation of treatment, with a median time to response of only two months. Grade 3 or higher AEs occurred in 75% of patients and led to dose reductions in 67% and discontinuation of treatment in 14% of patients. The most frequent grade 3 or higher treatment-related AEs were hypertension (42%), proteinuria (10%), arterial and venous thromboembolic events (2.7% and 3.8%, respectively), acute renal failure (1.9%), QTc prolongation (1.5%), and hepatic failure (0.4%). Six deaths in the lenvatinib group were considered probably treatment related by the investigators: 3 cases resulted from unspecified causes and 3 were associated with pulmonary embolism, hemorrhagic stroke, and health deterioration. No significant OS benefit was demonstrated with lenvatinib, but after correction for the potential benefits of crossover in patients of the placebo group who were treated with lenvatinib upon progression with a prespecified method, the benefit in terms of OS became significant (3).

Direct comparison of these two treatments has not been performed, but lenvatinib seems to be more effective than sorafenib, both in improving PFS and in obtaining an objective tumor response (Table 2). These data are even more meaningful when considering that the SELECT trial enrolled patients with more advanced and more aggressive disease (as shown by a shorter median PFS in the placebo arm), some of whom had been previously treated with an MKI.

Table 2. Phase III trials

Patients (n)	207 vs. 210	261 vs. 131
CR	0% vs. 0%	1.5% (n = 4) vs. 0%
PR	12.2% vs. 0.5%	63.2% vs. 1.5%
SD > 23 weeks	41.8% vs. 33.2%	15.3% vs. 29.8%
PFS months (median)	10.8 vs. 5.8 (HR 0.59 p < 0.0001)	18.3 vs. 3.6 (HR 0.21 p < 0.001)
Grade 3-4 AEs	37.2% vs. 26.3%	75.9% vs. 9.9%
OS	NS*	NS*

CR: complete response; PR: partial response; SD: stable disease; PFS: progression free survival; HR: hazard ratio; AEs: adverse events; OS: overall survival; NS: not statistically significant.
* Probably related to the crossover that occurs in most patients who progressed from the placebo treatment to the therapy treatment.

Pazopanib

Pazopanib targets *VEGFR1-3, PDGFR-a* and *-b*, and *c-KIT*. In a phase II trial on involving 37 patients with previously treated advanced RAI-refractory thyroid cancer, a PR occurred in 49% of patients and SD occurred in 47% of patients. AEs included fatigue, hair and skin hypopigmentation, alopecia, diarrhea, nausea, vomiting, anorexia, weight loss, hypertension, elevated liver function tests, proteinuria, and hematologic cytopenias. Serious AEs were uncommon but included lower gastrointestinal hemorrhage (grade 3) and intracranial hemorrhage (grade 4). A dose reduction due to AEs was required in 43% of patients. Two deaths were potentially related to the drug. It is important to note that the patients included in this trial were allowed to be treated with up to two previous systemic treatment lines, and radiographic progression of the disease was requested in the 6 months preceding enrolment. These criteria led to the selection of highly aggressive RAI-refractory DTC patients (34).

Cabozantinib

Cabozantinib targets *c-MET, VEGFR2,* and *RET* kinases and is currently approved for the treatment of advanced medullary thyroid cancer. Among 15 patients with RAI-refractory DTC, a PR was achieved in 8 (53%). All patients experienced at least one AE, and nearly all were grade 3 or higher. The most common AEs were diarrhea, nausea, fatigue, and decreased appetite (35).

Sunitinib

Sunitinib targets *VEGFR, PDGFR, c-KIT, FLT3,* and *RET*. In a phase II trial of 28 patients with advanced RAI-refractory DTC, sunitinib induced a PR in 28%, a CR in 1 patient, and SD in 46%. The most common AEs included fatigue, neutropenia, hand–foot syndrome, hypertension, and diarrhea. Four patients discontinued treatment due to toxicity; there were two serious bleeding episodes (36).

Vandetanib

Vandetanib targets *RET, VEGFR,* and *EGFR*. A randomized, double-blind, phase II trial enrolled 72 patients to the vandetanib group and 73 patients to the placebo group. Patients who received vandetanib had longer median PFS than those who received the placebo (11 months vs. 5.9, $p < 0.05$). PR and SD were observed in 8% and 57% of patients in the vandetanib

arm, respectively. The incidence of grade 3 AEs was 53% in the vandetanib group. QTc prolongation and diarrhea were the most common AEs, and other frequent AEs included hypertension, rash, acne, and decreased appetite (37).

Motesanib

Motesanib targets *VEGF-R, PDGF-R,* and c-*KIT*. In a phase II study on 93 patients who had progressive, RAI-resistant DTC, PR was observed in 14% and SD longer than 23 weeks was observed in 35%. Nearly all patients (94%) had at least one AE, being grade 3 or more in half of them. The most commonly reported AEs were diarrhea, hypertension, fatigue, and weight loss (38).

Axitinib

Axitinib is an inhibitor of *VEGF-R 1-3, c-KIT,* and *PDGF-R*. In a phase II study on 52 patients with refractory DTC, a PR was observed in 38% and SD in 30%. Almost all patients experienced AEs, the most common grade 3-4 being hypertension, proteinuria, diarrhea, weight loss, and fatigue (39,40). Similar results were found in another phase II trial (41).

Nintedanib

Nintedanib targets *VEGF-R, FGF-R, PDGF-R* and *RET, Flt-3,* and *Src*. Based on promising efficacy and safety results in many other solid tumors, nintedanib is currently under investigation in DTC (42,26).

Other treatment modalities

Chemotherapy

The most frequently used agent is doxorubicin. Phase II studies provided low and transient partial responses of 0 to 20%. Too few data exist to recommend other specific cytotoxic regimens, and their use within the context of a therapeutic clinical trial should be preferred (2,5).

Inmunotherapy

Some tumors evade immunosurveillance, which can occur through an inhibition of T-cell function induced by the expression of molecules such as CTLA-4, PD-1, or PD-L1 (43,44). Treatment with antibodies directed against checkpoint inhibitors (*e.g.,* PD-1/PD-L1) has shown promise in other cancer types and is being investigated in advanced RAI-refractory thyroid cancer, used either alone or in combination with an MKI or an RAI (5,45).

Selective BRAF inhibitors

Vemurafenib: in a retrospective review of 15 patients with advanced PTC harboring the $BRAF^{V600E}$ mutation, a PR was observed in 47% (46).

Dabrafenib: among 14 patients, dabrafenib induced 4 (29%) PRs, and 64% of patients achieved at least a 10% reduction in tumor size (47).

Crizotinib

Crizotinib is an inhibitor of anaplastic lymphoma kinase (*ALK*) and *c-MET*. Recently, rearrangements involving the *ALK* gene were discovered in rare, poorly differentiated, and anaplastic thyroid cancers and, more frequently, in radiation-induced DTC (48,49). Crizotinib may be used in patients with a demonstrated *ALK- or c-MET*-activating mutation (50).

Everolimus

Everolimus is an inhibitor of *mTOR*. Activation of the PI3 kinase pathway occurs mostly in poorly differentiated thyroid cancers in addition to the activation of the MAP kinase pathway (51). In a phase II study on 38 patients with advanced thyroid cancer of any histology, only 2 (5%) patients achieved a PR. The AEs were predominantly grade 1 or 2, and the most common was mucositis (84%) (52). Another trial investigating everolimus's combination with sorafenib is ongoing, and preliminary results have shown a synergistic effect, with PR in 58% of patients (33).

Selumetinib

Selumetinib is an MEK inhibitor that blocks the MAPK signaling pathway. It was used as a redifferentiating agent and increased the uptake of I^{124} in 12 (60%) of 20 patients with advanced refractory thyroid cancer; 8 of these 12 patients reached the dosimetry threshold for RAI therapy, and 5 of them achieved a PR after RAI treatment. It seems to be more effective in patients with *RAS*-mutated disease (53). Similar results were achieved in a phase II study with dabrafenib on 10 patients with $BRAF^{V600E}$ mutated thyroid cancers: 60% developed RAI uptake and 83% of patients showed a decrease in the size of target lesions after 6 months of RAI treatment, but only 2 patients met criteria for partial response (54).

Combined therapies

Most patients eventually progress after responding to a first-line treatment, though some must discontinue the drugs due to toxicity. As a consequence, a number of studies have looked at sequencing MKI administration or the use of MKIs in the second-line setting for RAI-refractory DTC in patients whose cancers have progressed while receiving a first-line agent. These data suggest that a second-line TKI can be effective, with similar benefits in terms of PFS (55,56).

Adverse events

Education should be provided to each patient and to care providers. After initiation of treatment, it is highly recommended that clinicians follow-up with patients at 2-week intervals for the first 2-3 months and then once a month in order to proactively manage AEs.

The most common AEs and their management are presented in Table 3 (57-59). Less common but serious AEs are hypertension, arterial and venous thrombotic events, bleeding, gastrointestinal fistula and perforation, acute myocardial infarction, heart failure, secondary malignancies (squamous cell carcinoma), cytopenias, hepatotoxicity, renal failure, and reversible posterior leukoencephalopathy syndrome (3,4).

WHEN TO STOP AN MKI TREATMENT?

Therapy should be continued as long as the net benefit exceeds the net detriment (5). There is no general consensus, and the decision to withdraw any MKI is made on a case-by-case basis. These situations are listed in Table 4 (25,59,60).

CONCLUSION

RAI refractoriness is an uncommon situation, and many patients may survive in the absence of treatment for years or even decades with a stable or slowly progressive disease. However, a few patients may require treatment when the tumor burden is large and when progression has been documented. MKIs represent the first-line treatment for advanced refractory DTC: they significantly prolong PFS, and some induce a high objective response rate. However, at present there is no demonstrated benefit regarding overall survival, and the quality of life is altered during treatment. For these reasons, it is important to adequately select patients who should be treated and then manage them with an interdisciplinary approach.

Table 3. Common adverse events of MKIs

Fatigue and loss of weight	All (26-59%)	Increase or at least maintain physical activity; take pills in the evening Monitor other causes (*e.g.*, anemia, depression, electrolyte disturbance, hypothyroidism)
Diarrhea	All (30-68%)	Loperamide and/or codeine Dietary changes (eat low-fiber foods; avoid high-fat or spicy foods, alcohol, and caffeinated or carbonated drinks)
HTA	All (30-67%)	Monitor blood pressure at least once a week Diuretics, ACEIs, ARBs, BBs, or CCBs alone or in combination Avoid diltiazem, verapamile, and nifedipine
Rash	All (20-50%)	Use perfume-free soaps and wear loose, natural-fabric clothing; avoid hot or cold water Topical corticosteroids or antihistamines
TSH increase	All (30-60%)	Monitor TSH levels monthly and adjust thyroid-replacement medication dose
Hand-foot syndrome	Sorafenib (76%)	Prevention: local care of feet and hands, urea cream 10% on hands and feet, use cotton socks Treatment: Thick urea-based cream (30%), topical lidocaine Use comfortable shoes and avoid hot/cold water NSAIDs, codeine, or pregabalin
Alopecia	Sorafenib (67%)	Inform the patient that it is temporary, usually recovering after the treatment, and does not require any treatment
Proteinuria	Lenvatinib (31%)	If ≥ 2 g/24 hours: withhold treatment Resume at reduced dose when proteinuria is < 2 g/24 hours Discontinue if nephrotic syndrome
Mucositis	All (30%)	Mouthwash with lidocaine + sucralfate, salt and sodium bicarbonate, or chlorhexidine
Hypocalcemia	Sorafenib (18%)	Monitor blood calcium levels at least monthly and replace calcium + vitamin D as necessary
QTc prolongation	Vandetanib (23%, G > 3 in 14%)	Serially monitor ECG and electrolytes and correct any abnormality Avoid drugs known to prolong QTc Discontinue MKIs if QTc ≥ 500 msec

AEs: adverse events; ACEI: angiotensin converting enzyme inhibitor; ARB: angiotensin II receptor blockers; BB: beta-blockers; CCB: calcium channel blockers; NSAID: non steroidal anti-inflammatory drugs.

Table 4. Factors that lead to MKI continuation or withdrawal

Benefits of continuing treatment	Maintain stable disease or slow disease progression
Magnitude of tumor reduction	If after an initial significant tumor response, a slow disease progression occurs, treatment may be continued as long as the clinical benefit is maintained
Size and location of tumor foci	Evaluate risk of local complications if the tumor progresses
Feasibility of focal treatments	In patients with dissociated responses, treatment may be maintained in those who progress in a single or in a few metastases that may benefit from focal treatment modalities. This may occur with bone metastases that progress and may then benefit from focal treatment, whereas metastases in lungs, lymph nodes, or liver respond
Tolerance	AEs are significant and may lead to a dose reduction in 11-73% of patients and to MKI withdrawal in 7-25%. However, AEs can frequently be managed without the need for dose reduction or discontinuation of treatment. Also, the tolerance is highly variable from patient to patient and between different MKIs
Availability of other treatment modalities	Availability of other drugs or possibility to include patients in international protocols of new drugs

REFERENCES

1. Durante C, Haddy N, Baudin E, Leboulleux S, Hartl D, Travagli JP, et al. Long-term outcome of 444 patients with distant metastases from papillary and follicular thyroid carcinoma: Benefits and limits of radioiodine therapy. JCEM. 2006;91(8):2892-9.

2. Albero A, Lopez JE, Torres A, de la Cruz L, Martin T. Effectiveness of chemotherapy in advanced differentiated thyroid cancer: a systematic review. Endocr Relat Cancer. 2016;23(2):R71-84.

3. Schlumberger M, Tahara M, Wirth LJ, Robinson B, Brose MS, Elisei R, et al. Lenvatinib versus Placebo in Radioiodine-Refractory Thyroid Cancer. NEJM. 2015;372(7):621-30.

4. Brose MS, Nutting CM, Jarzab B, Elisei R, Siena S, Bastholt L, et al. Sorafenib in locally advanced or metastatic, radioactive iodine-refractory, differentiated thyroid cancer: a randomized, double-blind, phase 3. DECISION trial. Lancet. 2014;384(9940):319-28.

5. Haugen BR, Alexander EK, Bible KC, Doherty G, Mandel SJ, Nikiforov YE, et al. 2015 American Thyroid Association Management Guidelines for Adult Patients with Thyroid Nodules and Differentiated Thyroid Cancer: The American Thyroid

Association Guidelines Task Force on Thyroid Nodules and Differentiated Thyroid Cancer. Thyroid. 2016;26(1):1-133.

6. Schlumberger M, Brose M, Elisei R, Leboulleux S, Luster M, Pitoia F, et al. Definition and management of radioactive iodine-refractory differentiated thyroid cancer. Lancet Diabetes Endocrinol. 2014;2(5):356-8.

7. Rubino C, de Vathaire F, Dottorini ME, Hall P, Schvartz C, Couette JE, et al. Second primary malignancies in thyroid cancer patients. Br J Cancer. 2003;89(9):1638-44.

8. Sacks W, Braunstein G. Evolving approaches in managing radioactive iodine-refractory differentiated thyroid cancer. Endocr Pract. 2014;20(3):263-75.

9. Sabra MM, Grewal RK, Tala H, Larson SM, Tuttle RM. Clinical Outcomes Following Empiric Radioiodine Therapy in Patients with Structurally Identifiable Metastatic Follicular Cell – Derived Thyroid Carcinoma with Negative Diagnostic. Thyroid. 2012;22(9):877-82.

10. Sgouros G, Kolbert KS, Sheikh A, Pentlow KS, Mun EF, Barth A, et al. Patient-specific dosimetry for 131I thyroid cancer therapy using 124I PET and 3-dimensional-internal dosimetry (3D-ID) software. J Nucl Med. 2004;45(8):1366-72.

11. Wang W, Larson SM, Tuttle RM, Kalaigian H, Kolbert K, Sonenberg M, et al. Resistance of [18f]-fluorodeoxyglucose-avid metastatic thyroid cancer lesions to treatment with high-dose radioactive iodine. Thyroid. 2001;11(12):1169-75.

12. Vaisman F, Tala H, Grewal R, Tuttle RM. In differentiated thyroid cancer, an incomplete structural response to therapy is associated with significantly worse clinical outcomes than only an incomplete thyroglobulin response. Thyroid. 2011;21(12):1317-22.

13. Eisenhauer EA, Therasse P, Bogaerts J, Schwartz LH, Sargent D, Ford R, et al. New response evaluation criteria in solid tumours: Revised RECIST guideline (version 1.1). Eur J Cancer. 2009;45(2):228-47.

14. Robbins RJ, Wan Q, Grewal RK, Reibke R, Gonen M, Strauss HW, et al. Real-time prognosis for metastatic thyroid carcinoma based on 2-[18F]fluoro-2-deoxy-D-glucose-positron emission tomography scanning. JCEM. 2006;91(2):498-505.

15. Deandreis D, Al Ghuzlan A, Leboulleux S, Lacroix L, Garsi JP, Talbot M, et al. Do histological, immunohistochemical, and metabolic (radioiodine and fluorodeoxyglucose uptakes) patterns of metastatic thyroid cancer correlate with patient outcome? Endocr Relat Cancer. 2011;18(1):159-69.

16. Salvatori M, Biondi B, Rufini V. Imaging in endocrinology: 2-[18F]-fluoro-2-deoxy-D-glucose positron emission tomography/computed tomography in differentiated thyroid carcinoma: clinical indications and controversies in diagnosis and follow-up. Eur J Endocrinol. 2015;173(3):R115-30.

17. Feine U, Lietzenmayer R, Hanke J, Held J, Wä H. Fluorine-18-FDG and Iodine-131-Iodide Uptake in Thyroid Cancer. J Nucl Med. 1996;37(9):7-11.

18. Nikiforova MN, Nikiforov YE. Molecular genetics of thyroid cancer: implications for diagnosis, treatment and prognosis. Expert Rev Mol Diagn. 2008;8(1):83-95.

19. Bunone G, Vigneri P, Mariani L, Butó S, Collini P, Pilotti S, et al. Expression of angiogenesis stimulators and inhibitors in human thyroid tumors and correlation with clinical pathological features. Am J Pathol. 1999;155(6):1967-76.

20. Klein M, Vignaud JM, Hennequin V, Toussaint B, Bresler L, Plénat F, et al. Increased expression of the vascular endothelial growth factor is a pejorative prognosis marker in papillary thyroid carcinoma. JCEM. 2001;86(2):656-8.

21. Carneiro RM, Carneiro BA, Agulnik M, Kopp PA, Giles FJ. Targeted therapies in advanced differentiated thyroid cancer. Cancer Treat Rev. 2015;41(8):690-8.

22. Schlumberger M. Prise en charge des cancers réfractaires de la thyroïde. Bull Cancer. 2011;72:149-57.

23. Miyauchi A, Kudo T, Miya A, Kobayashi K, Ito Y, Takamura Y, et al. Prognostic impact of serum thyroglobulin doubling-time under thyrotropin suppression in patients with papillary thyroid carcinoma who underwent total thyroidectomy. Thyroid. 2011;21(7):707-16.

24. Brose MS, Smit J, Capdevila J, Elisei R, Nutting C, Pitoia F, et al. Regional approaches to the management of patients with advanced, radioactive iodine-refractory differentiated thyroid carcinoma. Expert Ther. 2012;12(9):1137-47.

25. Schlumberger M, Sherman SI. Approach to the patient with advanced differentiated thyroid cancer. Eur J Endocrinol. 2012;166(1):5-11.

26. Vaisman F, Carvalho DP, Vaisman M. A new appraisal of iodine refractory thyroid cancer. Endocr Relat Cancer. 2015;22(6):R301-10.

27. Worden F. Treatment strategies for radioactive iodine-refractory differentiated thyroid cancer. Ther Adv Med Oncol. 2014;6(6):267-79.

28. Ito Y, Suzuki S, Ito K, Imai T, Okamoto T, Kitano H, et al. Tyrosine-kinase inhibitors to treat radioiodine-refracted, metastatic, or recurred and progressive differentiated thyroid carcinoma [Review]. Endocr J [Internet]. 2016;63(1):1-6. Available at: <https://www.jstage.jst.go.jp/article/endocrj/advpub/0/advpub_EJ16-0064/_article>.

29. Carhill AA, Cabanillas ME, Jimenez C, Waguespack SG, Habra MA, Hu M, et al. The noninvestigational use of tyrosine kinase inhibitors in thyroid cancer: Establishing a standard for patient safety and monitoring. JCEM. 2013;98(1):31-42.

30. Marotta V, Ramundo V, Camera L, Prete M Del, Fonti R, Esposito R, et al. Sorafenib in advanced iodine-refractory differentiated thyroid cancer: efficacy, safety and exploratory analysis of role of serum thyroglobulin and FDG-PET. Clin Endocrinol (Oxf). 2013;78(5):760-7.

31. McFarland DC, Misiukiewicz KJ. Sorafenib in radioactive iodine-refractory well-differentiated metastatic thyroid cancer. OncoTargets Ther. 2014;7:1291-9.

32. Brose MS, Nutting CM, Jarzab B, Elisei R, Siena S, Bastholt L, et al. Sorafenib in radioactive iodine-refractory, locally advanced or metastatic differentiated thyroid cancer: a randomised, double-blind, phase 3 trial. Lancet. 2014;384(9940):319-28.

33. Yeung KT, Cohen EEW. Lenvatinib in advanced, radioactive iodine-refractory, differentiated thyroid carcinoma. Clin Cancer Res. 2015;21(24):5420-6.

34. Bible K, Suman V, Molina J, Smallridge R, Maples W, Menefee M, et al. Efficacy of pazopanib in progressive, radioiodine-refractory, metastatic differentiated thyroid cancers: results of a phase 2 consortium study. Lancet Oncol. 2010;11(10):962-72.

35. Cabanillas ME, Brose MS, Holland J, Ferguson KC, Sherman SI. A phase I study of cabozantinib (XL184) in patients with differentiated thyroid cancer. Thyroid. 2014;24(10):1508-14.

36. Carr LL, Mankoff DA, Goulart BH, Eaton KD, Capell PT, Kell EM, et al. Phase II study of daily sunitinib in FDG-PET-positive, iodine-refractory differentiated thyroid cancer and metastatic medullary carcinoma of the thyroid with functional imaging correlation. Clin Cancer Res. 2010;16(21):5260-8.

37. Leboulleux S, Bastholt L, Krause T, de la Fouchardiere C, Tennvall J, Awada A, et al. Vandetanib in locally advanced or metastatic differentiated thyroid cancer: a randomised, double-blind, phase 2 trial. Lancet Oncol. 2012;13(9):897-905.

38. Sherman S, Wirth L, Droz J, Hofmann M, Bastholt L, Martins RG, et al. Motesanib Diphosphate in Progressive Differentiated Thyroid Cancer. NEJM. 2008;359(1):31-42.

39. Cohen EEW, Rosen LS, Vokes EE, Kies MS, Forastiere AA, Worden FP, et al. Axitinib is an active treatment for all histologic subtypes of advanced thyroid cancer: Results from a phase II study. J Clin Oncol. 2008;26(29):4708-13.

40. Cohen EEW, Tortorici M, Kim S, Ingrosso A, Pithavala YK, Bycott P. A phase II trial of axitinib in patients with various histologic subtypes of advanced thyroid cancer: Long-term outcomes and pharmacokinetic/pharmacodynamic analyses. Cancer Chemother Pharmacol. 2014;74(6):1261-70.

41. Locati LD, Licitra L, Agate L, Ou SHI, Boucher A, Jarzab B, et al. Treatment of advanced thyroid cancer with axitinib: Phase 2 study with pharmacokinetic/pharmacodynamic and quality-of-life assessments. Cancer. 2014;120(17):2694-703.

42. Awasthi N, Schwarz R. Profile of nintedanib in the treatment of solid tumors : the evidence to date. Onco Targets Ther. 2015;8:3691-701.

43. French JD. Revisiting immune-based therapies for aggressive follicular cell–derived thyroid cancers. Thyroid. 2013;23(5):529-42.

44. Cunha LL, Marcello MA, Ward LS. The role of the inflammatory microenvironment in thyroid carcinogenesis. Endocr Relat Cancer. 2014;21(3):85-103.

45. Bernet V, Smallridge R. New therapeutic options for advanced forms of thyroid cancer. Expert Opin Emerg Drugs. 2014;19(2):225-41.

46. Dadu R, Shah K, Busaidy NL, Waguespack SG, Habra MA, Ying AK, et al. Efficacy and tolerability of vemurafenib in patients with BRAFV600E positive papillary thyroid cancer: M.D. Anderson Cancer center off label experience. JCEM. 2015;100(1):77-81.

47. Falchook GS, Millward M, Hong D, Naing A, Piha-Paul S, Waguespack SG, et al. BRAF inhibitor dabrafenib in patients with metastatic BRAF-mutant thyroid cancer. Thyroid. 2015;25(1):71-7.

48. Hamatani K, Mukai M, Takahashi K, Hayashi Y, Nakachi K, Kusunoki Y. Rearranged anaplastic lymphoma kinase (ALK) gene in adult-onset papillary thyroid cancer amongst atomic bomb survivors. Thyroid. 2012;22(11):1153-9.

49. Kelly LM, Barila G, Liu P, Evdokimova VN, Trivedi S, Panebianco F, et al. Identification of the transforming STRN-ALK fusion as a potential therapeutic target in the aggressive forms of thyroid cancer. PNAS. 2014;111(11):4233-8.

50. Zhou Y, Zhao C, Gery S, Braunstein G, Okamoto R, Alvarez R, et al. Off Target Effects of c-MET Inhibitors on Thyroid Cancer Cells. Mol Cancer Ther. 2014;13(1):134-43.

51. Landa I, Ibrahimpasic T, Boucai L, Sinha R, Knauf JA, Shah RH, et al. Genomic and transcriptomic hallmarks of poorly differentiated and anaplastic thyroid cancers. J Clin Invest. 2016;126(3):1-16.

52. Lim SM, Chang H, Yoon MJ, Hong YK, Kim H, Chung WY, et al. A multicenter, phase II trial of everolimus in locally advanced or metastatic thyroid cancer of all histologic subtypes. Ann Oncol. 2013;24(12):3089-93.

53. Pezzulo AA, Tang XX, Hoegger MJ, Alaiwa MHA, Ramachandran S, Moninger TO, et al. Selumetinib-Enhanced Radioiodine Uptake in Advanced Thyroid Cancer. NEJM. 2013;487(7405): 109-13.

54. Rothenberg SM, McFadden DG, Palmer EL, Daniels GH, Wirth LJ. Redifferentiation of iodine-refractory BRAF V600E-mutant metastatic papillary thyroid cancer with dabrafenib. Clin Cancer Res. 2015;21(5):1028-35.

55. Dadu R, Devine C, Hernandez M, Waguespack SG, Busaidy NL, Hu MI, et al. Role of salvage targeted therapy in differentiated thyroid cancer patients who failed first-line sorafenib. JCEM. 2014;99(6):2086-94.

56. Massicotte M-H, Brassard M, Claude-Desroches M, Borget I, Bonichon F, Giraudet A-L, et al. Tyrosine kinase inhibitor treatments in patients with metastatic thyroid carcinomas: a retrospective study of the TUTHYREF network. Eur J Endocrinol. 2014;170(4):575-82.

57. Walko CM, Grande C. Management of common adverse events in patients treated with Sorafenib: Nurse and pharmacist perspective. Semin Oncol. 2014;41(Suppl. 2):S17-28.

58. Cabanillas ME, Hu MI, Durand JB, Busaidy NL. Challenges associated with tyrosine kinase inhibitor therapy for metastatic thyroid cancer. J Thyroid Res. 2011;2011(985780):1-9.

59. Pitoia F, Jerkovich F. Selective use of sorafenib in the treatment of thyroid cancer. Drug Des Ther. 2016;10:1119-31.

60. Brose MS, Frenette CT, Keefe SM, Stein SM. Management of Sorafenib-related adverse events: a clinician's perspective. Semin Oncol. 2014;41:S1-16.

20

Prevalence of metabolic syndrome in pre- and postmenopausal women

Ricardo de Marchi[1], Cátia Millene Dell'Agnolo[2], Tiara Cristina Romeiro Lopes[1], Angela Andréia França Gravena[1], Marcela de Oliveira Demitto[2], Sheila Cristina Rocha Brischiliari[2], Deise Helena Pelloso Borghesan[1], Maria Dalva de Barros Carvalho[1], Sandra Marisa Pelloso[1,2]

ABSTRACT

Objective: The objective of this study was to determine the prevalence of metabolic syndrome (MS) and its components among pre- and postmenopausal women, as well as the association between menopausal status and MS. **Materials and methods:** A retrospective study was conducted at a reference cardiology outpatient clinic in a city located in Northwestern Paraná State, Brazil. A total of 958 medical records of symptomatic climacteric women evaluated between 2010 and 2014 were analyzed. The study consisted of two groups: pre- and post-menopausal women. MS was characterized according to the criteria of the National Cholesterol Education Program's Adult Treatment Panel III – NCEP-ATP III-2005. **Results:** MS was observed in 18.5% of the total study population; 9.4% of the premenopausal women and 22.2% of the postmenopausal women displayed MS, corresponding to a relative risk of 2.75. In addition, the frequency of MS increased with age. Regarding the components of MS, postmenopausal women were more likely to have high density lipoprotein (HDL-C) levels < 50 mg/dL; systolic blood pressure (SBP) values ≥ 130 mmHg or diastolic blood pressure (DBP) values ≥ 85 mmHg; and fasting glucose levels ≥ 100 mg/dL. **Conclusion:** MS was more prevalent among postmenopausal women than among premenopausal women. Arch Endocrinol Metab. 2017;61(2):160-6.

Keywords
Metabolic syndrome; menopause; climacteric; cardiovascular disease

[1] Departamento de Ciências da Saúde, Pós-Graduação em Ciências da Saúde, Universidade Estadual de Maringá (UEM), PR, Brasil.
[2] Departamento de Enfermagem, Pós-Graduação em Enfermagem, Universidade Estadual de Maringá (UEM), PR, Brasil.

Correspondence to:
Cátia Millene Dell'Agnolo
Av. Colombo, 5790
87020-900 – Maringá, PR, Brasil
catiaagnolo@gmail.com

INTRODUCTION

Cardiovascular diseases (CVDs) are the leading cause of death among women in the United States. According to the American Heart Association (AHA), approximately one in three female adults has some form of CVD (1).

The cardiovascular risk profile coincides with menopause and it is characterized by the occurrence or worsening of some risk factors associated with this period such as abdominal obesity, hypertension, and dyslipidemia (2,3). These risk factors, in combination with insulin resistance, hyperinsulinemia, and hyperglycemia, compose metabolic syndrome (MS). Patients with MS are at increased risk of CVD and type 2 diabetes mellitus (2).

Postmenopausal status is associated with an increased incidence of MS and CVD, which is mainly associated with the reduction in the levels of female sex hormones (4). Studies have reported that menopause is an independent predictor of MS in females (5,6).

Several studies have identified risk factors for MS and CVD in menopausal women (7,8). However, few studies address this topic in the Brazilian population. Therefore, the objective of this study was to determine the prevalence of MS and its components in pre- and postmenopausal women, as well as the association between menopausal status and MS.

MATERIALS AND METHODS

This retrospective study was performed in a reference cardiology outpatient clinic in a city located in Northwestern Paraná State, Southern Brazil. A total of 958 medical records of women aged 40-65 years evaluated between 2010 and 2014 were analyzed. All of the women seen in the clinic during the study period were included in the study, except for hysterectomized women.

The study consisted of two groups: a premenopausal group composed of women who were still having either regular or irregular menstrual cycles and a postmenopausal group composed of women who had not experienced menstrual cycles in more than one year, according to the definition of the guideline on the diagnosis and management of menopause (9).

The presence of MS is considered a disorder associated with a set of cardiovascular risk factors including abdominal fat deposition, hypertension, low levels of high density lipoprotein cholesterol (HDL-C), elevated levels of low density lipoprotein cholesterol (LDL-C), hypertriglyceridemia, increased fasting glucose levels diagnosed according to the criteria of the National Cholesterol Education Program's Adult Treatment Panel III – NCEP-ATP III-2005 (2), and an increased body mass index (BMI) calculated by dividing the body weight (kg) by the height squared (m²). The subjects were classified as non-obese (BMI up to 29.9 kg/m²) and obese (BMI equal to or greater than 30 kg/m²) according to the World Health Organization (WHO) standards (10). According to the NCEP-ATP III, MS represents the combination of three of the following variables (2):

1) Abdominal obesity: waist circumference ≥ 88 cm;

2) Hypertriglyceridemia: serum TG levels ≥ 150 mg/dL;

3) Serum HDL-c, low: < 50 mg/dL;

4) Hypertension: systolic blood pressure (SBP) ≥ 130 mmHg and/or diastolic blood pressure (DBP) ≥ 85 mmHg or receiving treatment for hypertension; and

5) Elevated fasting glucose: glucose level > 100 mg/dL or receiving treatment for diabetes.

The following variables were analyzed: age, stratified into age groups (40-45 years, 46-50 years, 51-55 years, and 56-65 years); color (white and non-white); civil status (with or without a partner); paid occupation (yes or no); physical activity (yes or no); tobacco and alcohol use (yes or no); systolic and diastolic blood pressure values; waist circumference (WC); and an analysis of fasting glucose, HDL-C, LDL-C, and triglycerides levels and the BMI (obese or non-obese).

The values for WC, blood pressure and laboratory tests were obtained from the medical records of the participants. The outpatient clinic uses a standardized procedure for measuring blood pressure; namely, after a 5-min rest, blood pressure is measured in the left arm both at the beginning and end of the examination using an aneroid sphygmomanometer, and the patient is in a seated position. The WC corresponds to the midpoint between the lower margin of the last rib and the top of the iliac crest. The laboratory tests were performed in different laboratories, always after a 12-h fasting period.

For the statistical analysis, a descriptive analysis and a crude analysis were performed using the chi-square test. The risk of MS and its components was analyzed with the crude odds ratio (OR) using the chi-square test. The program Epi Info 3.5.1 was used, and a significance level of 5% and confidence interval (CI) of 95% were adopted.

The research project was approved by the Standing Committee on Research Ethics of the State University of Maringa (Universidade Estadual de Maringá – UEM), under decision number 856.300. A waiver of signed informed consent was requested because the data were obtained from medical records without patient identification.

RESULTS

The medical records of 958 climacteric women, including 277 premenopausal women (28.9%) and 681 postmenopausal women (71.1%), were analyzed. The overall mean age was 53.6 ± 7.52 years, with a large percentage of women aged 56-65 years (46.0%). The mean ages of the pre- and postmenopausal women were 44.5 ± 2.9 and 57.3 ± 5.33 years, respectively. According to the socio-demographic variables, 71.3% of the women had a partner, 95.4% were white, and 57.4% had a paid occupation.

MS was observed in 18.5% of women. MS was more prevalent among postmenopausal and the oldest women. A total of 9.4% of premenopausal women presented MS, while 22.2% of postmenopausal women presented this syndrome, with a relative risk of 2.75 (CI 1.76-4.28). Regarding the age groups, MS was more frequent with increasing age (Table 1).

Table 2 shows the association between the components of MS according to menopausal status. Postmenopausal women were more likely to have HDL-C levels < 50 mg/dL (OR 1.53; CI 1.08-2.18); SBP values ≥ 130 or DBP values ≥ 85 mmHg (OR 2.47; CI 1.85-3.31); and fasting glucose levels ≥ 100 mg/dL (OR 2.04; CI 1.30-3.21).

Table 1. Prevalence of metabolic syndrome according to menopausal status, sociodemographic data, and lifestyle. Sarandi, Paraná, Brazil, 2015

	n	% MS Yes n (%)	% MS No n (%)	OR	95% CI	p
Menopausal status	958					
Premenopausal		26 (9.4)	251 (90.6)	1		
Postmenopausal		151 (22.2)	530 (77.8)	2.75	1.76-4.28	< 0.001
Age group (years)	958					
40-45		10 (5.4)	174 (94.6)	1		
46-50		20 (12.7)	137 (87.3)	2.54	1.15-5.60	0.01
51-55		36 (19.9)	145 (80.1)	4.32	2.07-9.00	< 0.001
56-65		111 (25.5)	325 (74.5)	5.94	3.03-11.64	< 0.001
Skin color	951					
White		166 (18.3)	742 (81.7)	1		
Non-white		9 (20.9)	34 (79.1)	1.18	0.55-2.51	0.66
Marital status	937					
With partner		125 (18.5)	552 (81.5)	1		
Without partner		49 (18.8)	211 (81.2)	1.02	0.71-1.47	0.89
Paid occupation	951					
Yes		92 (16.5)	464 (83.5)	1		
No		84 (21.3)	311 (78.7)	1.36	0.98-1.89	0.06
Physical activity	294					
Yes		24 (16.1)	125 (83.9)	1		
No		21 (14.5)	124 (85.5)	0.88	0.46-1.66	0.69
Tobacco use	581					
Yes		12 (19.0)	51 (81.0)	1.18	0.60-2.31	0.62
No		86 (16.6)	432 (83.4)	1		
Alcohol use	845					
Yes		3 (15.8)	16 (84.2)	0.87	0.25-3.08	1.00
No		82 (17.6)	384 (82.4)	1		

MS: metabolic syndrome; OR: odds ratio; CI: confidence interval.

DISCUSSION

Few Brazilian studies address the correlation between MS and menopause, which sets the present study apart. However, some study limitations should be considered. Data were obtained from electronic medical records that were entered only once during medical visits and may have been incomplete. In fact, because the present study evaluated medical records, some relevant factors associated with MS were missing, such as lifestyle, physical activity, tobacco use, and obesity. The frequency and intensity of physical activity were not reported. Similarly, the tobacco use data were incomplete, as the time and frequency of use were not collected. Another important limitation of this study is that the sample comprised women who were observed at a reference cardiology outpatient clinic, and thus, they had a greater likelihood of presenting with cardiovascular risk factors and other comorbidities.

In this study, MS was present in 18.5% of the studied women. Another Brazilian study found a higher prevalence (34.7%) of MS in this group of women in the state of Maranhão (11). In studies from different countries, the prevalence of MS in women has ranged from 15.9% in Thai women (12) to 26.4% in Iranian women (5) and 33.8% in *Puerto Rican* women (13).

Our study found that MS was more prevalent among postmenopausal women (22.2%) than among premenopausal women (9.4%). The prevalence of MS among postmenopausal women has been reported to

Table 2. Presence of metabolic syndrome and its components according to menopausal status. Sarandi, Paraná, 2015

	N	Premenopause		Postmenopause		OR	95% CI	p
		N	%	N	%			
WC ≥ 88 cm	213							
Yes		31	23.3	102	76.7	1.32	0.70-1.49	0.37
No		23	28.8	57	71.3	1		
TGL ≥ 150 mg/dL	673							
Yes		40	21.5	146	78.5	1.44	0.96-3.15	0.07
No		138	28.3	349	71.7	1		
HDL-C < 50 mg/dL	661							
Yes		71	22.2	249	77.8	1.53	1.08-2.18	0.01
No		104	30.5	237	69.5	1		
LDL-C ≥ 130 mg/dL	629							
Yes		57	25.6	166	74.4	1.10	0.74-1.62	0.62
No		111	27.3	295	72.7	1		
SBP ≥ 130 or DBP ≥ 85 mmHg	932							
Yes		134	22.3	468	77.7	2.47	1.85-3.31	< 0.001
No		137	41.5	193	58.5	1		
Fasting glucose levels > 100 mg/dL	501							
Yes		32	17.2	154	82.8	2.04	1.30-3.21	0.001
No		94	29.8	221	70.2	1		
BMI (kg/m²)	204							
< 29.9		28	26.7	77	73.3	1		
≥ 30		30	30.3	69	69.7	0.84	0.43-1.61	0.56

WC: waist circumference; TGL: triglycerides; SBP: systolic blood pressure; DBP: diastolic blood pressure; BMI: body mass index; OR: odds ratio; CI: confidence interval.

vary by country, ranging between 16.9% in Thailand (12), 29.0% in Puerto Rico (13), 31.0% in Iran (14), 49.8% in Brazil (11), 53.5% in Iran (5), 55.5% in India (15), and 64.3% in Iran (16). MS is one factor that increases the mortality rate in both men and women (17). A meta-analysis confirmed this information by describing a higher prevalence of MS during the postmenopausal stage than the premenopausal stage, regardless of population (18).

There was a statistically significant relationship between postmenopausal stage and increased age with the presence of MS. Older women (older than 56 years of age) were 5.95 (CI: 3.03-11.64) times more likely than younger women to be diagnosed with MS. Some authors have identified age as the main risk factor for increased MS prevalence (10,19). The prevalence of MS varies among studies; however, several Brazilian (11,20) and international studies (15,16,21) found

a greater MS prevalence among postmenopausal women than among premenopausal women. A study performed in women aged 40-65 years in Argentina, another South American country, demonstrated a relative risk of 1.61 (CI: 1.18-2.19) of developing MS during post-menopause (22). The Third National Health and Nutrition Examination Survey (NHANES) III study described the association between MS and increased risk of mortality among postmenopausal women compared to premenopausal women (23).

Unfavorable cardiovascular risk factor levels are observed during menopause, including changes in body fat distribution from a gynaecoid pattern to an android pattern, abnormal blood lipid levels, increased sympathetic tone, endothelial dysfunction, vascular inflammation, and increased blood pressure. Postmenopausal women are at greater risk for CVDs than men (matched by age) due to the failure and reduction of the gonads and steroid production (24). Estrogens play a key role in maintaining adequate levels of HDL-C (8).

In our study, the prevalence of all MS components was higher in postmenopausal women, with a statistically significant association for low HDL-c levels, hypertension, and high fasting glucose levels. These components were also described as prevalent in postmenopausal women in Iran (5,6), South Korea (25), and Poland (26), as well as in Brazil (20). A study conducted in the state of Maranhão revealed that increased blood pressure was also prevalent (73.4%) among postmenopausal women (11). However, a recent study found no significance differences for body weight, BMI, WC, blood pressure, total cholesterol, LDL cholesterol, triglycerides and glucose levels between premenopausal and postmenopausal women (27).

Some researchers consider post-menopause as a period of hyperandrogenism that results from the greater reduction in estrogen, due to ovarian failure, than in androgens, with increased levels of LDL and decreased levels of HDL cholesterol, which characterize an atherogenic profile (28,29), compatible with MS. Estrogen seems to have a positive effect on the inner layer of artery wall, which helps to maintain blood vessels flexible (30). Conversely, the cause of hypertension is not well defined in postmenopausal women. It is believed that an increased androgen/estrogen ratio can alter the renin-angiotensin system (31). Other possible causes for hypertension are increased endothelin levels, oxidative stress, obesity and stimulation of the sympathetic nervous system (32). Whether administered chronically, endothelin causes increases in sodium reabsorption in the kidney and consequent increase in blood pressure (33), and in postmenopausal women, plasma endothelin levels are increased (34), suggesting that endothelin can play a part in increasing blood pressure after menopause (35). In conclusion, both endothelin and angiotensin II may contribute to oxidative stress (36). The oxidative stress markers are increased in women after menopause (37), and oxidative stress has caused the increase of blood pressure by decreasing the bioavailability of vasodilator (36). However, antioxidant therapy did not produce a reduction in blood pressure, in humans (38). The role of oxidative stress in hypertension in women after menopause has not been completely elucidated (35).

However, some authors found that although HDL cholesterol levels decrease with increased visceral fat and total weight, low HDL cholesterol levels are not a main feature of MS in postmenopausal women. HDL cholesterol levels appear to increase, not decrease, with age (27). Moreover, higher HDL cholesterol levels were found in postmenopausal women compared to premenopausal women (27,39).

In our study, we found a higher risk of glucose levels > 100 mg/dL. A study conducted with diabetic women found a high prevalence of MS in both premenopausal (87.5%) and postmenopausal (87.7%) women (24). Insulin resistance is described as a key factor implicated in the pathophysiology of MS (40). It contributes to increased glucose intolerance and diabetes, hypertension, increased triglyceride levels, and reduced HDL levels (41).

Another study revealed that postmenopausal women were more likely to present elevated total cholesterol levels, poor glycemic control (OR = 2.92; 95% CI = 1.32-6.33), and lower HDL levels (OR = 0.36; 95% CI = 0.19-0.68) than premenopausal women (42).

Although the BMI was not correlated with menopausal status in the present study, a previous study demonstrated that a BMI > 30 kg/m^2 (obese subjects) had a significant negative effect on blood pressure (increase), triglycerides, and fasting glucose levels, in addition to being associated with low HDL-C levels compared to a normal BMI (non-obese subjects). These data indicate that "obese" individuals have more cardiovascular risk factors (43).

Finally, some authors report that the prevention of metabolic diseases in menopause requires changes in lifestyle, including the performance of moderate physical activity and consumption of a healthy diet, as the main recommendation to prevent metabolic diseases during menopause. In some cases, after an individual evaluation, hormone replacement therapy was recommended (44), which could have a positive effect on lipids by reducing total and LDL cholesterol and by slightly increasing HDL levels, as demonstrated in a meta-analysis (45).

Thus, our data suggest that the prevalence of MS was higher among postmenopausal women than premenopausal women and increased with increasing age. The components of MS that were prevalent in postmenopausal women included low HDL-C levels (< 50 mg/dL), hypertension (SBP values ≥ 130 mmHg or DBP values ≥ 85 mmHg), and high fasting glucose levels (≥ 100 mg/dL).

REFERENCES

1. Sanders GD, Patel MR, Chatterjee R, Ross AK, Bastian LA, Coeytaux RR, et al. Noninvasive Technologies for the Diagnosis of Coronary Artery Disease in Women: Future Research Needs: Identification of Future Research Needs From Comparative Effectiveness Review No. 58. Agency for Healthcare Research and Quality (US). Report No.: 13-EHC072-EF, 2013.

2. Grundy SM, Cleeman JI, Daniels SR, Donato KA, Eckel RH, Franklin BA, et al. American Heart Association; National Heart, Lung, and Blood Institute. Diagnosis and management of the metabolic syndrome: an American Heart Association/National Heart, Lung, and Blood Institute Scientific Statement. Circulation. 2005;112:2735-52.

3. Alberti KG, Zimmet P, Shaw J. Metabolic syndrome: a new world-wide definition: a consensus statement from the International Diabetes Federation. Diabet Med. 2006;23:469-80.

4. Qader SS, Shakir YA, Nyberg P, Samsioe G. Sociodemographic risk factors of metabolic syndrome in middle-aged women: results from a population-based study of Swedish women, The Women's Health in the Lund Area (WHILA) Study. Climacteric. 2008;11(6):475-82.

5. Eshtiaghi R, Esteghamati A, Nakhjavani M. Menopause is an independent predictor of metabolic syndrome in Iranian women. Maturitas. 2010;65(3):262-6.

6. Ainy E, Mirmiran P, Zahedi AS. Prevalence of metabolic syndrome during menopausal transition in Tehranian women: Tehran Lipid and Glucose Study (TLGS). Maturitas. 2007;58:150-5.

7. Sallam T, Watson KE. Predictors of cardiovascular risk in women. Womens Health (Lond). 2013;9(5):491-8.

8. Dowling NM, Gleason CE, Manson JE, Hodis HN, Miller VM, Brinton EA, et al. Characterization of vascular disease risk in postmenopausal women and its association with cognitive performance. PLoS One. 2013;8(7):e68741.

9. Chaplin S. NICE guideline: diagnosis and management of the menopause. 2016.

10. WHO. World Health Organization. Global database on Body Mass Index. BMI classification, Washington, 2006. Available at: <http://apps.who.int/bmi/index.jsp?introPage=intro_3.html>. Acessed on: Aug. 24, 2009.

11. Figueiredo-Neto AA, Figuerêdo ED, Barbosa JB, Barbosa FF, Costa GRC, Nina VJS, et al. Síndrome metabólica e menopausa: estudo transversal em ambulatório de ginecologia. Arq Bras Cardiol. 2010;91:1-23.

12. Indhavivadhana S, Rattanachaiyanont M, Wongvananurak T, Kanboon M, Techatraisak K, Leerasiri P, et al. Predictors for metabolic syndrome in perimenopausal and postmenopausal Thai women. Climacteric. 2011;14:58-65.

13. Romaguera J, Ortiz AP, Roca FJ, Cólon G, Suárez E. Factors associated with metabolic syndrome in a sample of women in Puerto Rico. Menopause. 2010;17:388-92.

14. Marjani A, Moghasemi S. The metabolic syndrome among postmenopausal women in Gorgan. Int J Endocrinol. 2012;2012:953627.

15. Pandey S, Srinivas M, Agashe S, Joshi J, Galvankar P, Prakasam CP, et al. Menopause and metabolic syndrome: a study of 498 urban women from western India. J Midlife Health. 2010;1:63-9.

16. Heidari R, Sadeghi M, Talaei M, Rabiei K, Mohammadifard N, Sarrafzadegan N. Metabolic syndrome in menopausal transition: Isfahan Healthy Heart Program, a population based study. Diabetol Metab Syndr. 2010;2:59.

17. Meirelles RMR. Menopausa e síndrome metabólica. Arq Bras Endocrinol Metab. 2014;58:2.

18. Mendes CG, Theodoro H, Rodrigues AD, Olinto MTA. Prevalência de síndrome metabólica e seus componentes na transição menopáusica: uma revisão sistemática. Cad Saúde Pública. 2012;28:1423-37.

19. Nakhjavani M, Imani M, Larry M, Aghajani-Nargesi A, Morteza A, Esteghamati A. Metabolic syndrome in premenopausal and postmenopausal women with type 2 diabetes: loss of protective effects of premenopausal status. J Diabetes Metab Disord. 2014;13(1):102.

20. Mendes KG, Theodoro H, Rodrigues AD, Busnello F, Lorenzi DRS de, Olinto MTA. Menopausal status and metabolic syndrome in women in climacteric period treated at a clinic in Southern Brazil. Open J Endocr Metab Dis. 2013;3:31-41.

21. Jouyadeh Z, Nayebzadeh F, Qorbani M, Asadi M. Metabolic syndrome and menopause. J Diabetes Metab Disord. 2013;12:1.

22. Coniglio RI, Nellem J, Gentili R, Sibechi N, Agusti E, Torres M. Metabolic syndrome in employee in Argentina. Medicina (B Aires). 2009;69:246-52.

23. Lin JW, Caffrey JL, Chang MH, Lin YS. Sex, menopause, metabolic syndrome, and all-cause and cause-specific mortality-cohort analysis from the Third National Health and Nutrition Examination Survey. J Clin Endocrinol Metab. 2010;95:4258-67.

24. Narayanaswamy N, Moodithaya S, Halahalli H, Miratkar AM. Assessment of Risk Factor for Cardiovascular Disease Using Heart Rate Variability in Postmenopausal Women: A Comparative Study between Urban and Rural Indian Women Clinical Study. ISRN Cardiol. 2013(2013):ID858921.

25. Sieminska L, Wojciechowska C, Foltyn W, Kajdanivk D, Kos-Kudla B, Marek B, et al. The relation of serum adiponectin and leptin levels to metabolic syndrome in women before and after the menopause. Endokrynol Pol. 2006;57:15-22.

26. Kim HM, Park J, Ryu SY, Kim J. The effect of menopause on the metabolic syndrome among Korean women: the Korean National Health and Nutrition Examination Survey, 2001. Diabetes Care. 2007;30:701-6.

27. Fernandez ML, Murillo AG. Postmenopausal Women have higuer HDL and Decreased Incidence of low HDL than premenopausal women with metabolic syndrome. Healthcare. 2016;4:20.

28. Banks AD. Women and heart disease: missed opportunities. J Midwifery Womens Health. 2008;53:430-9.

29. Weinberg ME, Manson JE, Buring JE, Cook NR, Seely EW, Ridker PM, et al. Low sex hormone-binding globulin is associated with the metabolic syndrome in postmenopausal women. Metabolism. 2006;55:1473-80.

30. American Heart Association. Conditions. Menopause and Heart Disease, 2015. Available at: <http://www.heart.org/HEARTORG/Conditions/More/MyHeartandStrokeNews/Menopause-and-Heart-Disease_UCM_448432_Article.jsp#.V7t0s1cmXC4>. Acessed on: Aug. 22, 2016.

31. Fernandez-Vega F, Abellan J, Vegazo O, De Vinuesa SG, Rodriguez JC, Maceira B, et al. Angiotensin II type 1 receptor blockade to control BP in postmenopausal women: influence of hormone replacement therapy. Kidney Int. 2002;(Suppl):S36-41.

32. Reckelhoff JF, Fortepiani LA. Novel mechanisms responsible for postmenopausal hypertension. Hypertension. 2004;43:918-23.

33. Wilkins FC Jr, Alberola A, Mizelle HL, Opgenorth TJ, Granger JP. Systemic hemodynamics and renal function during long-term pathophysiological increases in circulating endothelin. Am J Physiol. 1995;268:R375-81.

34. Komatsumoto S, Nara M. Changes in the level of endothelin-1 with aging. Nihon Ronen Igakkai Zasshi. 1995;32:664-9.

35. Lima R, Wofford M, Reckelhoff JF. Hypertension in postmenopausal women. Curr Hypertens Rep. 2012;14:254-60.

36. Reckelhoff JF, Romero JC. Role of oxidative stress in angiotensin-induced hypertension. Am J Physiol Regul Integr Comp Physiol. 2003;284:R893-912.

37. Castelao JE, Gago-Dominguez M. Risk factors for cardiovascular disease in women: relationship to lipid peroxidation and oxidative stress. Med Hypotheses. 2008;71:39-44.

38. Yanes LL, Romero DG, Cucchiarelli VE, Fortepiani LA, Gomez-Sanchez CE, Santacruz F, et al. Role of endothelin in mediating postmenopausal hypertension in a rat model. Am J Physiol Regul Integr Comp Physiol. 2005;288:R229-333.

39. Derby CA, Crawford SL, Pasternak RC, Sowers M, Sternfeld B, Matthews KA. Lipid changes during the menopause transition in relation to age and weight. Am J Epidemiol. 2009;169:1352-61.

40. Gaspard U. Hyperinsulinaemia, a key factor of the metabolic syndrome in postmenopausal women. Maturitas. 2009;62:362-5.

41. Reaven G. Metabolic syndrome: pathophysiology and implications for management of cardiovascular disease. Circulation. 2002;106:286-8.

42. Udo T, McKee SA, White MA, Macheb RM, Barnes RD, Grilo CM. Menopause and metabolic syndrome in obese individuals with binge eating disorder. Eating Behaviors. 2014;15:182-5.

43. Bagnoli VR, Fonseca AM, Arie WM, Das Neves EM, Azevedo RS, Sorpreso IC, et al. Metabolic disorder and obesity in 5027 Brazilian postmenopausal women. Gynecol Endocrinol. 2014;30:717-20.

44. Stachowiak G, Pertyński T, Pertyńska-Marczewska M. Metabolic disorders in menopause. Prz Menopauzalny. 2015;14:59-64.

45. Xu Y, Lin J, Wang S, Xiong J, Zhu Q. Combined estrogen replacement therapy on metabolic control in postmenopausal women with diabetes mellitus. Kaohsiung J Med Sci. 2014;30: 350-61.

21

Low glycemic index diet reduces body fat and attenuates inflammatory and metabolic responses in patients with type 2 diabetes

Júnia Maria Geraldo Gomes[1], Sabrina Pinheiro Fabrini[2],
Rita de Cássia Gonçalves Alfenas[3]

[1] Instituto Federal de Educação, Ciência e Tecnologia do Sudeste de Minas Gerais, Campus Barbacena, Barbacena, MG, Brasil
[2] Centro Universitário de Belo Horizonte, Campus Estoril, Belo Horizonte, MG, Brasil
[3] Departamento de Nutrição e Saúde, Universidade Federal de Viçosa, Viçosa, MG, Brasil

ABSTRACT

Objective: The aim of this study was to verify the effects of glycemic index (GI) on body composition, and on inflammatory and metabolic markers concentrations in patients with type 2 diabetes. **Subjects and methods:** In this randomized controlled parallel trial, twenty subjects (aged 42.4 ± 5.1 years, BMI 29.2 ± 4.8 kg.m^{-2}) were allocated to low GI (LGI) (n = 10) or high GI (HGI) (n = 10) groups. Body composition, inflammatory and metabolic markers were assessed at baseline and after 30 days of intervention. Food intake was monitored during the study using three-day food records completed on two non-consecutive weekdays and on a weekend day. **Results:** Body fat reduced after the LGI intervention compared with baseline (P = 0.043) and with the HGI group (P = 0.036). Serum fructosamine concentration (P = 0.031) and TNF-α mRNA expression (P = 0.05) increased in the HGI group. Serum non-esterified fatty acids were greater in the HGI than in the LGI group (P = 0.032). IL-6 mRNA expression tended to decrease after the consumption of the LGI diet compared to baseline (P = 0.06). **Conclusion:** The LGI diet reduced body fat and prevented the negative metabolic and inflammatory responses induced by the HGI diet. Arch Endocrinol Metab. 2017;61(2):137-44.

Keywords
Glycemic index; inflammation; metabolic profile; diabetes mellitus; body fat

Correspondence to:
Júnia Maria Geraldo Gomes
Instituto Federal de Educação, Ciência e Tecnologia do Sudeste de Minas Gerais –
Campus Barbacena
Rua Monsenhor José Augusto, 204
36205-018 – Barbacena, MG, Brasil
junianut@yahoo.com.br

INTRODUCTION

The glycemic index (GI) has been used in clinical practice for more than three decades to classify the glycemic impact of foods, meals or diets on glycemic response (1). Its use is supported by the World Health Organization and American Diabetes Association, which recommend the preferential consumption of low GI diets to provide health benefits (1).

Chronic ingestion of low GI diets can prevent and control obesity (2), cardiovascular diseases (3), and type 2 diabetes mellitus (T2DM) (4). By contrast, consumption of high GI diets is related to hyperglycemia and hyperinsulinemia, favoring an increase in glucose uptake by the adipocytes, leading to weight gain and body fat accumulation (5). On the other hand, it has been claimed that daily consumption of two low GI meals can result in beneficial effects on body weight and body composition (6).

High GI diets seem to negatively affect insulin sensitivity and subclinical inflammation, contributing to the pathogenesis of T2DM (7,8). Low GI diets may decrease concentrations of pro-inflammatory biomarkers, especially ultra-sensitive C-reactive protein (CRP), fibrinogen, interleukin-6 (IL-6) and tumor necrosis factor-alpha (TNF-α) (3,7,9). However, there is no consensus among authors regarding these effects (10).

Some studies that evaluated the effect of GI on inflammatory markers are epidemiological (2,11). These studies can detect an association between the variables of interest, but are unable to prove causation (2,11). By contrast, the main limitation of the many clinical trials published is the different macronutrients and dietary fiber contents of the test meals (7). The consumption of diets differing in protein and fat content can lead to different glycemic responses (12).

Dietary fiber may also reduce the glycemic response, increasing glucose tolerance (13). Thus, the test meals in such studies must contain the same quantity of fiber and macronutrients so that the observed effect can be attributed to the GI. Due to the lack of consensus in the results of previous studies, we evaluated the effect of the consumption of high or low GI diets for 30 consecutive days on anthropometric, body composition, food intake, glycemic and lipid control, inflammatory marker in concentrations in patients with type 2 diabetes.

SUBJECTS AND METHODS

Subjects

Subjects were recruited via advertisements in local newspapers, in the university website and flyers distributed around the city of Viçosa, Minas Gerais, Brazil. Data collection took place between April and September 2007. An initial screening was conducted by phone calls and then in the laboratory. Eligible participants were men or premenopausal women between 18 and 55 years old with type 2 diabetes who were receiving biguanides therapy (metformin), which did not change their medications in the previous three months and who had body fat percentage values higher than 16% for men and 24% for women. The exclusion criteria were tobacco use, consumption of > 50 g/day of alcohol (14), pregnancy or lactation, menopause or postmenopause, regular use of hormones, anti-inflammatory medications or other medications that might interfere with outcome measures, recent change (in the previous three months) in the level of physical activity (15) or diet, weight instability (> 3 kg in the previous three months), on a therapeutic diet, dietary allergies or intolerances, cancer, or cardiovascular, renal, or liver disease. Of 102 individuals interested to participate in the study, 55 met the inclusion criteria in the initial screening (via telephone). However, only 41 fully met all the inclusion criteria after screening in the laboratory. Among these, 18 refused to participate due to unavailability to attend daily twice a day to the laboratory during the study. Therefore, 23 subjects were included in the study, and 20 completed the study (Figure 1). This study had a statistical power of 80% (16), considering the baseline mean and standard deviation data presented by the subjects that completed the study, a difference of 2% in body fat content (main variable), and an alpha level of 0.05.

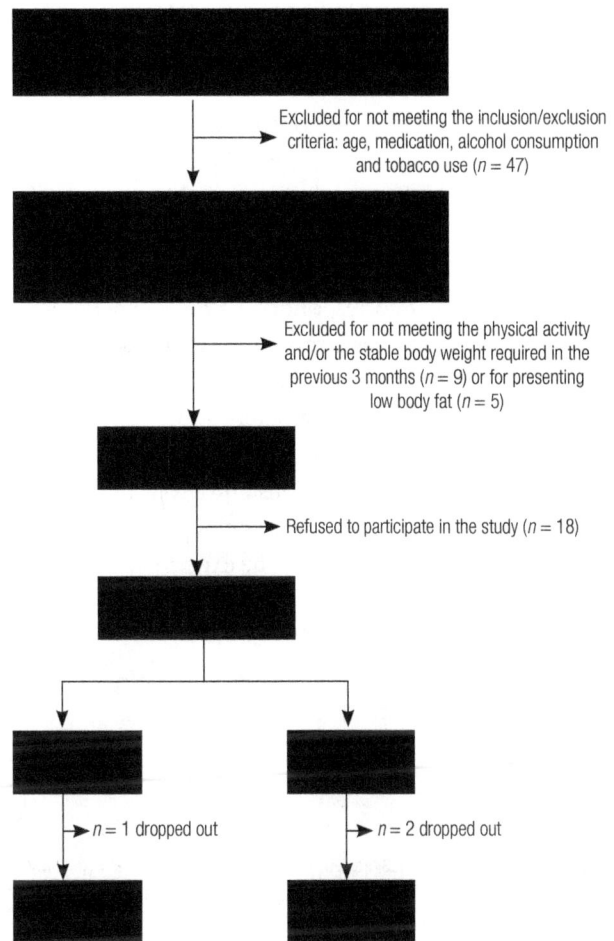

Excluded for not meeting the inclusion/exclusion criteria: age, medication, alcohol consumption and tobacco use ($n = 47$)

Excluded for not meeting the physical activity and/or the stable body weight required in the previous 3 months ($n = 9$) or for presenting low body fat ($n = 5$)

Refused to participate in the study ($n = 18$)

$n = 1$ dropped out　　　$n = 2$ dropped out

Figure 1. Screening fluxogram.

This study was conducted according to the guidelines laid down in the Declaration of Helsinki and all procedures involving human subjects were approved by the Federal University of Viçosa Ethics Committee, Viçosa, Minas Gerais, Brazil (UFV 0382007). Written informed consent was obtained from all subjects. The present trial was registered at www.clinicaltrials.gov, as "Effects of Low- or High-glycemic Index Diets on Metabolic and Inflammatory Responses in Diabetics" (ID no. NCT02383784).

Experimental design

This was a randomized, single blind (only the subjects were blind), parallel-arm clinical trial. During screening, subjects completed a form to provide demographic, health and habitual physical activity level data. Once selected, subjects were submitted to anthropometric, body composition, food intake and biochemical assessments. Next, they were allocated, according to the order of inclusion and based on the ABBA counter balancing design, to either a high GI (HGI) or low GI (LGI) group.

Two daily high or low GI test meals (breakfast and an afternoon snack) were consumed in the laboratory during 30 consecutive days. Other meals were consumed in free-living conditions. Subjects received a list discriminating the foods according to their GI values and were instructed to preferentially consume high or low GI foods that corresponded to their experimental group. Food intake was assessed at baseline and weekly throughout the study. Anthropometric, biochemical and body composition parameters were reassessed at the end of the intervention (Figure 2). Subjects were instructed to maintain a constant level of physical activity and to maintain the same type/dose of oral antidiabetic medication during the experimental period.

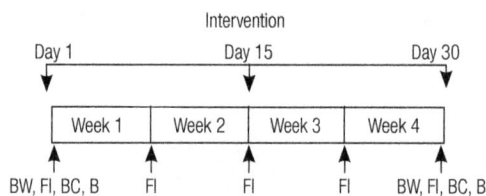

Figure 2. Experimental design. Body weight (BW), food intake (FI), body composition (BC) and biochemical parameters (B) were assessed at baseline and after the experimental period. Food intake was assessed weekly.

Test meals

The test meals' GIs were determined in a pilot study and it involved 15 healthy subjects (seven men and eight women, mean age of 23 ± 3.2 years, body mass index [BMI] 21.1 ± 2.3 kg/m^2, nondiabetic, normoglycemic, no family history of diabetes, and not taking medications regularly [except birth control pills]). After 12 hours of overnight fasting, the subjects consumed a portion of the test meals or a glucose solution (reference food) containing 50 g of available carbohydrates within 15 minutes. All subjects consumed the test meals once and the glucose solution was consumed on three different test days by each subject. The test days were separated by a washout period of at least four days (17).

Capillary blood glucose was obtained by a finger-prick at 0 (immediately before meal consumption), 15, 30, 45, 60, 90 and 120 minutes after the start of the consumption of the test meals or glucose solution. The positive area under the glycemic response curve for each test meal was computed by the trapezoidal method and

then expressed as a percentage of the average glycemic response of glucose obtained for the same subject. The resulting values were used to calculate the GI of each test meal (12).

The test meals (14 HGI [GI > 70] and 14 of LGI [GI < 55]) (18) had similar energy density, dietary fiber, and macronutrients contents (19) (Table 1). These meals provided 15% of the Estimated Energy Requirements (EER) for each subject (20). The meals' nutritional compositions were calculated using Diet Pro 5.1i software and based on food label information.

Table 1. Mean ± SE test meals glycemic index, available carbohydrate, protein, fat and dietary fiber contents

	Test meals		P value
	High GI	**Low GI**	
GI	74.1 ± 2.9^a	35.8 ± 3.3^b	0.010
Energy density (kcal/g)	1.5 ± 0.2	1.5 ± 0.2	1.000
Available carbohydrate (g)	53.7 ± 4.5	53.0 ± 1.1	1.000
Protein (g)	4.9 ± 1.6	4.8 ± 1.5	0.787
Fat (g)	6.4 ± 2.3	6.3 ± 2.3	0.854
Dietary fiber (g)	3.6 ± 1.5	3.0 ± 1.0	0.723

Different letters in the same line indicate statistical difference between groups (t-Student test, $P < 0.05$).
Test meals' GIs (14 types per group) were determined in the laboratory (FAO, 1998). Nutritional composition was obtained using Diet Pro 5.1i Software and food labels. Test meals provided 15% of the Estimated Energy Requirements (EER) for each subject.
GI: glycemic index.

Test meals were composed of a drink, a starchy food, and a fruit. While Corn Flakes® cereal, whole milk, sports drinks, white bread, margarine and papaya were used to prepare the high GI meals, All Bran® cereal, fat free strawberry yogurt, grape juice, multi-grain bread, margarine and apples were the food types used for the low GI versions. Benefiber® (added to high GI meals), glucose (added to HGI meals) and fructose (added to LGI meals) were used to make the test meals nutritionally similar in composition.

Food intake

Food intake was assessed at baseline and weekly throughout the study, using three-day food records, which were completed on two non-consecutive weekdays and on a weekend day. During the first visit to the laboratory, subjects were instructed on how to complete the food records. Each food record was reviewed with the subjects to ensure data accuracy and completeness. Data was assessed by a single investigator using Diet Pro 5.1i software.

The GI and the glycemic load (GL) of the daily consumed diet (in the laboratory and outside the laboratory) were calculated considering glucose as the reference food (1). For foods not listed in Atkinson and cols. (1), we used GI values of foods presenting similar nutritional composition. Dietary GI and GL were obtained using the following equations (21):

$$GI = \Sigma GI_a \times (CHO_a/CHO_{a-n}) \ (A)$$
$$GL = \Sigma GI_a \times CHO_a/100 \ (B)$$

Where GI_a represents the GI of a given food; CHO_a, the available carbohydrate of that same food, and CHO_{a-n}, the meal total available carbohydrate content.

Anthropometry and body composition

Anthropometric and body composition parameters were assessed at baseline and at the end of the intervention. These assessments were conducted by the same investigator, which was trained to ensure precision on data collection. Subjects were asked to wear light clothes, use no accessories, to be barefoot, not to consume water or any other type of food 4 hours before the test, refrain from intense physical activity, avoid caffeine consumption, not use diuretics or drugs that cause water retention in the 24 hours before the test, and not to consume alcohol 48 hours before the test. The assessments were not done in subjects presenting fever, edema or on their menstrual period (women). Upon arriving at the laboratory, participants were instructed to urinate (at least 30 minutes prior to body composition assessment).

Body weight was assessed using a digital electronic scale, with 150 kg capacity and 0.05 kg accuracy (22). Height was determined using an anthropometer fixed to the wall, with 2 m extension and 0.5 cm scale (22). In both procedures, participants stood up barefoot, in erect position, with relaxed arms and head in the horizontal plan. BMI was calculated by dividing body weight (kg) by height squared (m²). Waist circumference (WC) was measured with a non-elastic, 2 m extension, 1 mm precision flexible tape measure. WC was assessed in a standing position at the midpoint between the last rib and the iliac crest, and hip was measured at the maximum circumference of the buttocks (23).

Body composition was assessed by tetrapolar bioelectrical impedance (Biodynamics, model 310, TMB). Measurements were taken in the right hemibody, with subjects laid in dorsal decubitus on an isolating surface, without shoes, socks or accessories. The subject's skin was cleaned with alcohol before placing the electrodes to the hand, wrist, foot and ankle.

Biochemical assays

Biochemical parameters were assessed at baseline and at the end of the intervention. Serum samples (glucose, total cholesterol, HDL cholesterol, triglycerides, non-esterified free fatty acids (NEFA), ultra-sensitive CRP, insulin, fructosamine, and high molecular weight adiponectin analyses), plasma samples (fibrinogen) and buffy coat (IL-6 and TNF-α) were collected after 12 hours of overnight fasting at baseline and after the experimental period. Samples were centrifuged at 4°C and stored at -80°C for later batch analyses.

Glucose, total cholesterol, HDL cholesterol and triglycerides were determined by enzymatic colorimetric tests (autoanalyzer BS200 model, Mindray Bio-Medical Electronics Co., Ltda. Shenzhen, China). Ultra-sensitive CRP was assessed by the immunoturbidimetric method, using the same biochemical analyzer. LDL cholesterol was estimated using Friedewald equation (24).

NEFA were determined by the enzymatic colorimetric method described in the kit Wako® NEFAC (Neuss, Germany). Insulin concentration was measured by the electrochemiluminescence immunoassay (ECLIA) using the Immulite 2000 (DPC®) device. High molecular weight adiponectin was evaluated using ELISA kit (EZHMWA-64K, Millipore, Missouri, USES). Fibrinogen analysis was based on Clauss automated method (Fibriquik, brand Organon Teknika). Insulin resistance (IR) was assessed using the HOMA-IR index (Homeostasis Model Assessment-Insulin Resistance) (25).

Quantitative RT-PCR

Inflammatory markers were assessed at baseline and at the end of the intervention. Analyses of IL-6 and TNF-α were conducted through real-time polymerase chain reaction technique (RT-PCR). Briefly, total RNA (ribonucleic acid) was isolated from buffy coat using TRIZOL reagent (Invitrogen, Paisley, Renfrewshire, UK). High-Capacity cDNA Reverse Transcription Kit (Applied Biosystems, Foster City, California, USA) was used for reverse transcription. Real-time detection of target gene complementary DNA amplification was performed using TaqMan Gene Expression Assays

(Applied Biosystems, Foster City, California, USA) for IL-6 (Hs.654458) and TNF-α (Hs.241570). RN18S1 (Hs.03928985_g1) was used as an endogenous reference gene to calculate comparative/delta cycle threshold (DCt) values for IL-6 complementary DNA and TNF-α complementary DNA amplification. The DCt values of target gene amplification were compared with those of an in-house calibrator sample for relative values of gene expression.

Statistical analysis

Statistical analysis was performed using SPSS software (version 18.0, SPSS Inc., Chicago, IL). The Shapiro-Wilk test (1% significance) was used to evaluate the normality of data distribution. Student's t-test or the Mann-Whitney U test was used for between groups comparisons, while for paired t-test or Wilcoxon rank sum test was used for within groups comparisons (at baseline and after intervention). Data are presented as mean ± standard deviation (SD) or median (minimum/maximum). The criterion for statistical significance was $P < 0.05$.

RESULTS

Twenty patients with type 2 diabetes (10 men and 10 women), aged 42.4 ± 5.1 years old (38 to 49 years old), and mean BMI 29.2 ± 4.8 kg.m^{-2} (22.5 to 37.5 kg.m^{-2}) participated in the study. The subjects' baseline sociodemographic and clinical characteristics are presented in Table 2.

Table 2. Baseline sociodemographic and clinical[1] characteristics presented by the subjects[2]

Characteristic	HGI diet (n = 10)	LGI diet (n = 10)	P value*
Age (years)	41.1 ± 3.2	44.3 ± 4.8	0.665
Males (%)	5 (50%)	5 (50%)	---
Educational level (years)	8.7 ± 2.5	8.3 ± 2.8	0.723
Disease duration (years)	4.9 ± 1.6	4.8 ± 1.5	0.821
Metformin dosage (mg/day)	655 + 194.2	640 + 171.5	0.671

HGI: high glycemic index; LGI: low glycemic index.
[1] Other clinical characteristics are presented in Table 3. [2] Values expressed as mean ± SD or n (%).
* No statistical difference between groups (student's t test).

The subjects conducted light to moderate physical activity and consumed diets presenting similar macronutrients and dietary fiber contents (50-60% carbohydrate, 15-20% protein, 20-35% fat, and 20-25 g fiber). The diet consumed differed only in term of

GI and GL (Table 3). Macronutrient intake was not affected during the study (Table 3).

There were no differences in anthropometric measures, body composition and biochemical parameters between the HGI and LGI groups at baseline. Body fat reduced in the LGI group compared with baseline (P = 0.043) and the HGI group (P = 0.036). LGI group body fat reduced by 1.8% and in the HGI group by 0.4% (Table 3).

All subjects presented ultra-sensitive CRP concentrations below 10 mg/dL, indicating absence of infection (26). Serum NEFA concentration increased in the HGI group compared to the LGI group after the intervention (P = 0.032). Serum fructosamine concentration (P = 0.031) and TNF-α mRNA expression (P = 0.05) increased in the HGI group at the end of the study. The other biochemical parameters remained unchanged during the study (Table 3, Figure 3).

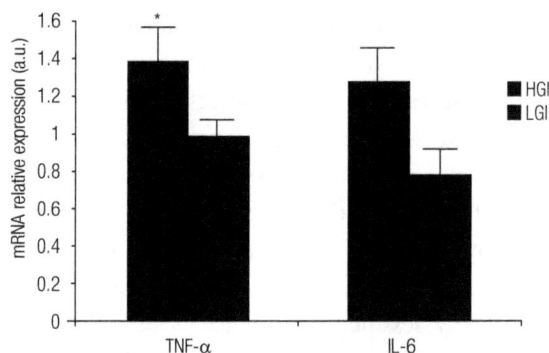

HGI: high glycemic index diet; LGI: low glycemic index diet; TNF-α: tumor necrosis factor-alpha; IL-6: interleukin-6; a.u.: arbitrary units.

* TNF-α mRNA expression increased in the HGI group after intervention (P = 0.05, Wilcoxon test). There is not a significant difference between the changes in TNF-α and Il-6 expression between the groups.

Figure 3. Mean delta ± SD (final – initial values) inflammatory markers expression according to experimental group (n = 10).

DISCUSSION

Consumption of a low GI diet for 30 consecutive days led to greater body fat reduction (1.8%) compared to high GI diet (0.4%). This reduction is desirable, especially among patients with type 2 diabetes, since body fat is positively correlated with cardiovascular disease risk (27). Bouché and cols. (28) also verified a reduction of ~700 g in total fat mass in 11 healthy men after five weeks of LGI. Similar results were observed by Costa and Alfenas (6) in 17 glucose intolerant and excessive body weight subjects in response to 30 consecutive days of LGI hypocaloric diet. In that study, WC decreased after the low GI session (6).

Table 3. Body composition, anthropometry and biochemical outcomes presented by the subjects at baseline and after 30 days of intervention

Outcomes	HGI diet (n = 10)		P-value[2]	LGI diet (n = 10)		P-value[3]	P-value[4]	P-value[5]
	Baseline	30 days		Baseline	30 days			
Body composition and anthropometry[1]								
Body fat (%)	30.1 ± 5.6	29.7 ± 4.3	0.18	33.1 ± 4.9	31.3 ± 4.7	0.043*	0.22	0.036[†]
BMI (kg.m[-2])	28.6 (25.4/37.5)	28.2 (25.5/36.8)	0.79	28.8 (22.5/33.9)	28.5 (22.5/34.6)	0.83	0.86	0.91
WC (cm)	101 ± 8.7	101 ± 13.4	0.85	99 ± 7.5	98.7 ± 8.5	0.84	0.85	0.61
WHR	0.98 (0.85/1.04)	0.95 (0.86/1.02)	0.89	0.98 (0.86/1.07)	0.97 (0.86/1.04)	0.78	0.97	0.72
Biochemical parameters[1]								
Fasting glycemia (mg/dL)	147.8 ± 10.7	157.8 ± 10.4	0.20	148.9 ± 8.2	150.8 ± 8.7	0.36	0.43	0.43
Fructosamine (mmol/L)	1.90 ± 0.05	2.21 ± 0.08	0.031*	1.93 ± 0.04	1.96 ± 0.03	0.23	0.13	0.09
Total cholesterol (mg/dL)	210.1 (180/273.5)	211 (172/284)	0.54	200.4 (123/248.1)	214.1 (145/288.5)	0.15	0.10	0.38
HDL cholesterol (mg/dL)	43 (30/59)	40 (30/54)	0.67	38 (27.6/45.2)	41 (24.5/47)	0.34	0.27	0.76
Triglycerides (mg/dL)	180.2 (88.7/287)	175.3 (132/311.2)	0.09	195 (68/372)	205.1 (63/384.1)	0.09	0.14	0.08
NEFA (mmol/L)	1.0 (0.5/1.5)	1.6 (0.6/1.5)	0.10	1.0 (0.4/1.2)	0.8 (0.6/5.0)	0.22	0.93	0.032[§]
HOMA-IR	4.8 (1.4/10.4)	4.7 (2.1/7.7)	0.87	4.2 (1.2/8.7)	4.3 (1.9/6.2)	0.76	0.34	0.57
Adiponectin (ng/mL)	30.9 (29.8/31.4)	30.8 (30.2/31.6)	0.90	30.1 (29.4/31.3)	30.5 (26.7/93)	0.81	0.78	0.74
Fibrinogen (mg/dL)	289.7 (213.5/333.9)	294.6 (193.6/413.4)	0.35	255.1 (118.5/395.2)	261.3 (141/374.7)	0.48	0.26	0.16
CRP (mg/L)	2.6 (0.8/7.3)	2.8 (0.6/6.13)	0.87	2.7 (0.5/5.5)	2.5 (0.1/6.9)	0.73	0.84	0.44
Food intake[1]								
GI	66 ± 4	72 ± 3	0.007*	63 ± 6	54 ± 4	0.005*	0.86	0.001[†]
GL	36.2 ± 10.1	39.3 ± 12.4	0.08	38.6 ± 11.1	32.5 ± 10.6	0.031*	0.75	0.025[†]
Dietary fiber (g)	18.5 ± 5.4	20.6 ± 6.1	0.92	19.6 ± 7.6	21.4 ± 7.2	0.08	0.43	0.53
Carbohydrate (%)	53.5 ± 8.4	57.9 ± 7.7	0.07	59.8 ± 9.3	57.0 ± 8.1	0.33	0.15	0.54
Protein (%)	13.2 ± 1.6	15 ± 2.7	0.09	14 ± 2.0	15.8 ± 2.7	0.67	0.81	0.91
Fat (%)	30.4 ± 3.9	34.0 ± 5.9	0.25	31.9 ± 5	34.3 ± 5.2	0.12	0.58	0.83
Energy (kcal/d)	2432.1 ± 581.4	2012.9 ± 591.4	0.08	2217.7 ± 602.4	1997.7 ± 596.2	0.11	0.73	0.85

HGI: high glycemic index; LGI: low glycemic index; BMI: body mass index; WC: waist circumference; WHR: waist-hip ratio; NEFA: non-esterified free fatty acids; CRP: ultra-sensitive C reactive protein; HOMA-IR: Homeostasis Model Assessment – Insulin Resistance; GI: glycemic index; GL: glycemic load. [1] Values expressed as mean ± SD or median (minimum/maximum). [2] Comparisons between baseline and 30 days after HGI diet. [3] Comparisons between baseline and 30 days after LGI diet. [4] Comparisons between baseline values (HGI x LGI diet). [5] Comparisons between final values (HGI x LGI diet). * $P < 0.05$ (t-paired test). [†] $P < 0.05$ (t test). [§] $P < 0.05$ (Mann Whitney test).

Wee and cols. (29) showed that the consumption of low GI diets favors fat instead of carbohydrate oxidation, leading to body fat reduction. Further, Bouché and cols. (28) observed a reduction on abdominal tissue hormone sensitive lipase (HSL) and on subcutaneous tissue lipoprotein lipase (LPL) gene expression after the consumption of low GI diets. Thus, these authors concluded that the decrease in body fat was not due to increased lipolysis mediated by the HSL, but instead to less fat deposition in the adipose tissue mediated by the LPL (28).

Human LPL promotes plasma triglycerides hydrolysis, increasing circulating NEFA concentrations and its uptake by the adipose tissue. The consumption of high GI diets decreases insulin sensitivity and increases LPL action, since insulinemia is positively correlated with the levels of this enzyme (30). Consequently, although LPL levels were not measured in our study, LPL may have contributed to the increased NEFA concentrations in the HGI group and also to reduce body fat in the LGI group. However, this is only a hypothesized mechanism to try to explain the effects observed in our study.

We verified that HGI diet increased NEFA's concentrations after the intervention compared to baseline. High concentrations of NEFA appear to inhibit the activity of phosphofructokinase and lead to glucose-6-phosphate accumulation inside the muscle cells, inhibiting cellular glucose uptake (31). The final effect of high serum NEFA concentrations is increased insulin secretion and its reduced action in peripheral tissues, causing beta cells depletion and IR (32). So, the increased serum NEFA and fructosamine concentrations after the intervention may indicate worse glycemic control in the HGI group subjects.

Opperman and cols. (33) assessed the effect of consuming diets differing in GI in a randomized clinical trials meta-analysis. The consumption of low GI diets led to a reduction of fructosamine concentrations compared to high GI diets (33). In our study, although the consumption of the high GI diet increased fructosamine concentrations, the opposite effect did not occur in response to the low GI diet. It is possible that the duration of the present study was not long enough to cause that reduction. Robert and Ismail (34) observed that the GI was useful to evaluate the glycemic response in patients with type 2 diabetes to individual high-carbohydrate foods and to mixed meals (n = 10). However, it must be highlighted that many factors can affect the GI value of foods, such as climate, soil, preparation, cooking time, temperature and acidity (12,13). Therefore, the values obtained in the laboratory under controlled conditions may not be reflected when these same foods are consumed in free living conditions. However, the consumption of two HGI or LGI meals associated with the instruction to preferentially consume foods presenting the same GI of each subject's study group was sufficient to ensure that diets consumed during our study differed in GI. We also verified elevated TNF-α mRNA expression in the HGI group. TNF-α action may dramatically increase IR and affect glycemic control. TNF-α production is usually increased in obese subjects and its production by adipose tissue is one of the causes of IR (35). This cytokine plays an important regulatory role on adipose tissue fat accumulation (36). TNF-α inhibits LPL action and induces HSL increase, stimulating lipolysis in the adipocytes (36), and consequently increasing circulating NEFA concentrations, as observed in our study. Moreover, TNF-α reduces glucose transporters GLUT 1 and 4 expressions, contributing to IR (35).

Frost and cols. (7) assessed the effect of the GI on insulin sensitivity and TNF-α production in women with a high risk of heart disease. Twenty-eight premenopausal women participated in the study and randomly consumed, for three weeks, isocaloric high or low GI diets presenting similar macronutrients and dietary fiber contents. At the end of the study, there was an increase in insulin sensitivity in response to the consumption of the low GI diet. Adipocyte TNF-α production was higher among people with a family history of cardiovascular disease, but was not affected by GI. However, the GI of the consumed diets was estimated based on food records completed only in the last week of the study, which may not reflect the diet consumed during the study. In that study, the GI was estimated considering the values presented in international tables of GI, instead of being determined

in the laboratory, as we did in our study. Consequently, there is no guarantee that the GI values assigned to the test diets were accurate. The GI can be affected by factors such as fruit ripeness, food processing and interactions between nutrients of a mixed meal (37). It has been verified that mixed meals' GI estimation based on such types of tables may not predict the GI directly measured in the laboratory (38).

The small sample size of our study limited the statistical power to conduct a multivariate statistical analysis. However, the randomization process was carefully conducted by us. Because of that, the intervention groups (HGI and LGI) presented similar baseline body composition, besides clinical, biochemical, and anthropometric data. The wide variance in BMI could also be considered another limitation of our study. Although there was a wide variance in the BMI of our subjects, the baseline values presented by groups was not statistically different. That is, the wide range of variation occurred in both groups. We also emphasize that high body fat percentage (up to 16% for men and 24% for women) instead of BMI was considered as a criterion for inclusion in the study.

In conclusion, while the consumption of a high GI diet for 30 consecutive days caused an increase in fructosamine, NEFA and TNF-α concentrations, consuming a low GI diet caused a significant reduction of approximately 2% in body fat among overweight patients with type 2 diabetes. These results suggest that the consumption of low GI diets can help reduce body fat and prevent the harmful inflammatory and metabolic changes induced by high GI diets.

REFERENCES

1. Atkinson FS, Foster-Powell K, Brand-Miller JC. International tables of glycemic index and glycemic load values: 2008. Diabetes Care. 2008;31:2281-3.

2. Mendez MA, Covas MI, Marrugat J, Vila J, Schroeder H. Glycemic load, glycemic index, and body mass index in Spanish adults. Am J Clin Nutr. 2009;89:316-22.

3. Ebbeling CB, Leidig MM, Sinclair KB, Seger-Shippee LG, Feldman HA, Ludwig DS. Effects of an ad libitum low-glycemic load diet on cardiovascular disease risk factors in obese young adults: a randomized trial. Am J Clin Nutr. 2005;81:976-82.

4. Jenkins DJ, Kendall CW, McKeown-Eyssen G, Josse RG, Silverberg J, Booth GL, et al. Effect of a Low-glycemic index or a high-cereal fiber diet on type 2 diabetes: a randomized trial. JAMA. 2008;300:2742-53.

5. Ludwig DS. The glycemic index: physiological mechanisms relating to obesity, diabetes, and cardiovascular disease. JAMA. 2002;287:2414-23.

6. Costa JA, Alfenas RCG. The consumption of low glycemic meals reduces abdominal obesity in subjects with excess body weight. Nutr Hosp. 2012;27:1178-83.

7. Frost G, Leeds A, Trew G, Margara R, Dornhorst A. Insulin sensitivity in women at risk of coronary heart disease and the effect of a low glycemic diet. Metabolism. 1998;47:1245-51.

8. Dickinson S, Hancock DP, Petocz P, Brand-Miller J. High glycemic index carbohydrate mediates an acute proinflammatory process as measured by NF-kappaB activation. Asia Pac J Clin Nutr. 2005;14 Suppl:S120.

9. Neuhouser ML, Schwarz Y, Wang C, Breymeyer K, Coronado G, Wang CY, et al. A low-glycemic load diet reduces serum C-reactive protein and modestly increases adiponectin in overweight and obese adults. J Nutr. 2012;142:369-74.

10. Raatz SK, Torkelson CJ, Redmon JB, Reck KP, Kwong CA, Swanson JE, et al. Reduced glycemic index and glycemic load diets do not increase the effects of energy restriction on weight loss and insulin sensitivity in obese men and women. J Nutr. 2005;135:2387-91.

11. Liu S, Manson JE, Buring JE, Bagshaw D, Kris-Etherton PM, Ulbrecht J, et al. Relation between a diet with a high glycemic load and plasma concentrations of high-sensitivity C-reactive protein in middle-aged women. Am J Clin Nutr. 2002;75:492-8.

12. Wolever TMS, Jenkins DJA, Jenkins AL, Josse RG. The glycemic index: methodology and clinical implications. Am J Clin Nutr. 1991;54:846-54.

13. Marsh K, Barclay A, Colagiuri S, Brand-Miller J. Glycemic index and glycemic load of carbohydrates in the diabetes diet. Curr Diab Rep. 2011;11:120-7.

14. O'Keefe JH, Bhatti SK, Bajwa A, DiNicolantonio JJ, Lavie CJ. Alcohol and cardiovascular health: the dose makes the poison... or the remedy. Mayo Clin Proc. 2014;89:382-93.

15. Craig CL, Marshall AL, Sjöström M, Bauman AE, Booth ML, Ainsworth BE, et al. International physical activity questionnaire: 12-country reliability and validity. Med Sci Sports Exerc. 2003;35:1381-95.

16. Mera R, Thompson H, Prasad C. How to calculate sample size for an experiment: a case-based description. Nutr Neurosci. 1998;1:87-91.

17. Brouns F, Bjorc I, Fray KN, Gibbs AL, Lang V, Slama G. Glycaemic index methodology. Nutr Res Rev. 2005;18:145-71.

18. Brand-Miller JC, Wolever TMS, Foster-Powell K, Colagiuri S. the new glycemic index revolution: the autoritative guide to the glycemic index. New York, NY: Marlowe e Company; 2003.

19. Universidade Estadual de Campinas – Unicamp. Tabela brasileira de composição de alimentos – TACO. 2. ed. Campinas: Unicamp/NEPA; 2006.

20. Institute of Medicine. Dietary reference intakes for energy, carbohydrate, fiber, fat, fatty acids, cholesterol, protein and amino acids, vitamin A, vitamin K, arsenic, boron, chromium, copper, iodine, iron, manganese, molybdenum, nickel, silicon, vanadium, zinc, vitamin C, vitamin E, selenium, and carotenoids (Macronutrients). Washington: National Academy Press; 2002.

21. Foster-Powell K, Holt SH, Brand-Miller JC. International table of glycemic index and glycemic load values. Am J Clin Nutr. 2002;76:5-56.

22. Jellife DB. Evolución del estado de nutrición de la comunidad. Organización Mundial de la Salud: Genebra, 1968.

23. Wang J, Thornton JC, Bari S, Williamson B, Gallagher D, Heymsfield SB, et al. Comparisons of waist circumferences measured at 4 sites. Am J Clin Nutr. 2003;77:379-84.

24. Friedewald WT, Levy RI, Fredrickson DS. Estimation of the concentration of low-density lipoprotein cholesterol in plasma, without use of the preparative ultracentrifuge. Clin Chem. 1972;18:499-502.

25. Matthews DR, Hosker JP, Rudenski AS, Naylor BA, Treacher DF, Turner RC. Homeostasis model assessment: insulin resistance and cell function from fasting plasma glucose and insulin concentrations in man. Diabetologia. 1985;28:412-9.

26. Pearson TA, Mensah GA, Alexander RW, Anderson JL, Cannon III RO, Criqui M, et al. Markers of inflammation and cardiovascular disease application to clinical and public health. Circulation. 2003;107:499-511.

27. American Diabetes Association (ADA) Standards of Medical Care in Diabetes – 2015. Diabetes Care. 2015;38 Suppl:S4.

28. Bouché C, Rizkalla SW, Luo J, Vidal H, Veronese A, Pacher N, et al. Five-week, low-glycemic index diet decreases total fat mass and improves plasma lipid profile in moderately overweight nondiabetic men. Diabetes Care. 2002;25:822-8.

29. Wee S, Williams S, Gray S, Horabin J. Influence of high and low glycemic index meals on endurance running capacity. Med Sci Sports Exerc. 1999;31:393-9.

30. Merkel M, Heeren J, Dudeck W, Rinninger F, Radner H, Breslow JL, et al. Inactive lipoprotein lipase (LPL) alone increases selective cholesterol ester uptake in vivo, whereas in the presence of active LPL it also increases triglyceride hydrolysis and whole particle lipoprotein uptake. J Biol Chem. 2002;277:7405-11.

31. Bays H, Mandarino L, DeFronzo RA. Role of the adipocyte, free fatty acids, and ectopic fat in pathogenesis of type 2 diabetes mellitus: peroxisomal proliferator-activated receptor agonists provide a rational therapeutic approach. J Clin Endocrinol Metab. 2004;89:463-78.

32. Poitout V, Robertson PR. Glucolipotoxicity: fuel excess and β-cell dysfunction. Endocrine Rev. 2008;29:351-66.

33. Opperman AM, Venter CS, Oosthuizen W, Thompson RL, Vorster HH. Meta-analysis of the health effects of using the glycaemic index in meal planning. Br J Nutr. 2004;92:367-81.

34. Robert SD, Ismail ALS. Glycemic responses of patients with type 2 diabetes to individual carbohydrate-rich foods and mixed meals. Ann Nutr Metab. 2012;60:27-32.

35. Moller DE. Potential role of TNF-alpha in the pathogenesis of insulin resistance and type 2 diabetes. Trends Endocrinol Metab. 2000;11:212-7.

36. Kern PA, Ranganathan S, Li C, Wood L, Ranganathan G. Adipose tissue tumor necrosis factor and interleukin-6 expression in human obesity and insulin resistance. Am J Physiol Endocrinol Metab. 2001;280:E745-51.

37. O'Dea K, Nestloe PJ, Antoff L. Physical factors influencing postprandial glucose and insulin responses to starch. Am J Clin Nutr. 1980;33:760-5.

38. Flint A, Moller BK, Raben A, Pedersen D, Tetens I, Holst JJ, et al. The use of glycaemic index tables to predict glycaemic index of composed breakfast meal. Br J Nutr. 2004;91:979-89.

22

Waist circumference measurement sites and their association with visceral and subcutaneous fat and cardiometabolic abnormalities

Cláudia Porto Sabino Pinho[1], Alcides da Silva Diniz[1], Ilma Kruze Grande de Arruda[1], Ana Paula Dornelas Leão Leite[2], Marina de Moraes Vasconcelos Petribu[2], Isa Galvão Rodrigues[2]

ABSTRACT

Objectives: To estimate the degree of variability of the waist circumference (WC) when obtained in different anatomical sites and compare the performance of the measurement sites as predictors of visceral adipose tissue (VAT) and subcutaneous adipose tissue (SAT) and cardiometabolic abnormalities. Subjects and methods: Cross-sectional study involving 119 individuals with overweight (50.3 ± 12.2 years), in which six WC measurement sites were evaluated (minimal waist, immediately below the lowest rib, midpoint between the lowest rib and the iliac crest, 2 cm above the umbilicus, immediately above the iliac crest, umbilicus level), in addition to the VAT and SAT (quantified by computed tomography) and cardiometabolic parameters. Results: The differences between the measurements ranged from 0.2 ± 2.7 cm to 6.9 ± 6.7 cm for men, and from 0.1 ± 3.7 cm to 10.1 ± 4.3 cm for women. The minimum waist showed significant correlation with VAT (r = 0.70) and with a higher number of cardiometabolic parameters among men. Regarding women, the WC measurement showed high correlation with SAT and moderate correlation with VAT, not being found superiority of one measurement protocol in relation to the others when assessed the correlation with VAT and with cardiometabolic parameters. Conclusions: Greater variability between the measuring sites was observed among women. With respect to men, the minimum waist performed better as a predictor of VAT and cardiometabolic alterations. Arch Endocrinol Metab. 2018;62(4):416-23

Keywords
Waist circumference; visceral fat; subcutaneous fat; abdominal fat

[1] Universidade Federal de Pernambuco (UFPE), Recife, PE, Brasil
[2] Pronto-Socorro Cardiológico Universitário de Pernambuco, Recife, PE, Brasil

Correspondence to:
Cláudia Porto Sabino Pinho
Universidade Federal de Pernambuco,
Departamento de Nutrição
Prof. Morais Rego Ave, 1235
Cidade Universitária
50670-901 – Recife, PE, Brasil
claudiasabinopinho@hotmail.com

INTRODUCTION

The waist circumference (WC) measurement has been recommended in clinical guidelines and by the leading authority in health and societies as a cardiometabolic risk predictor associated with central adiposity, both in clinical practice and in epidemiological studies (1-6). Despite the widespread use of this anthropometric parameter, there is no consensus on the evaluation protocol and the measurement standardization due to lack of consistent evidence justifying the superiority of one measurement site in relation to others, resulting in a wide variety of techniques reported in the literature.

A systematic review of 120 studies showed eight different protocols for WC measurement (7), some endorsed by international bodies and other experimental protocols adopted to a lesser extent in the publications on the subject. The World Health Organization (8) and the International Diabetes Federation (4) recommend the measurement at the midpoint between the iliac crest and the lowest rib. The National Institutes of Health (9), in turn, establishes the superior border of the iliac crest as the anatomical site of WC measurement. Other anatomical sites such as the minimal waist and the umbilicus are also commonly adopted (7,10).

Although these measurement sites present close correlation, significant differences between the WC measures obtained at different locations have been reported (11-14). Previous studies comparing the different protocols showed a profound influence of the measurement site on the absolute values of WC (11,13,15). Those differences, even if subtle, could potentially affect the utility of the WC measurement for assessing the cardiometabolic risk, particularly when the stratification of the risk depends on dichotomous thresholds, with possible repercussion on the clinical decision making (16). In addition, little attention has been given to the method for determining the WC when comparing data from different studies (13,14).

This study aimed to estimate the degree of variability of the WC when obtained from different anatomical sites and compare the performance of the measurement sites as predictors of visceral and subcutaneous fat and cardiometabolic abnormalities.

SUBJECTS AND METHODS

Cross-sectional study developed in a nutrition clinic of a public university hospital, reference in cardiology, in northeastern Brazil, involving individuals with overweight, of both sexes and age ≥ 20 years. In this clinic, the patients are predominantly individuals with non-communicable chronic diseases: obesity, hypertension, diabetes mellitus, metabolic syndrome and dyslipidemia.

Overweight was established based on the body mass index (BMI) ≥ 25 kg/m² for adults (8) and ≥ 27 kg/m² for the elderly (17).

The sample was built based on voluntary adhesion, being picked up patients in first consultation. Individuals with hepatomegaly and/or splenomegaly, ascites and recent abdominal surgery were excluded, as well as pregnant women and those who had children up to 6 months prior to the screening for the study, characteristics that may influence the intra-abdominal fat measurement and/or the anthropometric measurements.

Assuming a 5% α error, a β error of 20%, an estimated average correlation between the WC measures and the metabolic changes of 0.4 (p) and a variability of 0.1 (d²), it was obtained a minimum sample size of 108 individuals. To correct possible losses, that number was increased by 10% [100/(100-10)], with a total sample of n = 119.

The visceral adipose tissue (VAT) and the subcutaneous adipose tissue (SAT) were assessed by computed tomography (CT), using the Philips Brilliance CT-10 slice tomoghaph (VMI *Indústria e Comércio Ltda.,* Lagoa Santa, MG, Brazil). The survey was conducted in four hours fasting with the patient in supine position. The tomographic cut was obtained with radiographic parameters of 140 kV and 45 mA, at the L4 level, having a thickness of 10 mm. The total area of total abdominal fat and the visceral fat area were manually outlined with free cursor contouring each region. The entire surface of the skin was excluded

from the marking area. The area of the VAT was determined using as limits the inner borders of the rectus abdominis, internal oblique and square lumbar muscles, excluding the vertebral body and including the retroperitoneal, mesenteric and omental fat. The subcutaneous fat area was calculated by subtracting the VAT from the total fat area. All areas of fat were described in cm². For identification of the adipose tissue, it was used the density values of -50 and -250 Hounsfield units (18-20).

The WC was obtained by inelastic tape measure, with accuracy of 0.1 cm, directly on the skin, in six anatomical regions: 1) at the minimal waist (narrowest region between the chest and hips) (WC1) (10); 2) immediately below the lowest rib (WC2) (10,11); 3) at the midpoint between the lowest rib and the iliac crest (WC3) (4,8); 4) 2 cm above the umbilicus (WC4) (21); 5) immediately above the iliac crest (WC5) (9); at the umbilicus level (WC6) (7,22).

The bony landmarks of the lowest rib and of the iliac crest were located and palpated by the examiner at the level of the middle axillary line. The measuring tape was placed on a horizontal plane around the abdomen in the locations described above and particular attention was given to ensure that the tape was parallel to the floor and perpendicular to the longitudinal axis of the body. The measurement was performed at the end of the normal expiration with the inelastic tape adjacent to the skin, without compressing it, keeping the participant standing up, straight, with parallel legs and arms hanging down on the sides. For each evaluated anthropometric point, a double measurement was obtained by a trained examiner (12,23). When the measure difference between measurements was greater than 0.1 cm, a third measurement was performed. The final measure considered was the average of the two closest values.

It were evaluated the following cardiometabolic parameters: fasting blood glucose, glycated hemoglobin (HbA1C), lipid profile (triglycerides (TG), total cholesterol (TC) and fractions, non-HDL cholesterol and TG/HDL-c ratio), C-reactive protein (CRP) and uric acid. Samples were collected with 9-12 hours fasting, considering a preparation protocol (24). Blood glucose, lipid profile and uric acid were analyzed by the enzymatic method, and HbA1c and CRP by turbidimetry. Biochemical analyses were carried out using a Cobas Integra 400® analyzer (Roche Diagnostics) in the Laboratory of Clinical Analyses in the service facilities.

The non-HDL cholesterol fraction, calculated by subtracting HDL-c from TC (non-HDL cholesterol = TC - HDL-c), was adopted as the estimate of the total number of atherogenic particles in the plasma (VLDL + IDL + LDL) (24). The TG/HDL-c ratio was used as atherogenicity index for reflecting the size of LDL-c particles (25).

Data were analyzed using the Statistical Package for Social Sciences, version 13.0 (SPSS Inc., Chicago, IL, USA). Continuous variables were tested for normal distribution using the Kolmogorov-Smirnov test, being described as mean and standard deviation or median and interquartile range, according to the distribution pattern. CRP was the only variable that showed non-normal distribution.

The Student t test for independent samples was used for comparison of the WC means between the sexes. The one-way ANOVA test was used for comparison of the six WC measurement sites, using the Bonferroni test *a posteriori*. Proportions were compared by Pearson Chi Square.

The Pearson or Spearman correlation was used to evaluate the relationship between the different anatomical sites of WC measurement with VAT, SAT and biochemical parameters. To analyze the correlation between WC and lipid profile, it were excluded subjects who reported use of lipid-lowering medications, and to verify the association between the WC sites and the glycemic parameters (fasting and HbA1c), it were excluded diabetic subjects. Statistical significance was considered when $p < 0.05$.

RESULTS

Were included 124 individuals, but after discarding the losses for refusal or information inconsistency (n = 5), 119 patients were included in the final sample of the study. The mean age was 50.3 ± 12.2 years and women predominated (68.1%; $CI_{95\%}$: 59.2-75.8). Although men and women have displayed similar characteristics regarding age, nutritional status, subcutaneous fat and prevalence of diabetes mellitus and arterial hypertension, there were higher averages of visceral fat in men ($p < 0.001$) (Table 1).

BMI averages were similar between sexes (p = 0.715), however, WC averages were higher among men, expressing, between sexes, a different distribution pattern of the body fat (Table 2).

Table 1. Sample characteristics, stratified by sex (n = 119)

Variables	Males (n = 38)	Females (n = 81)	p-value*
Age, years (mean/SD)	49.9 (±13.7)	50.5 (±11.8)	0.817*
Arterial hypertension (%, $CI_{95\%}$)	68.4 (52.5-80.9)	59.3 (47.8-70.0)	0.420§
Diabetes mellitus (%, $CI_{95\%}$)	26.3 (15.0-42.0)	21.0 (12.7-31.5)	0.659§
BMI, kg/m² (mean/ SD)	33.1 (±4.9)	33.5 (±5.3)	0.715*
VAT (cm²)	378.9 (±118.7)	258.6 (±75.4)	< 0.001*
SAT (cm²)	506.3 (±162.2)	540.9 (±145.6)	0.294*

* Student t test for independent samples; § Pearson Chi Square. SD: standard deviation; CI95%: confidence interval of 95%; BMI: body mass index; VAT: visceral adipose tissue; SAT: subcutaneous adipose tissue.

Table 2. Comparative analysis of the averages of six anatomical sites of measurement of the waist circumference in individuals with overweight, according to sex

Variables	Males (n = 38)	Females (n = 81)	p-value*
WC1 (cm)	106.2 (±10.6)	96.8 (±10.0) cm[a]	< 0.001
WC2 (cm)	107.5 (±11.4)	97.6 (±11.3) cm[a]	< 0.001
WC3 (cm)	112.9 (±12.5)	103.2 (±11.0) cm[b]	< 0.001
WC4 (cm)	112.3 (±11.5)	104.6 (±11.5) cm[b,c]	0.003
WC5 (cm)	109.9 (±13.7)	106.7 (±10.7) cm[c]	0.273
WC6 (cm)	113.1 (±12.5)	106.8 (±10.7) cm[c]	0.012
p-value**	0.143	< 0.001	

* Student t Test for independent samples. ** ANOVA *one way*. [a,b,c] Different letters mean statistical diferences by the Bonferroni test. WC1: minimal waist; WC2: immediately below the lowest rib; WC3: at the midpoint between the lowest rib and the iliac crest; WC4: 2 cm above the umbilicus; WC5: immediately above the iliac crest; WC6: at the umbilicus level.

It was observed significant difference in the absolute values of the WC obtained in six anatomical sites of women (p < 0.001). Notwithstanding, among men, the difference was not observed (p = 0.143) and may suggest that they have uniformity in the waist circumference along the upper body (Table 2).

The maximum absolute difference among the various protocols examined was observed when compared the WC obtained at the umbilicus (WC6) and at the minimal waist (WC1) in both sexes. The average differences between the measurements ranged from 0.2 ± 2.7 cm to 6.9 ± 6.7 cm among men, and from 0.1 ± 3.7 cm to 10.1 ± 4.3 cm among women.

In men, the minimal waist (WC1) showed better correlation with VAT and lower correlation with subcutaneous fat, unlike other measurement sites, which showed a higher correlation with SAT than with VAT. Furthermore, the minimal waist (WC1) was the only measurement site that showed correlation with triglycerides (r = 0.595, p < 0.05) and with the TG/HDL-c ratio (r = 0.506, p < 0.05).

The measures of the circumferences obtained at the bony landmark of the iliac crest (WC5) and at the umbilicus (WC6) showed higher correlation coefficients with SAT and lower correlation with VAT in both sexes. In women, these two anatomical sites have higher absolute values, expressing that the higher abdominal circumference can be much more represented by the SAT than by the VAT (Table 3).

Table 3. Pearson correlation (r) between waist circumference measures obtained at six anatomical sites with visceral and subcutaneous fat and cardiometabolic profile in subjects with overweight, according to sex

Parameters	Males					
	WC1	WC2	WC3	WC4	WC5	WC6
VAT	0.701*	0.598*	0.531*	0.566*	0.358	0.426*
SAT	0.621*	0.700*	0.800*	0.712*	0.836*	0.863*
TC	-0.012	-0.147	-0.197	-0.207	-0.380	-0.300
HDL-c	-0.267	-0.336	-0.421	-0.431	-0.177	-0.415
LDL-c	-0.245	-0.301	-0.316	-0.347	-0.464	-0.401
TG	0.595*	0.425	0.377	0.421	0.139	0.305
Non HDL-c	0.039	-0.082	-0.115	-0.124	-0.345	-0.219
TG/HDL	0.506*	0.324	0.313	0.351	0.012	0.234
Glucose	-0.244	-0.253	-0.243	-0.258	-0.215	-0.264
HbA1C	-0.380	-0.500*	-0.529*	-0.555*	-0.484*	-0.553*
CRP#	-0.131	-0.193	-0.235	-0.230	-0.281	-0.248
Uric acid	0.032	-0.011	-0.022	0.017	-0.183	-0.032
Parameters	Females					
	WC1	WC2	WC3	WC4	WC5	WC6
VAT	0.462*	0.425*	0.397*	0.383*	0.332*	0.359*
SAT	0.714*	0.732*	0.758*	0.776*	0.783*	0.809*
TC	-0.265	-0.199	-0.198	-0.234	-0.240	-0.241
HDL-c	-0.189	-0.130	-0.126	-0.086	-0.121	-0.110
LDL-c	-0.254	-0.193	-0.199	-0.225	-0.244	-0.229
TG	-0.021	-0.030	-0.037	-0.100	-0.113	-0.143
Non HDL-c	-0.232	-0.177	-0.177	-0.224	-0.222	-0.226
TG/HDL	0.027	0.022	0.032	-0.054	0.000	-0.074
Glucose	0.240	0.251	0.162	0.144	0.131	0.112
HbA1C	0.049	0.032	0.102	-0.012	0.068	0.000
CRP#	0.239	0.205	0.238	0.293*	0.241*	0.246*
Uric acid	0.340*	0.238*	0.313*	0.325*	0.395*	0.362*

* p < 0,05. # Spearman correlation. VAT: visceral adipose tissue; SAT: subcutaneous adipose tissue; TC: total cholesterol; TG: triglycerides; HbA1C: glycated hemoglobin; CRP: C-reactive protein. WC1: minimal waist; WC2: immediately below the lowest rib; WC3: at the midpoint between the lowest rib and the iliac crest; WC4: 2 cm above the umbilicus; WC5: immediately above the iliac crest; WC6: at the umbilicus level.

It was found, for females, that the six evaluated protocols for obtaining the WC showed similar correlation with VAT (moderate correlation) and with SAT (high correlation). Regarding the metabolic abnormalities, it was observed, in females, that the uric acid correlated directly with the measures obtained at all measurement sites and that the CRP correlated with the three major measures observed among women (WC4, WC5, WC6).

DISCUSSION

Although much progress has been made with respect to the use of the WC as a predictor of the cardiometabolic risk, up to now there is no ideal and uniform definition for using the WC measurement. One major objective of developing a definition is to minimize measurement errors and thus improve the efficiency in the estimates in studies of association and comparison involving this parameter. Lack of standards regarding anatomical site, posture, breathing phase and other factors contribute to measurement errors. Several protocols have been recommended, but the comparison between them has not been sufficiently explored.

The results of this study indicate that the choice of the measurement protocol influences the magnitude of the WC measurement, especially in women. The substantial differences in the absolute values of the measures obtained for females were not reproduced in males. Similar result was reported by other authors (14,26), who indicated greater impact of the measurement site among women.

These results observed for different genders may reflect sex differences in the abdominal fat distribution pattern. Similar measures among men indicate uniformity in the total fat accumulation deposited throughout the abdomen. Nonetheless, in women, the changes observed in the abdominal girth suggest a more curvilinear structure and with greater accumulation of adiposity in the lower torso.

The maximum differences between the measures observed in this study (6.9 cm for men and 10.1 cm for women) reveal profound influence of the measurement site on the WC value. This result was relatively similar to the findings reported by Willis and cols. (12), who showed differences of 4.5 cm and 10.6 cm for males and females, respectively, when evaluating patients with an average BMI of 30 kg/m². Agarwal and cols. (13) reported mean differences between the measures of 5.3

cm for men and 5.5 cm for women, when evaluating 123 Asian subjects, with a mean age of 34 ± 8.7 years and average BMI of 23.9 ± 4.9 kg/m². Other studies (23,26) have indicated differences of approximately 2.0 cm for men and 5.5 cm for women. The variability in the differences between the measurement sites reported among diverse populations suggests that these differences may vary depending on the sample characteristics, including age, sex, race/ethnicity and level of adiposity. What seems to be consensus is that the results indicate greater influence of the measurement site on females.

The differences in the measures, even if slight, can have particular effect on the abdominal obesity classification. The abdominal fat as a proxy of the cardiometabolic risk depends on dichotomized thresholds, and subtle variations can exert influence when this risk is stratified. Willis and cols. (12) reported that the estimates of prevalence of abdominal obesity (> 88 cm/> 102 cm) drastically varied according to the measurement site. In women, the measure taken at the minimal waist resulted in lower prevalence (31%) when compared to the measures obtained at the umbilicus (55%). In men, a small average difference between measures (2.5 cm) had a noticeable impact on the prevalence of abdominal obesity (34% when considering the measure taken at the umbilicus and 23% when using the minimal waist). Consequently, the choice of the measurement site can result in significant repercussions on the interpretation of epidemiological data. Therefore, small differences can be amplified when dichotomous cutoff points are used to define abdominal obesity. Despite the risks of using different protocols in the abdominal obesity classification, a systematic review of 120 studies demonstrated similar pattern of association of the different sites of obtention of the WC with cardiovascular diseases, diabetes mellitus and mortality (7).

This study, by engaging a group of individuals with overweight and obesity, did not assess the impact of using different WC evalution protocols on the prevalence of abdominal obesity.

Although some results elect the WC as a better indicator of the visceral fat and of the cardiovascular risk in comparison with the BMI and the waist-hip ratio (WHR) (27-29), few studies (12,23,26) compared the performance of different WC measurement sites as predictors of visceral fat accumulation. Furthermore, the available studies compared the use of only two

(12,26) or three measurement protocols (23), different from our study that compared six anatomical sites.

This study showed among men that the minimal waist was a better marker of visceral fat than of subcutaneous fat, unlike other measurement protocols, which showed better correlation with the subcutaneous fat. This observation, coupled with the fact that no significant difference was observed in the WC measures for males, allows us to infer that the visceral fat is more concentrated in the upper abdomen and that VAT and SAT are not evenly disposed over the abdominal wall of males.

Furthermore, the minimal waist was directly correlated with a greater number of cardiometabolic parameters (two) compared to the other measurement sites (one or zero). A similar result was produced by other research (12) that, when evaluating American adults with overweight and obesity, found that the minimal waist showed stronger correlation with VAT ($r = 0.64$; $p < 0.001$) and a higher number of metabolic parameters (three) compared to the measure obtained at the umbilicus, which presented lower correlation coefficient with VAT ($r = 0.54$; $p < 0.001$) and association with only two metabolic parameters.

It is plausible to suppose that the measure offering the best correlation with VAT would have higher correlation with metabolic changes. It is well established the connection of the visceral obesity with a pro-atherogenic state (30,31) and the epicenter of most of the hypotheses postulated to explain this association (32,33) refers to the portal drainage of VAT, which provides direct access of free fatty acids and adipokines to the liver, by activating immune hepatic mechanisms for the production of inflammatory mediators, and thus promoting greater insulin resistance and increased production of triglycerides (34,35).

Among women, it was found that the WC, regardless of the measurement site, was predominantly a subcutaneous fat index, corroborating the findings of another investigation (23). The minimal waist also showed a slight superiority in the correlation with VAT, when compared to the other measurements, while the larger abdominal circumferences (at the level of the umbilicus or the iliac crest) had lower correlation coefficients. These findings demonstrate that the larger perimeters reflect much more the excess subcutaneous fat than the excess visceral fat and corroborate the indication that the visceral fat would be proportionally more concentrated in the upper abdomen than in the lower abdômen (23,36).

WC reflects the abdominal adipose tissue, not being able to distinguish the deposits of visceral and subcutaneous fat (23,37). However, being used as a cardiometabolic risk predictor, it should better predict the VAT than the SAT, but this is not what the literature has shown (23,26,37), being very important the reflection on the widespread use of WC as a single parameter of risk screening.

Some potential limitations need to be considered when interpreting the data presented. It was not a random sample and the participants of the study were taken from a hospital center which is reference in cardiology. In addition, it were included only individuals with overweight and obesity and therefore the data presented may not be generalized to individuals with low levels of adiposity. The small number of subjects included can also be a limitation in the statistical power of the study and compromise its external validity. Moreover, given that the racial characteristics influence the distribution of body fat, the extrapolation of data for individuals of different ethnic groups should be carried out with due caution.

Another aspect that should be discussed within the framework of the topic and that has not been explored in this research refers to the technical issues of evaluation of the WC. Although the standardization for obtaining the WC is relevant, the reproducibility of the technique should be an aspect considered in the definition of the protocol for obtaining the measure. External landmarks (minimal waist and umbilicus) are widely used and may be more reproducible as they require less experience from the evaluator. Notwithstanding, the adoption of internal bony landmarks (iliac crest and lowest rib) as a reference shows advantages in the clinical follow-up of measurements, since they remain unaltered with changing adiposity (16). Thus, these aspects should be considered in future research and in the selection of the best assessment protocol.

It should be noted that the comparison of the performance of six measurement sites and the use of a method considered "gold standard" for quantifying visceral fat are important aspects of the study.

In summary, the magnitude of the WC is influenced by the anatomical site of measurement, particularly in women, indicating the need for standardization of protocols for obtaining the measurement and thus allowing valid comparisons between the studies.

In conclusion, among men, the minimal waist showed better correlation with VAT and with cardiometabolic parameters. In women, the WC seems to be a more accurate indicator of subcutaneous fat than of visceral fat. The findings of this study do not provide clear evidence of the superiority of a single measurement to predict the cardiometabolic risk. It would be important to conduct longitudinal studies involving a larger number of participants to compare the predictive ability of different WC measures for the development of cardiovascular and metabolic disorders.

Therefore, data on the preference of a measurement protocol are still limited and more studies need to be developed in order to outline more conclusive evidence on the anatomical site of measurement that should be adopted as a clinical tool to assess the cardiometabolic risk. Replicating this approach in different populations will facilitate global comparisons.

Transparency declaration: the lead author affirms that this manuscript is an honest, accurate, and transparent account of the study being reported. The reporting of this work is compliant with CONSORT1/STROBE2/PRISMA3 guidelines. The lead author affirms that no important aspects of the study have been omitted and that any discrepancies from the study as planned have been explained.

Authors' contributions: CPSP conceived of the study, carried out the studies and data analyses and drafted the manuscript. ASD and IKGA conceived of the study, and participated in its design and coordination to draft the manuscript. APDLL, MMVP and IGR performed the measurements. All authors read and approved the final manuscript.

Funding: this research did not receive any specific grant from funding agencies in the public, commercial, or not-for-profit sectors.

REFERENCES

1. Alberti KG, Zimmet P, Shaw J. IDF Epidemiology Task Force Consensus Group. The metabolic syndrome-a new worldwide definition Lancet. 2005;366(9491):1059-62.
2. Executive Summary of The Third Report of The National Cholesterol Education Program (NCEP) Expert Panel on Detection, Evaluation, And Treatment of High Blood Cholesterol In Adults (Adult Treatment Panel III). JAMA. 2001;285(19):2486-97.
3. WHO. Definition, diagnosis and classification of diabetes mellitus and its complications: report of a WHO consultation. Geneva: WHO; 1999.
4. International Diabetes Federation: The IDF consensus worldwide definition of the metabolic syndrome. Available from: <http://www.idf.org/webdata/docs/Metabolic_syndrome_definition.pdf>. Accessed on: Aug 2, 2015.
5. Klein S, Allison DB, Heymsfield SB, Kelley DE, Leibel RL, Nonas C, et al. Waist circumference and cardiometabolic risk: a consensus statement from Shaping America's Health: Association for Weight Management and Obesity Prevention; NAASO, The Obesity Society; the American Society for Nutrition; and the American Diabetes Association. Am J Clin Nutr. 2007;85(5):1197-202.
6. Yusuf S, Hawken S, Ounpuu S, Bautista L, Franzosi MG, Commerford P, et al. INTERHEART Study Investigators. Obesity and the risk of myocardial infarction in 27,000 participants from 52 countries: a case-control study. Lancet. 2005;366(9497):1640-9.
7. Ross R, Berentzen T, Bradshaw AJ, Janssen I, Kahn HS, Katzmarzyk PT, et al. Does the relationship between waist circumference, morbidity and mortality depend on measurement protocol for waist circumference? Obes Rev. 2008;9(4):312-25.
8. World Health Organization. Obesity: Preventing and Managing the Global Epidemic. Technical Report Series no. 894. Geneva: World Health Organization, 2000.
9. National Health and Medical Research Council. Clinical practice guidelines for the management of overweight and obesity in adults 2003. Available from: <http://www.health.gov.au/internet/main/publishing.nsf/Content/obesityguidelinesguidelines-adults.htm>. Accessed on: Aug 2, 2015.
10. Lohman TG. Anthropometric standardization reference manual. Champaign, IL: Human Kinetics, 1988. p. 28-80.
11. Wang Z, Hoy WE. Waist circumference, body mass index, hip circumference and waist-to-hip ratio as predictors of cardiovascular disease in aboriginal people. Eur J Clin Nutr. 2004;58(6):888-93.
12. Willis LH, Slentz CA, Houmard JA, Johnson JL, Duscha BD, Aiken LB, et al. Minimal versus umbilical waist circumference measures as indicators of cardiovascular disease risk. Obesity (Silver Spring). 2007;15(3):753-9.
13. Agarwal SK, Misra A, Aggarwal P, Bardia A, Goel R, Vikram NK, et al. Waist circumference measurement by site, posture, respiratory phase, and meal time: implications for methodology. Obesity (Silver Spring). 2009;17(5):1056-61.
14. Mason C, Katzmarzyk PT. Effect of the site of measurement of waist circumference on the prevalence of the metabolic syndrome. Am J Cardiol. 2009;103(12):1716-20.
15. Zhu S, Heymsfield SB, Toyoshima H, Wang Z, Pietrobelli A, Heshka S. Race-ethnicity-specific waist circumference cutoffs for identifying cardiovascular disease risk factors. Am J Clin Nutr. 2005;81(2):409-15.
16. Mason C, Katzmarzyk PT. Variability in waist circumference measurements according to anatomic measurement site. Obesity (Silver Spring). 2009;17(9):1789-95.
17. Lipschitz DA. Screening for nutritional status in the elderly. 1994:21(1):55-67.
18. Borkan GA, Gerzof SG, Robbins AH, Hults DE, Silbert CK, Silbert JE. Assessment of abdominal fat content by computed tomography. Am J Clin Nutr. 1982;36(1):172-7.
19. Rockall AG, Sohaib SA, Evans D, Kaltsas G, Isidori AM, Monson JP, et al. Computed tomography assessment of fat distribution in male and female patients with Cushing's syndrome. Eur J Endocrinol. 2003;149(6):561-7.
20. Seidell JC, Oosterlee A, Thijssen MA, Burema J, Deurenberg P, Hautvast JG, et al. Assessment of intra-abdominal and subcutaneous abdominal fat: relation between anthropometry and computed tomography. Am J Clin Nutr. 1987;45(1):7-13.
21. Rossen J, Yngve A, Hagströmer M, Brismar K, Ainsworth BE, Iskull C, et al. Physical activity promotion in the primary care setting in pre- and type 2 diabetes – the Sophia step study, an RCT. BMC Public Health. 2015 Jul 12;15:647.
22. Klein S, Allison DB, Heymsfield SB, Kelley DE, Leibel RL, Nonas C, Kahn R; Association for Weight Management and Obesity Prevention; NAASO, The Obesity Society; American Society for Nutrition; American Diabetes A, et al. Waist circumference and

cardiometabolic risk: a consensus statement from Shaping America's Health: Association for Weight Management and Obesity Prevention; NAASO, The Obesity Society; the American Society for Nutrition; and the American Diabetes Association. Am J Clin Nutr. 2007;85(5):1197-202.

23. Bosy-Westphal A, Booke CA, Blöcker T, Kossel E, Goele K, Later W, et al. Measurement site for waist circumference affects its accuracy as an index of visceral and abdominal subcutaneous fat in a caucasian population. J Nutr. 2010;140(5):954-61.

24. Jellinger PS, Smith DA, Mehta AE, Ganda O, Handelsman Y, Rodbard HW, et al. AACE Lipid and Atherosclerosis Guidelines. American Association of Clinical Endocrinologists' Guidelines for Management of Dyslipidemia and Prevention of Atherosclerosis. Endocr Pract. 2012;18 Suppl 1:1-78.

25. Maruyama C, Imamura K, Teramoto T. Assessment of LDL particle size by triglyceride/HDL-cholesterol ratio in non-diabetic, healthy subjects without prominent hyperlipidemia. J Atheroscler Thromb. 2003;10(3):186-91.

26. Ma WY, Yang CY, Shih SR, Hsieh HJ, Hung CS, Chiu FC, et al. Measurement of Waist Circumference: midabdominal or iliac crest? Diabetes Care. 2013;36(6):1660-6.

27. Cornier MA, Després JP, Davis N, Grossniklaus DA, Klein S, Lamarche B, et al. American Heart Association Obesity Committee of the Council on Nutrition; Physical Activity and Metabolism; Council on Arteriosclerosis; Thrombosis and Vascular Biology; Council on Cardiovascular Disease in the Young; Council on Cardiovascular Radiology and Intervention; Council on Cardiovascular Nursing, Council on Epidemiology and Prevention; Council on the Kidney in Cardiovascular Disease, and Stroke Council. Assessing adiposity: a scientific statement from the american heart association. Circulation. 2011;124(18):1996-2019.

28. Pouliot MC, Després JP, Lemieux S, Moorjani S, Bouchard C, Tremblay A, et al. Waist circumference and abdominal sagittal diameter: best simple anthropometric indexes of abdominal visceral adipose tissue accumulation and related cardiovascular risk in men and women. Am J Cardiol. 1994;73(7):460-8.

29. Rankinen T, Kim SY, Pérusse L, Després JP, Bouchard C. The prediction of abdominal visceral fat level from body composition and anthropometry: ROC analysis. Int J Obes Relat Metab Disord. 1999;23(8):801-9.

30. Tchernof A, Després JP. Pathophysiology of human visceral obesity: an update. Physiol Rev. 2013;93(1):359-404.

31. Cartier A, Côté M, Lemieux I, Pérusse L, Tremblay A, Bouchard C, et al. Age-related differences in inflammatory markers in men: contribution of visceral adiposity. Metabolism. 2009;58(10):1452-8.

32. Bélanger C, Luu-The V, Dupont P, Tchernof A. Adipose tissue intracrinology: potential importance of local androgen/estrogen metabolism in the regulation of adiposity. Horm Metab Res. 2002;34(11-12):737-45.

33. Bergman RN, Van Citters GW, Mittelman SD, Dea MK, Hamilton-Wessler M, Kim SP, et al. Central role of the adipocyte in the metabolic syndrome. J Investig Med. 2001;49(1):119-26.

34. Jensen MD. Role of body fat distribution and the metabolic complications of obesity. J Clin Endocrinol Metab. 2008;93(11 Suppl 1):S57-63.

35. Korenblat KM, Fabbrini E, Mohammed BS, Klein S. Liver, muscle, and adipose tissue insulin action is directly related to intrahepatic triglyceride content in obese subjects. Gastroenterology. 2008;134(5):1369-75.

36. Shen W, Punyanitya M, Wang Z, Gallagher D, St-Onge MP, Albu J, et al. Visceral adipose tissue: relations between single-slice areas and total volume. Am J Clin Nutr. 2004;80(2):271-8.

37. Kullberg J, von Below C, Lönn L, Lind L, Ahlström H, Johansson L. Practical approach for estimation of subcutaneous and visceral adipose tissue. Clin Physiol Funct Imaging. 2007;27(3):148-53.

23

Efficacy and safety of a single radiofrequency ablation of solid benign non-functioning thyroid nodules

Roberto Cesareo*[1], Andrea Palermo*[2], Valerio Pasqualini[3],
Carla Simeoni[4], Alessandro Casini[1], Giuseppe Pelle[3],
Silvia Manfrini[2], Giuseppe Campagna[1], Roberto Cianni[3]
* These authors contributed equally to this paper as first author

ABSTRACT

Objective: The objective of our study is to evaluate the clinical outcomes and safety of radiofrequency thermal ablation (RFA) for benign thyroid nodules (BTNs) over a 1-year follow-up. **Subjects and methods:** This is a monocentric retrospective study. Forty-eight patients with solid, non-functioning BTNs were treated by RFA using a 17G internally cooled electrode. We categorized thyroid nodules as small ($\leq$ 12 mL), medium (12 to 30 mL), or large (over 30 mL). BTNs volume reduction, thyroid function, cosmetic and compressive score changes and side effect evaluation at 6 and 12 months were evaluated. **Results:** BTN volume decreased significantly from baseline to 6 (mean percentage decrease of BTN volume was 66.8 ± 13.6%, p < 0.001). At 12 months, the mean percentage reduction of BTN volume compared to six months was 13.7 ± 17.1% (p < 0.001). At 6-month, symptom score had improved significantly (p < 0.001) while it does not change significantly between 6 and 12 months. In particular, symptom score improved significantly in the medium (p < 0.001) and large (p < 0.01) subgroups. Cosmetic score improved significantly between baseline and 6 months (p < 0.001) and between 6 and 12 months (p < 0.01). In all the subgroups, cosmetic score improved significantly between baseline and 6 months, while between 6 and 12 months it improved significantly only in the large group (p < 0.05). RFA was well tolerated. Only one patient experienced permanent right paramedian vocal cord palsy. **Conclusions:** A single RFA treatment was effective in reducing BTNs volume, in particular small and medium nodules. Cosmetic score improved in all treated BTNs while symptom score only got better in the medium and large BTNs. Arch Endocrinol Metab. 2017;61(2):173-9.

[1] Department of Internal Medicine "S. M. Goretti" Hospital, Latina, Italy
[2] Department of Endocrinology, University Campus Bio-Medico, Rome, Italy
[3] Department of Radiology, "S. M. Goretti" Hospital, Latina, Italy
[4] Compensatory authority (INAIL), Monte Porzio Catone, Rome, Italy

Correspondence to:
Andrea Palermo
Department of Endocrinology and Diabetes, University Campus Bio-Medico of Rome
Via Alvaro del Portillo, 21
00128 – Rome, Italy
a.palermo@unicampus.it

Keywords
Radiofrequency ablation; thyroid nodules; ultrasounds; cosmetic score; symptom score

INTRODUCTION

Over the last decade, non-surgical minimally invasive US-guided debulking techniques have been proposed to reduce the volume of thyroid nodules when surgery is contraindicated or refused (1). US-guided percutaneous ethanol injection (PEI) therapy is currently considered one of the first-line treatment modality for cystic and predominantly cystic nodules (2,3). Laser ablation (LA) has been proposed as a safe outpatient procedure that effectively reduces the volume of solid nodules and the clinical outcomes in the majority of patients (4-9).

Although it is a newer technique compared to LA, radiofrequency ablation (RFA) has been gaining popularity as a minimally invasive treatment for thyroid nodules (10-12). Indications for RFA of benign thyroid nodules (BTNs) are nodule-related clinical symptoms such as neck pain, dysphasia, foreign body sensation, discomfort, cough, cosmetic problems, or thyrotoxicosis in cases of autonomously functioning thyroid nodules (10-12).

The real impact of RFA of benign thyroid nodules in terms of efficacy is still controversial because most of the published studies are compromised by several bias such as trials not controlled, small thyroid nodule volume or short follow-up period (13-20). Moreover, a few authors have treated large thyroid nodules and, in these patients, further RFA treatments were needed to obtain a significant volumetric reduction (14,15).

Furthermore, there are contrasting evidence on the role of thyroid nodule function (15,16,21), as it may affect the volumetric response to the RFA treatment.

Two retrospective studies have shown the ability of the RFA to reduce the thyroid nodule volume but the authors enrolled patients with cystic nodules and sometimes re-treatment was provided (22,23).

Our retrospective study aims to evaluate the clinical outcomes and safety of a single RFA treatment for benign non-functioning thyroid solid nodules over a 1-year follow-up. In particular, we categorized thyroid nodules in small (≤ 12 mL), medium (12 to 30 mL), or large (over 30 mL) and BTN volume reduction, thyroid function, cosmetic and compressive score changes and side effects were evaluated.

SUBJECTS AND METHODS

Study population

From June 2012 to November 2015, a total of 90 patients affected by thyroid nodules were treated and enrolled. Ninety thyroid nodules were treated with US-guided RF ablation at the Thyroid Center of "S. M. Goretti" Hospital.

Subjects were enrolled if they fulfilled all the following criteria:
- Older than 18 years;
- Reported cosmetic and/or symptomatic problems;
- Solid thyroid nodule (solid portion over 70%);
- Thyroid nodules with maximum diameter > 2 cm steadily growing over time;
- Cytologically confirmed benign nodule on two separate US-guided FNAB;
- Serum thyroid hormone (free T4 and free T3), thyrotropin levels (TSH), calcitonin, thyroid peroxidase and thyroglobulin antibodies within normal ranges;
- No history of radioiodine therapy or thermal ablation;
- No previous neck or trunk external beam radiotherapy;
- Refusal of or ineligible for surgery;
- One single RFA treatment.

Exclusion criteria were:
- Pregnancy;
- Malignant or suspicious thyroid nodules;
- Nodules that were confluent in a compressive lobar mass;
- Hot nodule at 99mTc-pertechnetate scintigraphy.

Subjects with small nodules and cosmetic score less than 3 (see section below on the Thyroid nodule classification according to the volume).

Finally, we enrolled 48 patients (17 men, 31 women; age 57.7 ± 14 yrs, range 24-80) who were followed up for 1 year after treatment.

Thyroid nodule classification according to the volume

We classified nodules according to baseline volume as small (≤ 12 mL), medium (12 to 30 mL), or large (over 30 mL), as previously shown in a recent randomized control trial (24). One single nodule per patient was treated with RFA. In patients with multiple thyroid nodules, the largest and/or most symptomatic one was treated. All patients were clinically, biochemically, and morphologically evaluated at 6 and 12 months.

Procedure

US was performed using a 7.5–12MHz linear probe equipped with Color Doppler and Power Doppler modules (Technos MPX; Esaote My Lab 50, Italy). We recalculated the nodule volume and percentage of volume reduction (PVR) with the following equations: volume percentage (ellipsoid equation): V = length x width x depth x 0.525; volume reduction percentage: PVR = [initial volume – final volume] ×100)/initial volume (24).

A single BTN volume was measured in case of uninodular goiter or in case of multinodular goiter when characterized by one predominant nodule associated with other non-clinically significant thyroid nodules. We took photos of all enrolled patients at baseline and at 1, 6 and 12 months after RFA. A radiofrequency generator (Cool-tip, E-Series Covidien) and a 17 gauge, 15 cm electrode with a 1 cm active tip was used. All RF procedures were carried out by the same operator under US control with the same scanner used for the initial diagnostic evaluation. The intra- and inter-observer coefficients of variation for sonographic volume assessment were previously defined as 4% and 6%, respectively (24). The patients were treated with 2% Mepivacain 2-5 mL (Carbosen) and 3 mL of Ropivacaine (Naropine, Fresenius Kabi, USA) for local anesthesia at the puncture site. Four mg of dexamethasone IV before RFA of large thyroid nodule were prescribed to reduce post-treatment oedema. On the basis of previous experience, the procedure utilized included the trans-isthmic approach along the short axis of the nodule, and the nodules were managed with the "moving-shot technique" as described elsewhere by Baek and cols. (14).

We adopted a variant of the aforementioned technique, using 60 W of radiofrequency outpower and exposure time needed to obtain a transient multiple hyperechoic zones as a sign of the manoeuvre. All the patients were informed and treated after written informed consent was obtained.

Clinical evaluation

We classified symptom and cosmetic scores, as described in a previous consensus statement (10). All patients were asked to rate pressure symptoms on a 10-cm visual analogue scale (grade 0-10 cm) at enrolment and during follow-up. A cosmetic score was obtained according to the following scale: 1, no palpable mass; 2, no cosmetic problem but palpable mass; 3, a cosmetic problem on swallowing only; 4, easily visible mass. According to this classification, we decide to treat subjects with small nodules with cosmetic score more than 2 or nodules with symptoms score ≥ 3.

Biochemical evaluation

The laboratory studies included chemiluminescent enzyme immunoassay (Architect i4000 SR, Abbott) for serum thyrotropin (normal range, 0.5–4.9 mIU/L), serum free triiodothyronine (normal range, 1.7-3.7 pg/mL), serum-free thyroxine (normal range, 0.7-1.7 pg/mL), and serum antithyroid peroxidase antibodies (normal range, 0–35 IU/mL); immunoradiometric assay (Architect i4000 SR, Abbott) for serum calcitonin (normal range, 0–10 pg/mL) and blood coagulation tests (prothrombin time, activated partial thromboplastin time).

Statistical analysis

Statistical analysis was performed using IBM-SPSS Statistics version 21. Descriptive statistics (median, mean, standard deviation, range) were computed on thyroid volume and other clinical variables. To compare group mean values, appropriate parametric test of statistical significance (t test) was used, where a Shapiro–Wilk test indicated that the data conformed to a log-normal distribution. Otherwise, an equivalent non parametric test was employed (Kruskal–Wallis test, Wilcoxon for paired sample). The significance level was defined as $p \leq 0.05$.

RESULTS

Nodule volume

Characteristics and clinical data are summarized in Table 1. BTN volume decreased significantly (Table 2) from baseline to 6 months (23.5 ± 18.6 at baseline to 8.5 ± 9 at 6 months; p < 0.001); the mean percentage decrease of BTN volume was 66.8 ± 13.6% at 6 months.

Table 1. Main characteristics of the study population and clinical data at baseline

Parameter	
N	48
Sex (males/females)	17/27
Age in years	56 ± 14 (24 – 80)
Thyroid nodule volume (mL)	23.5 ± 18.6 (3.4 – 89)
TSH (mIU/mL)	2.0 ± 0.9 (0.6 – 4.1)
FT3 (pg/mL)	2.6 ± 0.6 (1.2 – 3.7)
FT4 (pg/mL)	1.3 ± 0.2 (0.8 – 1.7)

Table 2. Thyroid nodule volume (mL) in radiofrequency ablation group

	Baseline	6 months	12 months
Whole group (n = 48)			
TN vol.	23.5 ± 18.6	8.5 ± 9.0***	7.6 ± 8.7***
TN vol. variation (%) from baseline		-66.8 ± 13.6	-71.1 ± 14.3
TN vol. variation (%) from 6 months			-13.7 ± 17.1
Small (n = 12)			
TN vol.	7.4 ± 2.6	2.0 ± 1.1***	1.6 ± 0.9*
TN vol. variation (%) from baseline		-73.5 ± 10.8	-78.7 ± 1
TN vol. variation (%) from 6 months			-18.7 ± 18.8
Medium (n = 24)			
TN vol.	18.3 ± 42	6.2 ± 2.6***	5.6 ± 2.7***
TN vol. variation (%) from baseline		-65.8 ± 13.7	-69.0 ± 14.4
TN vol. variation (%) from 6 months			-10.8 ± 13.4
Large (n = 12)			
TN vol.	49.8 ± 18.4	19.7 ± 11.6***	17.5 ± 12.3*
TN vol. variation (%) from baseline		-62.0 ± 14.3	-67.7 ± 15.9
TN vol. variation (%) from 6 months			-14.7 ± 21.8

Differences are considered between baseline and 6 months and between 6 and 12 months.

* p ≤ 0.05; *** p ≤ 0.001.

At 12 months, BTN volume was 7.6 ± 8.7 mL and the mean percentage reduction of BTN volume compared to six months was 13.7 ± 17.1% (p < 0.001).

The mean percentage of volumetric reduction differed in the three classes of nodules: for small nodules, the mean percentage decrease was 73.5 ± 10.8% at 6 months and 78.7 ± 10% at 12 months; for medium nodules, it was 65.8 ± 13.7% at 6 months and 69 ± 14.4% at 12 months and for large nodules it was 62 ± 14.3% at 6 months and 67.7 ± 15.9% at 12 months.

Hormonal evaluation

All patients were euthyroid at baseline (Table 1) and serum thyroid function tests after 1, 6 and 12 months did not show significant modification. No significant changes were observed either in TgAb and TPOAb titers or in calcitonin serum concentrations during the follow-up period except for two patients who developed autoimmune thyroid diseases with hyperthyroidism six and twelve months after RF ablation.

Symptom and cosmetic score evaluation

At 6-month evaluation (Table 3), symptom score improved significantly (p < 0.001) while it doesn't change significantly between 6 and 12 months (0.5 ± 0.8 at 6 months and 0.4 ± 0.8 at 12 months (p = ns). Between baseline and 6 months, symptom score significantly improved in the medium (p < 0.001) and large subgroups (p < 0.01), whereas, of course, no improvement was observed in the small subgroup. The overall cosmetic score improved significantly between baseline and 6 months (p < 0.001) and between 6 and 12 months (p < 0.01). In all subgroups cosmetic score improved significantly between baseline and 6 months, while between 6 and 12 months it decreased significantly only in large group (p < 0.05).

Complications and safety

RFA was generally safe and well tolerated in all patients, who were placed under observation for 4 hours after the procedure. No patient needed hospitalization after treatment. During the RFA procedure, 8 (21%) of the 48 patients experienced mild local pain, occasionally radiating to the ear or jaw or chest, but it was limited and resolved quickly after the power was switched off. In one patient, however, the procedure was stopped due to severe chest pain (it was resolved quickly after the power was switched off). The most feared complication is voice change after RFA. Only 2 patients (4.7%) had voice change immediately after the RFA session but it resolved completely 2 or 3 hours after the procedure. One patient experienced permanent right paramedian vocal cord palsy with inspiratory stridor without dysphonia.

DISCUSSION

This one year retrospective study has demonstrated that one single RFA treatment was effective in reducing benign non-functional thyroid nodules volume in particular small and medium nodules.

In order to avoid some confounding factors, we previously excluded from our analysis patients with thyroid cystic nodule or thyroid nodules with a solid portion less than 70%. Indeed a large quantity of fluid may affect the "volumetric" response to RFA and PEI should be used to manage thyroid cystic lesions (2,3).

Up to now, there is no univocal and shared classification that divides the thyroid nodules according to size. Compressive symptoms are usually linked to large nodules, while cosmetic problems can be due to smaller nodules that are located in a superficial part of the gland. In this study, as previously reported (24), we arbitrarily divided the thyroid nodules into small, medium and large (see materials and methods section). According to this distribution, we have noticed that the

Table 3. Cosmetic score and symptom score groups

	All		Small n = 12		Medium n = 24		Large n = 12	
	Cosmetic score	Symptom score	Cosmetic score	Symptom score	Cosmetic score	Symptom score	Cosmetic score	Symptom score
Baseline	2.8 ± 0.7	3.4 ± 3	3 ± 0	0 ± 0	2.5 ± 0.7	3.6 ± 2.8	3.3 ± 0.8	6.2 ± 1.3
6 months	1.6 ± 0.6***	0.5 ± 0.8***	1.0 ± 0**	0 ± 0	1.6 ± 0.6***	0.4 ± 0.9***	2.2 ± 0.6**	1.0 ± 1.0**
12 months	1.5 ± 0.7**	0.4 ± 0.8°	1.0 ± 0	0 ± 0	1.6 ± 0.6	0.3 ± 0.8°	1.8 ± 0.8*	0.9 ± 1.0°

Differences are considered between baseline and 6 months and between 6 and 12 months.

* p ≤ 0.05; ** p ≤ 0.01; *** p ≤ 0.001; °n.s.

percentage decrease for the small nodules was larger compared to the other groups, as already shown by other authors (15,23,25).

In particular, according to these findings, multi-RFA treatments would be needed to achieve a clinically significant volume reduction for larger nodules (15,26) therefore, when not contraindicated, surgical treatment or more than a single RFA treatment should be recommended.

We have obtained the maximum volume reduction after 6-month treatment even if we have recorded a further reduction (14,16) at the end of the study period. Only 2 subjects have experienced an increase of the thyroid volume from 6 to 12 months (11.6 mL vs 12.6 mL and 17.3 mL vs 20.0 mL) but none of them exceeded 50% at 1-year post RFA treatment (volume increases after the last follow-up of 8.6 and 15.6% respectively). In another retrospective study, the authors found that 5.6 % subjects (7/126) experienced > 50% increase in nodule volume compared to the previous follow-up volume (23). Probably, the longer follow-up period (4 years) of the Hyun's study (23) can explain the difference in terms of regrowth rate.

Moreover, our study population is homogenous. Indeed, as previously reported (20,24), thyroid nodules have been treated by one single RFA using the same radiofrequency outpower in order to better evaluate the efficacy of this technique.

We enrolled only patients with non-functioning thyroid nodules because it cannot be fully excluded that their functional state could affect the volumetric response to the RFA treatment (15,16,21,27).

Only two other retrospective studies were published investigating the efficacy of RFA on thyroid nodules (22,23). These authors also took into consideration nodules with a large amount of liquid, sometimes multi-RFA treatments were needed to achieve a significant volume reduction and the basal mean volume was significant lower compared to our study population one (22,23). In previous clinical trials (13,14,18,19,21), it has always been found that there is a significant amelioration of both symptoms and cosmetic score regardless of the thyroid nodule volume and location.

Conversely, we have shown that RFA is able to suddenly improve the symptom score in patients with medium or large nodules and this improvement remained stable until the end of the study period. However, no improvement in the symptom score was observed in the small nodule subgroup.

Moreover, we have shown that, in the overall study population, the cosmetic score improved significantly between baseline and 6 months and between 6 and 12 months while between 6 and 12 months it decreased significantly only in large group.

More than 20% of patients experienced local mild neck pain but it was not necessary to stop the treatment. Two people, a man and a woman, developed an autoimmune hyperthyroidism at 6 and 12 months after RFA treatment respectively. Graves' disease or autoimmune hyperthyroidism is a complication that can be expected after laser ablation or PEI, probably due to the extensively damage of follicular thyroid cells. The mechanism for causality between these treatments and Graves' disease is not completely known. Regalbuto and cols. had been issued a theory contend that the destruction of thyroid tissue after ablation therapy or injection of ethanol, among subjects genetically predisposed to autoimmune reactions, could release a large quantity of antigenic material (including TSHr protein) from follicular thyroid cells, that may trigger an autoimmune inflammatory response thought thyroid and orbital soft tissues (28). Anyway, we cannot surely state if, in these 2 subjects, the onset of autoimmune hyperthyroidism is due to the previous radiofrequency ablation treatment. One patient experienced major complication – permanent right paramedian vocal cord palsy with inspiratory stridor without dysphonia.

In our study, we did not perform a particular cost analysis comparing RFA to surgical procedure. Anyway, we agree with Bernardi's findings (29). She has clearly shown that RFA may be a cost-effective technique to treat the thyroid nodules compared to surgery. Indeed, she performed a cost analysis included the procedures (RFA or surgery) and the respective pre- and post-procedural exams. The length of RFA session was short and was set in an outpatient regimen with an overall cost of about 1,660 € compared to surgical procedure (the operative time was longer, the length of the hospital stay was 1-2 days and the mean cost was about 4,550 €). However, a recent study (30) did not confirm these findings. Indeed, Che and cols. stated that compared with surgery, the advantages of radiofrequency ablation include fewer complications, preservation of thyroid function, and fewer hospitalization days but the cost difference was not significant.

The strength of our study is that compared to the previous published evidence, the study population is homogeneous regarding thyroid function, thyroid nodule volume, radiofrequency out-power and number of RFA sessions. In particular:

- We enrolled only patients with non-functioning thyroid nodules because it cannot be fully excluded that their functional state could affect the volumetric response to the RFA treatment.
- We previously excluded from our analysis patients with thyroid cystic nodule or thyroid nodules with a solid portion less than 70%.
- Thyroid nodules have been treated by one single RFA using the same radiofrequency outpower. Furthermore, our mean baseline nodule volume is significant higher compared to the other studies (much more close to what we face in the the real life when we suggest the RFA technique). Moreover, compared to the previous publication (24), this study confirms the significant volume reduction at 6 months after RFA treatment and demonstrates further significant volume decline at 12 months after RFA in this homogeneous study population.

This study has a few major limitations. In particular, this is a retrospective study and the follow-up period is quite short.

In conclusion our study has shown that a single RFA treatment was effective in reducing benign thyroid nodules volume. Moreover, larger BTNs seem to be less responsive and perhaps in these cases a further RFA treatment should be used to get all the desired clinical and radiological outcomes. Cosmetic score improved in all treated BTNs, while symptom score got better only in medium and large BTN. RF ablation can be a valuable and generally safe tool for the non-surgical management of BTNs. Other large and prospective studies are needed to confirm these findings.

Funding: no competing financial interests exist.

REFERENCES

1. Hegedus L. Therapy: a new nonsurgical therapy option for benign thyroid nodules? Nat Rev Endocrinol. 2009;5:476-8.
2. Del Prete S, Caraglia M, Russo D, Vitale G, Giuberti G, Marra M, et al. Percutaneous ethanol injection efficacy in the treatment of large symptomatic thyroid cystic nodules: ten-year follow-up of a large series. Thyroid. 2002;12:815-21.
3. Guglielmi R, Pacella CM, Bianchini A, Bizzarri G, Rinaldi R, Graziano FM, et al. Percutaneous ethanol injection treatment in benign thyroid lesions: role and efficacy. Thyroid. 2004;14:125-31.
4. Pacella CM, Bizzarri G, Guglielmi R, Anelli V, Bianchini A, Crescenzi A, et al. Thyroid tissue: US-guided percutaneous interstitial laser ablation-a feasibility study. Radiology. 2000:217:673-7.
5. Døssing H, Bennedbaek FN, Karstrup S, Hegedüs L. Benign solitary solid cold thyroid nodules: US-guided interstitial laser photocoagulation--initial experience. Radiology. 2002;225:53-7.
6. Pacella CM, Bizzarri G, Spiezia S, Bianchini A, Guglielmi R, Crescenzi A, et al. Thyroid tissue: US-guided percutaneous laser thermal ablation. Radiology. 2004;232:272-80.
7. Papini E, Guglielmi R, Bizzarri G, Graziano F, Bianchini A, Brufani C, et al. Treatment of benign cold thyroid nodules: a randomized clinical trial of percutaneous laser ablation versus levothyroxine therapy or follow-up. Thyroid. 2007;17:229-35.
8. Valcavi R, Riganti F, Bertani A, Formisano D, Pacella CM. Percutaneous laser ablation of cold benign thyroid nodules: a 3-year follow-up study in 122 patients. Thyroid. 2010;20:1253-61.
9. Døssing H, Bennedbæk FN, Hegedüs L. Long-term outcome following interstitial laser photocoagulation of benign cold thyroid nodules. Eur J Endocrinol. 2011;165:123-8.
10. Na DG, Lee JH, Jung SL, Kim JH, Sung JY, Shin JH, et al. Radiofrequency ablation of benign thyroid nodules and recurrent thyroid cancers: consensus statement and recommendations. Korean J Radiol. 2012;13:117-25.
11. Baek JH, Lee JH, Sung JY, Bae JI, Kim KT, Sim J, et al. Complications encountered in the treatment of benign thyroid nodules with US-guided radiofrequency ablation: a multicenter study. Radiology. 2012;262:335-42.
12. Ha EJ, Baek JH, Kim KW, Pyo J, Lee JH, Baek SH, et al. Comparative efficacy of radiofrequency and laser ablation for the treatment of benign thyroid nodules: systematic review including traditional pooling and bayesian network meta analysis. J Clin Endocrinol Metab. 2015;100:1903-11.
13. Kim YS, Rhim H, Tae K, Park DW, Kim ST. Techniques in thyroidology radiofrequency ablation of benign cold thyroid nodules: initial clinical experience. Thyroid. 2006;16:361-7.
14. Baek JH, Kim YS, Lee D, Huh JY, Lee JH. Benign predominantly solid thyroid nodules: prospective study of efficacy of sonographically guided radiofrequency ablation versus control condition. AJR Am J Roentgenol. 2010;194:1137-42.
15. Spiezia S, Garberoglio R, Milone F, Ramundo V, Caiazzo C, Assanti AP, et al. Thyroid nodules and related symptoms are stably controlled two years after radiofrequency thermal ablation. Thyroid. 2009;19:219-25.
16. Deandrea M, Limone P, Basso E, Mormile A, Ragazzoni F, Gamarra E, et al. Us-guided percutaneous radiofrequency thermal ablation for the treatment of solid benign hyperfunctioning or compressive thyroid nodules. Ultrasound Med Biol. 2008;34:784-91.
17. Turtulici G, Orlandi D, Corazza A, Sartoris R, Derchi LE, Silvestri E, et al. Percutaneous radiofrequency ablation of benign thyroid nodules assisted by a virtual needle tracking system. Ultrasound Med Biol. 2014;40:1447-52.
18. Che Y, Jin S, Shi C, Wang L, Zhang X, Li Y, et al. Treatment of Benign Thyroid Nodules: Comparison of Surgery with Radiofrequency Ablation. AJNR Am J Neuroradiol. 2015;36:1321-5.
19. Ugurlu MU, Uprak K, Akpinar IN, Attaallah W, Yegen C, Gulluoglu BM. Radiofrequency ablation of benign symptomatic thyroid nodules: prospective safety and efficacy study. World J Surg. 2015;39:961-8.
20. Deandrea M, Sung JY, Limone P, Mormile A, Garino F, Ragazzoni F, et al. Efficacy and Safety of Radiofrequency Ablation versus Control Condition for Nonfunctioning Benign Thyroid Nodules: A Randomized Controlled International Collaborative Trial. Thyroid. 2015;25:890-6.
21. Faggiano A, Ramundo V, Assanti AP, Fonderico F, Macchia PE, Misso C, et al. Thyroid nodules treated with percutaneous

radiofrequency thermal ablation: a comparative study. J Clin Endocrin Metab. 2012;97:4439-45.

22. Jeong WK, Baek JH, Rhim H, Kim YS, Kwak MS, Jeong HJ, et al. Radiofrequency ablation of benign thyroid nodules: safety and imaging follow-up in 236 patients. Eur Radiol. 2008;18:1244-50.

23. Lee JH, Ha EJ, Sung JY, Kim JK, Baek JH. Radiofrequency ablation of benign non-functioning thyroid nodules: 4-year follow-up results for 111 patients. Eur Radiol. 2013;23:1044-9.

24. Cesareo R, Pasqualini V, Simeoni C, Sacchi M, Saralli E, Campagna G, et al. Prospective study of effectiveness of ultrasound-guided radiofrequency ablation versus control group in patients affected by benign thyroid nodules. J Clin Endocrinol Metab. 2015;100:460-6.

25. Huh JY, Baek JH, Choi H, Kim JK, Lee JH. Symptomatic benign thyroid nodules: efficacy of additional radiofrequency ablation treatment session--prospective randomized study. Radiology. 2012;263:909-16.

26. Papini E, Pacella CM, Hegedus L. Thyroid ultrasound (US) and US-assisted procedures: from the shadows into an array of applications. Eur J Endocrinology. 2014;170:133-46.

27. Sung JY, Baek JH, Jung SL, Kim JH, Kim KS, Lee D, et al. Radiofrequency ablation for autonomously functioning thyroid nodules: a multicenter study. Thyroid. 2015;25:112-7.

28. Regalbuto C, Le Moli R, Muscia V, Russo M, Vigneri R, Pezzino V. Severe Graves' ophthalmopathy after percutaneous ethanol injection in a nontoxic thyroid nodule. Thyroid. 2012;22:210-3.

29. Bernardi S, Dobrinja C, Fabris B, Bazzocchi G, Sabato N, Ulcigrai V, et al. Radiofrequency Ablation Compared to Surgery for the Treatment of Benign Thyroid Nodules. Int J Endocrinol. 2014;2014:934595.

30. Che Y, Jin S, Shi C, Wang L, Zhang X, Li Y, et al. Treatment of benign thyroid nodules: comparison of surgery with radiofrequency ablation. AJNR Am J Neuroradiol. 2015;36:1321-5.

24

Lean mass as a determinant of bone mineral density of proximal femur in postmenopausal women

Rosangela Villa Marin-Mio[1], Linda Denise Fernandes Moreira[1],
Marília Camargo[1], Neide Alessandra Sansão Périgo[2],
Maysa Seabra Cerondoglo[2], Marise Lazaretti-Castro[1]

ABSTRACT

Objective: To verify which component of body composition (BC) has greater influence on postmenopausal women bone mineral density (BMD). Subjects and methods: Four hundred and thirty women undergoing treatment for osteoporosis and 513 untreated women, except for calcium and vitamin D. Multiple linear regression analysis was performed in order to correlated BMD at lumbar spine (LS), total femur (FT), femoral neck (FN) with body mass (BM), total lean mass (LM) and total fat mass (FM), all determined by DXA. Results: BM significantly correlated with all bone sites in untreated and treated women (r = 0.420 vs 0.277 at LS; r = 0.490 vs 0.418 at FN, r = 0.496 vs 0.414 at FT, respectively). In untreated women, the LM correlated better than FM with all sites, explaining 17.9% of LS; 32.3% of FN and 30.2% of FT; whereas FM explained 13.2% of LS; 27.7% of FN, 23.4% of FT. In treated women, correlations with BC were less relevant, with the LM explaining 6.7% of BMD at LS; 15.2% of FN, 16% of FT, whereas the FM explained 8.1% of LS; 17.9% of FN and 17.6% of FT. Conclusion: LM in untreated women was better predictor of BMD than FM, especialy for distal femur, where it explained more than 30% of the BMD, suggesting that maintaining a healthy muscle mass may contribute to decrease osteoporosis risk. Treatment with anti-osteoporotic drugs seems to mask these relationships. Arch Endocrinol Metab. 2018;62(4):431-7

Keywords
Osteoporosis; treatment; body weight; body composition

[1] Disciplina de Endocrinologia da Universidade Federal de São Paulo (Unifesp), São Paulo, SP, Brasil
[2] Disciplina de Geriatria e Gerontologia da Universidade Federal de São Paulo (Unifesp), São Paulo, SP, Brasil

Correspondence to:
Rosangela Villa Marin Mio
Av. Salgado Filho, 2844, ap. 708, Torre 2
07115-000 – Guarulhos, SP, Brasil
rosevillamarin@uol.com.br

INTRODUCTION

Osteoporosis is intimaly associated to the aging process and represents a social problem nowadays. Populational statistics shows that the situation can get even worse in the future due to the increase in longevity. Low bone mass is one of the main determinants of osteoporosis, which associates with bone microstructural changes resulting in a higher fracture risk. By comprehending what positively influences bone mass of individual health professionals will be able to create strategies to control bone loss throughout aging (1,2).

Total body mass is one of the biological variables that best correlates with bone mass. However, it remains unclear what would be the influence of the different body mass components on bone metabolism (1,3-6). Gillette-Guyonnet and cols. (5) studied older osteoporotic women (75 to 89 years old) and observed a significant correlation between bone mineral density and body composition (BC), which includes body mass, fat mass and lean mass. In this study, fat mass showed a better association with bone mass than lean mass, suggesting that fat mass could exert a protective effect on the proximal femur. On the other hand, Binder and Kohrt (7), studying elderly men and women, observed that the lean mass was the BC component that best correlated with bone mineral density (BMD). The authors suggested that the association of lean mass and fat mass with bone mass reflects not only the effects of total body mass mechanical loading on bone, but also the functional relation between muscles and bones.

It is believed that muscle contractions, as well as physical exercise, act as potent anabolic stimuli to strengthen bone tissue. On the other hand, low fat mass can represent especially relevant state of denutrition in elderly, which could reflect on the health of bone tissue, currently recognized as a tissue involved in energy metabolism (2,8).

As studies about BC and bone mass still show controversial results, our aim was to determine which of the components of BC would be better related to bone mass in a representative population of postmenopausal women both treatment and treatment näive for osteoporosis.

SUBJECTS AND METHODS

The sample consisted of 943 independent postmenopausal women, with age above 40 years old (average 66.9 ± 7.8 years old), who volunteered to participate in three different protocols to evaluate physical exercise effects on bone mass, conducted by the same group of researchers. The present cross-sectional study used the baseline data from all these women as they entered the study protocols, which were conducted by the same professionals and utilized the same methodology for measurement of antrhopometric and body composition parameteres. The selection criteria for choosing study participants are described in details in the publications resulting from these three studies (9-11). For further analysis, these women were divided into two groups: 430 that were undergoing treatment for osteoporosis (47 to 87 years old, average of 68.3 ± 8.2 years old) (10,11) and 513 never treated for osteoporosis (41 to 87 years old, average of 65.8 ± 7.4 years old) (9,11).

The study has the approval of the Ethics and Research Committee of *Universidade Federal de São Paulo* – Unifesp/EPM, numbered CEP: 32882/12, CAAE: 02252312.1.0000.5505. All the subjects signed an informed consent.

The methods selected to evaluate the total and the segmental BC, as well as the total and the compartmental anthropometric measurements and sites of bone mineral density are described as follows.

The total body mass was measured using a platform-type mechanical scale (Filizola, São Paulo, Brazil) with a maximum capacity of 150 kg and variation 0.1 kg. Height was measured using a vertical bar stadiometer with maximum range of 220 cm and accuracy of 0.1 cm. Body mass index – BMI (kg/m²), was calculated from weight and height measurements using the formula BMI = weight (in kg) divided by height (in m⁻²) (12).

The BC and the bone mineral density (BMD) analyzes were obtained by dual-energy X-ray absorptiometry (DXA), in a Hologic QDR 4500A equipment (Waltham, MA). This assessment was performed at the Bone Evaluation Laboratory of the Endocrinology Division, at Universidade Federal de Sao Paulo. In our hands the CV% for lumbar spine and

total femur is 1%, for trochanter is 1.2% and for femoral neck is 1.4%. The studied variables were: BMD in the sites of lumbar spine L1-L4 (LS), total femur (TF) and femoral neck (FN) in grams/cm² and the T-score values; in addition to the lean mass (LM) and fat mass (FM) in absolute values.

Statistical analysis

Normality of the data was assessed by using the Kolmogorov-Smirnov adherence test. When the groups were divided into treated and untreated women, they were compared by the "t" test of Student for independent samples in order to determine whether the groups presented any different characteristics.

The Pearson Linear correlation, as well as the univariate linear regression and the analysis of multiple linear regressions were performed, having the bone sites as the dependent variables and BC (total body mass, total lean mass) as the independent ones.

The studied variables that presented $p < 0.20$ in the Pearson linear correlation analysis were selected and included in the models and, further, considered for inclusion in the multiple linear regression model. For this model, the stepwise forward modeling strategy was used.

The variables that remained significant were kept in the final multiple linear regression model, always observing the possible collinearities. The variable age was considered as a control variable. All the analisys were made by using the Statistical Package for the Social Sciences – SPSS for Windows – version 19".

RESULTS

All studied variables were different between the two evaluated groups – women treated and untreated for osteoporosis, emphasizing that the treated participants were older, thinner, shorter, presented a worse bone mass and lower values of body composition components (Table 1).

In women not treated for osteoporosis, among all the studied variables, the total body mass was the one that best correlated with all sites of bone mass: LS r = 0.427 (p = 0.000), FN r = 0.490 (p = 0.000) and TF r = 0.496 (p = 0.000). The correlation between the different sites of bone mass with height or BMI showed values ranging from r = 0.120 to r = 0.430 (p = 0.000). For the same 513 women, the lean mass was the variable that best correlated with all sites of bone mineral density, r = 0.423 (p = 0.000) at LS, r = 0.505 (p = 0.000) at FN and r = 0.520 (p = 0.000) at TF (Figure 1). The associations with fat mass were also significant but showed less expressive results in all sites [r = 0.361 (p = 0.000) for LS; r = 0.433 (p = 0.000) for FN and r = 0.430 (p = 0.000) for TF].

After performing the individual analyzes, we started to build statistical models to determine the influence of lean and fat mass on bone mass in the 513 untreated women and the 430 women treated for osteoporosis.

In untreated women, the coefficients of BMD determination found for lean mass models were better than the ones found for the fat mass: 17.9% in BMD of LS; 32.3% for FN and 30.2% of TF. On the other hand, models showed that fat mass could explain 13.2% of LS BMD; 27.7% of FN BMD and 23.4% of TF BMD (Table 2).

In women treated with active drugs for osteoporosis, the correlation between BMD and body mass became

Table 1. Descriptive characteristics of bone mass and body composition of untreated and treated women for osteoporosis

Variables	Untreated n = 513				Treated n = 430			
	x	sd	min	max	x	sd	min	Max
Age (years)	65.8*	7.4	41	87	68.3	8.2	47	87
Weight (kg)	70.8*	13.4	36.0	111.6	60.7	11.3	35.0	104.0
Height (m)	1.55*	0.06	1.36	1.90	1.53	0.07	1.33	1.74
BMI (kg/m²)	29.5*	5.1	14.4	50.1	25.9	4.2	16.6	42.7
BMD LS (g/cm²)	0.933*	0.156	0.464	1.608	0.759	0.128	0.371	1.634
BMD FN (g/cm²)	0.764*	0.128	0.398	1.342	0.657	0.097	0.408	1.010
BMD TF (g/cm²)	0.878*	0.126	0.449	1.266	0.756	0.108	0.350	1.052
T score LS	- 1.0*	1.4	- 5.3	5.1	- 2.6	1.1	- 6.1	5.3
T score FN	- 0.8*	1.1	- 4.1	4.4	- 1.7	0.9	- 4.0	1.5
T Score TF	- 0.5*	1.1	- 4.0	2.7	- 1.5	0.9	- 4.9	0.9
Lean mass (kg)	42.1*	6.1	27.9	59.8	37.3	5.1	24.4	67.0
Fat mass (kg)	27.5*	8.1	9.5	50.9	21.9	6.9	7.5	48.5

* p < 0.05 treated vs untreated.

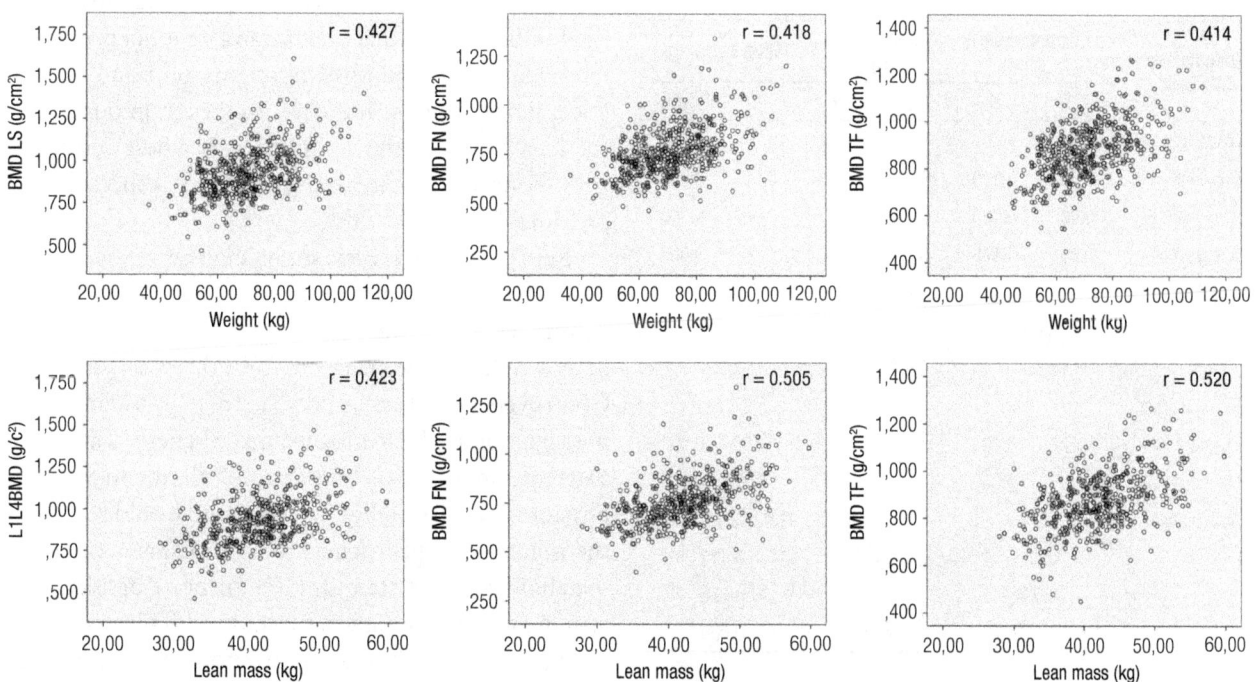

Figure 1. Correlation charts between the bone sites, total body mass and lean mass of untreated women for osteoporosis.

weaker. In this group, the models for lean mass explained only 6.7% of LS BMD; 15.2% of FN BMD and 16% of TF BMD (Table 3), while the model for fat mass explained 8.1% of LS BMD, 17.9% of FN

BMD and 17.6% of FT BMD. Therefore, treatment of osteoporosis appears to modify the relation between bone mass and the anthropometric variables, decreasing the great influence of these parameters on the BMD.

Table 2. Results of the multiple linear regression analysis between the sites of BMD and lean body mass and fat mass variables of 513 untreated women for osteoporosis

Independent variables	Lumbar spine (g)		Femural neck (g)		Total femur (g)	
	β	p	β	p	β	p
Model lean mass						
Constant	0.480	0.000	0.669	0.000	0.659	0.000
Lean mass (kg)	0.011	0.000	0.009	0.000	0.010	0.000
Age (years)*	- 4.508	0.996	- 0.005	0.000	- 0.003	0.000
r	0.423		0.558		0.549	
r²	0.179		0.323		0.302	
p	0.000		0.000		0.000	
Model fat mass						
Constant	0.795	0.000	0.936	0.000	0.956	0.000
Fat mass (kg)	0.007	0.000	0.006	0.000	0.006	0.000
Age (years)*	- 0.001	0.389	- 0.005	0.009	- 0.004	0.000
r	0.363		0.526		0.483	
r²	0.132		0.277		0.234	
p	0.000		0.000		0.000	

* All adjustments for age.

Table 3. Results of the multiple linear regression analysis between the sites of BMD and lean body mass and fat mass variables of 430 treated women for osteoporosis

Independent variables	Lumbar spine (g)		Femural neck (g)		Total femur (g)	
	β	p	β	p	β	p
Model lean mass						
Constant	0.453	0.000	0.498	0.000	0.637	0.000
Lean mass (kg)	0.006	0.000	0.007	0.000	0.007	0.000
Age (years)*	0.001	0.178	- 0.001	0.010	- 0.002	0.000
r	0.258		0.390		0.399	
r²	0.067		0.152		0.160	
p	0.000		0.000		0.000	
Model fat mass						
Constant	0,577	0.000	0.632	0.000	0.786	0.000
Fat mass (kg)	0.005	0.000	0.006	0.000	0.006	0.000
Age (years)*	0.001	0.191	- 0.001	0.009	- 0.002	0.000
r	0.285		0.423		0.419	
r²	0.081		0.179		0.176	
p	0.000		0.000		0.000	

* All adjustments for age.

DISCUSSION

The total body mass in adults is one of the biological variables that most consistently correlate with bone mass and fracture risk (8). In our study, this phenomenon was detected with greater relevance among women without treatment for osteoporosis. Treatment with specific drugs for osteoporosis made the relationship between BMD and body mass less relevant, probably because these drugs directly interfere on bone remodeling, mitigating the local influence of body mass (2). In a similar study with Italian Caucasian postmenopausal women, authors (13) concluded that both fat and lean masses might affect bone mass but depending on the osteoporotic status. In non-osteoporotic women, only lean mass was associated with BMD. In osteoporotic women treated for osteoporosis, however, the lean and fat masses had the same importance.

Lewin and cols. (14) also studied a population of Brazilian Caucasian women and observed that heavier girls reached bone mass peak earlier, besides having higher BMD values. In addition, the bone loss caused by aging was reduced in those women with higher total body mass.

In our study, the correlation of total body mass was more relevant with the proximal femur than with the lumbar spine, what could translate influence of the mechanical load and physical activity on bone mass of lower limbs. To contribute to this theory, in our results the lean mass was the component that best correlated with bone density in different places, especially the proximal femur.

Reid (3), in a review study, emphasizes that total body mass is a main determinant of bone mineral density as well as fracture risk, and concludes that fat mass would be the main contributor to this relation. Controversely, other authors (6,15-17) sustain that a higher amount of lean mass would be beneficial and have a stronger influence on bone mass. Both statements have physiological plausibility. The fat tissue would represent the influence of neuroendocrine factors, as well as the metabolism of sex steroids (17) on bone density. The lean mass, on the other hand, would represent the mechanical and physical stimulation effect on bone tissue. Li and cols. (17), analysing perimenopausal women (average of 49.6 years), revealed that both fat mass and lean mass had positive relations with BMD of lumbar spine and femur. However, using multiple regression analysis, authors observed that only lean mass and ethnicity remained significant predictors of BMD of femoral neck. The lean mass was the only predictor of BMD of the total femur, explaining in 38% the BMD at this site, while fat mass was not a significant predictor of BMD in any of the analyzed sites.

The influence of total body mass and its different components on bone mass apears to vary according to age, gender and skeletal site of the studied populations (Table 4). In most studies, the lean mass apears to have a greater influence on bone density than fat mass, specialy at proximal femoral sites. In younger men, however, fat mass can have negative effects on bone mass (4). With aging, changes in body composition components induce an increment of fat mass followed by a decrement of lean mass. Considering postmenopausal American women, Chen and cols. (18) also observed that lean mass exerts a stronger influence on the BMD of differente bone sites.

In a Korean rural population (19 to 80 years old, both genders), lean mass was an important determinant of BMD either for young and elderly population, but fat mass showed a dual effect. High fat mass showed negative influence on bone mass in younger, however, with positive influence in postmenopausal women and older men (4).

The physiological mechanisms that would explain this important correlation between bone mass and body mass are not completely defined yet. Some experimental studies suggest the existence of a bone remodeling central control that would work via neuropeptides and neurotransmitters, such as serotonin (21,22) in addition to adipokines, as leptin, which would connect fat tissue to bone metabolism (22). Karsenty (23) postulate that bone tissue has an endocrine role in the regulation of energy metabolism, especially decarboxylated osteocalcin, acting in the regulation of glucose homeostasis and insulin sensitivity (21-28).

It is well established that mechanical loading has a powerful anabolic effect on bone tissue, an effect coordinated by osteocytes (29). This can be confirmed by increased bone mass observed in athletes, when compared with sedentary controls (30). On the other hand, immobility and inactivity are considered great causes for low bone mass, risk of falls and fractures (31).

Table 4. Description of published studies which investigated relationships between body compartments and bone density in different populations

Author	Country	Population	Age (years)	Lean mass	Fat mass	Additional finding
Chen and cols., 1997 (18)	USA	50 postmenopausal Caucasian women	> 65	Strongest determinant of bone mass, especially total bone mass and bone content		The increase in body mass showed significant association with the increase in bone mass
Ho-Pham and cols., 2010 (15)	Vietnam	210 postmenopausal women	50 to 85	Positive influence on spine and femur bone mass	Positive influence on spine and femur bone mass	
Zhu and cols., 2015 (19)	Australia	915 men and 1014 women	45 to 66	Predicted bone mass in both genders	Predicted bone mass in both genders	
Gjesdal and cols., 2008 (16)	Norway	2214 men and 2991 women	47 to 50 and 71 to 75	Predicted bone mass in both genders	Predicted bone mass in both genders	
Cui and cols., 2007 (4)	South Korea	737 men and 867 women	19 to 80	**Younger:** positive influence on all bone mass sites	**Younger:** negative influence on all bone mass sites	Lean mass was considered an important predictor of bone mass; however, fat mass also positively contributed to bone mass in postmenopausal women and older men
				Older: positive influence on all bone mass sites	**Older:** positive influence on forearm and calcaneus bone mass	
				Premenopausal: positive influence with all bone sites	**Postmenopausal:** positive influence with all bone sites	
Gillette-Guyonnet and cols., 2000 (5)	France	129 healthy women	75 to 89	Positive influence on all bone mass sites	Positive influence on all bone mass sites	
Taaffe and cols., 2000 (20)	USA	54 women Non-Hispanic Caucasians and Mexican-Americans with BMI < 30 kg/m²	60 to 86	**Non Hispanic:** positive influence on bone mass of lumbar spine. **Mexican-Americans:** positive influence on bone mass of lumbar spine and trochanter	**Non Hispanic:** positive influence on femoral neck bone mass	

Thus, lean mass measured by DXA can be interpreted as a marker of bone health, which means a greater mechanical load on the skeleton and would justify our findings. This gives better basis for the importance of encouraging physical activity to maintain muscle mass in preventing osteoporosis (32).

In conclusion, revious studies, as well as the present one, confirm that several variables contribute to the association between lean mass, fat mass and bone mass. Among these variables we highlight the treatment for osteoporosis, different ages and stages of life, gender and ethnicity. Our data revealed an important relationship between total body mass and all bone mass sites in postmenopausal women without osteoporosis treatment. However, in women being treated for osteoporosis these correlations lose their relevance. Among the different BC components, we found that lean mass was the one that presented the best correlation with bone mineral density, mainly on the proximal femur. In multiple variables model, when lean mass was corrected by the age of women without treatment for osteoporosis it explained about 30% of proximal femur bone mass. These results suggest that maintaining a healthy muscle mass can contribute to decrese the risk for osteoporosis. Results like ours also stimulate the search for mechanisms that explain this phenomenon, as well as the relevance of BC parameters on bone mass during treatment of osteoporosis.

REFERENCES

1. Marin RV, Pedrosa MA, Moreira-Pfrimer LD, Matsudo SM, Lazaretti-Castro M. Association between lean mass and handgrip strength with bone mineral density in physically active postmenopausal women. J Clin Densitom. 2010;13(1):96-101.
2. Radominski SC, Bernardo W, Paula AP, Albergaria B, Moreira C, Fernandes CE, et al. Diretrizes brasileiras para o diagnóstico e tratamento da osteoporose em mulheres na pós-menopausa. Rev Bras Reumatol. 2017;57(2):452-66.
3. Reid IR. Fat and bone. Arch Biochem Biophys. 2010;503(1):20-7.
4. Cui LH, Shin MH, Kweon SS, Park KS, Lee YH, Chung EK. Relative contribution of body composition to bone mineral density at different sites in men and women of South Korea. J Bone Miner Metab. 2007;25(3):165-71.
5. Gillette-Guyonnet S, Nourhashemi F, Lauque S, Grandjean H, Vellas B. Body composition and osteoporosis in elderly women. Gerontology. 2000;46(4):189-93.
6. Xiang J, Chen Y, Wang Y, Su S, Wang X, Xie B, et al. Lean Mass and Fat Mass as Mediators of the Relationship Between Physical Activity and Bone Mineral Density in Postmenopausal Women. J Womens Health (Larchmt). 2017;26(5):461-6.
7. Binder EF, Kohrt WM. Relationships between body composition and bone mineral content and density in older women and men. Clinical Exercise Physiology. 2000;2:84-91.
8. Camargo MB, Cendoroglo MS, Ramos LR, de Oliveira Latorre Mdo R, Saraiva GL, Lage A, et al. Bone mineral density and osteoporosis among a predominantly Caucasian elderly population in the city of São Paulo, Brazil. Osteoporos Int. 2005;16(11):1451-60.
9. Moreira LD, Fronza FC, Dos Santos RN, Zach PL, Kunii IS, Hayashi LF, et al. The benefits of a high-intensity aquatic exercise program (HydrOS) for bone metabolism and bone mass of postmenopausal women. J Bone Miner Metab. 2014;32(4):411-9.
10. Camargo MB, Kunii LS, Hayashi LF, Muszkat P, Anelli CG, Marin-Mio RV, et al. Modifiable factors of vitamin D status among a Brazilian osteoporotic population attended a public outpatient clinic. Arq Bras Endocrinol Metabol. 2014;58(5):572-82.
11. Nascimento NA, Moreira PF, Marin RV, Moreira LD, Castro ML, Santos CA, et al. Relation among 25(OH)D, aquatic exercises, and multifunctional fitness on functional performance of elderly women from the community. J Nutr Health Aging. 2016;20(4):376-82.
12. Heyward V, Stolarczyk LM. Anthropometric method. Applied body composition assessment. Ed. Champaign: Human Kinetics; 1996. p. 76-85.
13. Gnudi S, Sitta E, Fiumi N. Relationship between body composition and bone mineral density in women with and without osteoporosis: relative contribution of lean and fat mass. J Bone Miner Metab. 2007;25(5):326-32.
14. Lewin S, Gouveia CH, Marone MMS, Wehba S, Malvestiti LF, Bianco AC. Densidade mineral óssea vertebral e femoral de 724 mulheres brancas brasileiras: influência da idade e do peso corporal. Rev Assoc Med Bras. 1997;43(2):127-36.
15. Ho-Pham LT, Nguyen ND, Lai TQ, Nguyen TV. Contributions of lean mass and fat mass to bone mineral density: a study in postmenopausal women. BMC Musculoskelet Disord. 2010;11:59.
16. Gjesdal CG, Halse JI, Eide GE, Brun JG, Tell GS. Impact of lean mass and fat mass on bone mineral density: The Hordaland Health Study. Maturitas 2008;59(2):191-200.
17. Li S, Wagner R, Holm K, Lehotsky J, Zinaman MJ. Relationship between soft tissue body composition and bone mass in perimenopausal women. Maturitas. 2004;47(2):99-105.
18. Chen Z, Lohman TG, Stini WA, Ritenbaugh C, Aickin M. Fat or lean tissue mass: which one is the major determinant of bone mineral mass in healthy postmenopausal women? J Bone Miner Res. 1997;12(1):144-51.
19. Zhu K, Hunter M, James A, Lim EM, Walsh JP. Associations between body mass index, lean and fat body mass and bone mineral density in middle-aged Australians: The Busselton Healthy Ageing Study. Bone. 2015;74:146-52.
20. Taaffe DR, Villa ML, Holloway L, Marcus R. Bone mineral density in older non-Hispanic Caucasian and Mexican-American women: relationship to lean and fat mass. Ann Hum Biol. 2000;27(4):331-44.
21. Borba VZC, Kulak CAM, Lazaretti-Castro M. Controle neuroendócrino da massa óssea: Mito ou verdade? Arq Bras Endocrinol Metab. 2003;47(4):453-7.
22. Ducy P, Amling M, Takeda S, Priemel M, Schilling AF, Beil FT, et al. Leptin inhibits bone formation through a hypothalamic relay: a central control of bone mass. Cell. 2000;100(2):197-207.
23. Karsenty G. Convergence between bone and energy homeostases: Leptin regulation of bone mass. Cell Metab. 2006;4(5):341-8.
24. Sharma S, Tandon VR, Mahajan S, Mahajan V, Mahajan A. Obesity: Friend or foe for osteoporosis. J Midlife Health. 2014;5(1):6-9.
25. Lee S, Rhee Y. Bone and energy metabolism. J Korean Diabetes. 2013;14(4):174-7.

26. Yadav VK, Karsenty G. Leptin-dependent co-regulation of bone and energy metabolism. Aging (Albany NY). 2009;1(11):954-6.

27. Araújo TF, Guimarães DF, Ferreira F, Luz JCM, Spini VBMG. Leptina e o controle neuroendócrino do peso corporal. Rev Bras Med. 2009;66(10):325-30.

28. Lee NK, Karsenty G. Reciprocal regulation of bone and energy metabolism. J Musculoskelet Neuronal Interact. 2008;8(4):351.

29. Ocarino NM, Serakides R. Efeito da atividade física no osso normal e na prevenção e tratamento da osteoporose. Rev Bras Med Esporte. 2006;12(3):164-8.

30. Lazzoli JK, Oliveira MAB, Leitão MB, Nóbrega ACL, Nahas RM, Rezende L, et al. Posicionamento Oficial da Sociedade Brasileira de Medicina do Esporte sobre: esporte competitivo em indivíduos acima de 35 anos. Rev Bras Med Esporte. 2001;7(3):83-92.

31. Zazula FC, Pereira MAS. Fisiopatologia da osteoporose e o exercício físico como medida preventiva. Arq Cienc Saúde Unipar. 2003;7(3):269-75.

32. Klein-Nulend J, Bacabac RG, Bakker AD. Mechanical loading and how it affects bone cells: the role of the osteocyte cytoskeleton in maintaining our skeleton. Eur Cell Mater. 2012;24:278-91.

25

Estimation of cardiovascular risk and detection of subclinical carotid atheromatosis in patients with diabetes without a history of cardiovascular disease

Walter Masson[1], Salvador De Francesca[1], Micaela Molinero[1], Daniel Siniawski[1], Andrés Mulassi[1], Frank Espinoza Morales[1], Melina Huerin[1], Martín Lobo[1], Graciela Molinero[1]

ABSTRACT

Objectives: Cardiovascular risk estimated by several scores in patients with diabetes mellitus without a cardiovascular disease history and the association with carotid atherosclerotic plaque (CAP) were the aims of this study. **Materials and methods:** Cardiovascular risk was calculate using United Kingdom Prospective Diabetes Study (UKPDS) risk engine, Framingham risk score for cardiovascular (FSCV) and coronary disease (FSCD), and the new score (NS) proposed by the 2013 ACC/AHA Guideline on the Treatment of Blood Cholesterol. Ultrasound was used to assess CAP occurrence. A receiver operating characteristic (ROC) analysis was performed. **Results:** One hundred seventy patients (mean age 61.4 ± 11 years, 58.8% men) were included. Average FSCV, FSCD and NS values were 33.6% ± 21%, 20.6% ± 12% and 24.8% ± 18%, respectively. According to the UKPDS score, average risk of coronary disease and stroke were 22.1% ± 16% and 14.3% ± 19% respectively. Comparing the risks estimated by the different scores a significant correlation was found. The prevalence of CAP was 51%, in patients with the higher scores this prevalence was increased. ROC analysis showed a good discrimination power between subjects with or without CAP. **Conclusion:** The cardiovascular risk estimated was high but heterogenic. The prevalence of CAP increased according to the strata of risk. Understanding the relationship between CAP and scores could improve the risk estimation in subjects with diabetes. Arch Endocrinol Metab. 2017;61(2):122-9.

Keywords
Diabetes; cardiovascular risk estimation; carotid atherosclerotic plaque

[1] Council of Epidemiology and Cardiovascular Prevention "Dr. Mario Ciruzzi" of the Argentine Society of Cardiology, Buenos Aires, Argentina

Correspondence to:
Walter Masson
Servicio de Cardiología,
Hospital Italiano de Buenos Aires
Pte. Perón 4190 – C1181ACH
Ciudad de Buenos Aires, Argentina
walter.masson@hospitalitaliano.org.ar

INTRODUCTION

The presence of type 2 diabetes mellitus approximately doubles the risk of cardiovascular mortality when compared with individuals without diabetes (1).

Previously, published studies showed that the cardiovascular prognosis of patients with diabetes without acute myocardial infarction (AMI) was similar to patients without diabetes but with a history of AMI (2-4). Consequently, the third National Cholesterol Education Program (NCEP) expert panel report on elevated blood cholesterol detection, assessment and treatment in adults (Adult Treatment Panel III – ATP III), considered the patient with diabetes as "coronary equivalent" (5). However, other reports have not confirmed these findings, generating controversy over what is the real cardiovascular risk of subjects with diabetes without coronary disease history (6-8).

A number of cardiovascular risk functions or scores have been developed from large epidemiological studies in general population (9-11). However, the low number of people with diabetes in the cohorts that originated these scores, puts limits its applicability. One of the few risk scores specifically developed in a population with diabetes came from the United Kingdom Prospective Diabetes Study (UKPDS risk engine) (12).

The estimation of cardiovascular risk in patients with diabetes would have clinical implications. Patients with diabetes, with or without additional risk factors or target organ damage, are considered "very high risk" or "high risk" respectively, with different LDL-C goal recommended in both groups, according to European guidelines for the management of cholesterol (13).

On the other hand, the 2013 American College of Cardiology/American Heart Association (ACC/AHA)

Guideline on the Treatment of Blood Cholesterol recommends a new risk score (NS) in the population with diabetes without cardiovascular disease, suggesting moderate or high doses of statins according to the estimated risk (< or ≥ 7.5% respectively) (14).

There is evidence that the presence or absence of subclinical carotid atherosclerotic detected by ultrasound, improve the prediction of cardiovascular events in general population as well as in diabetes population (15-17).

Cardiovascular stratification with several risk scores, the association with the presence of carotid atherosclerotic plaque (CAP) and their implications on the use of statins have been previously evaluated by our working group in a primary prevention population in our country, but this analysis did not include patients with diabetes (18).

Therefore, the aims of the study were: 1) To stratify the cardiovascular risk using four different risk scores in patients with diabetes without cardiovascular disease history; 2) To estimate the correlation and concordance between these risk scores; 3) To describe the prevalence of CAP in the different risk categories according to each score; 4) To establish the optimal cutoff point (OCP) of each score that allows us to discriminate between subjects with or without CAP.

MATERIALS AND METHODS

Subjects

A multicenter, descriptive, cross-sectional study was performed on consecutive samples obtained in the cardiovascular prevention outpatient clinics of five cardiology centers in Buenos Aires, Argentina.

Subjects with diagnostic of diabetes were included in the study (fasting plasma glucose concentration ≥ 126 mg/dL in two consecutive measurements or plasma glucose ≥ 200 mg/dL on a 2-hour oral glucose tolerance test). Exclusion criteria were: 1) previous cardiovascular disease defined as AMI, prior percutaneous coronary intervention or coronary artery bypass graft surgery, or stroke or peripheral artery disease history; 2) chronic renal disease stage 4-5 (creatinine clearance < 30 mL/min); 3) concomitant lipid lowering therapy. The variables age, gender, total cholesterol, cholesterol bound to high-density lipoproteins (HDL-C), cholesterol bound to low-density lipoproteins (LDL-C), triglycerides, body mass

index, systolic and diastolic blood pressure, duration of diabetes, hemoglobin glycosylate (HbA1c), family history of early coronary heart disease, smoking, presence of atrial fibrillation, and pharmacotherapy were collected.

Cardiovascular scores and CAP

Four risk scores were calculated: 1) The Framingham 10-year risk score for cardiovascular disease (coronary death, AMI, coronary insufficiency, angina, ischemic stroke, hemorrhagic stroke, transient ischemic attack, peripheral artery disease, heart failure) based on lipids (FSCV) (19). 2) The Framingham 10-year risk score for coronary disease (FSCD) (9). 3) The NS for cardiovascular disease (AMI and stroke, fatal and nonfatal) used by the 2013 ACC/AHA Guideline on the Treatment of Blood Cholesterol (14). We consider indication of statins at moderate or high doses according to the estimated risk (< or ≥ 7.5% respectively). 4) The UKPDS 10-year risk score. The risk of coronary heart disease and stroke (fatal and nonfatal) was calculated. The UKPDS risk engine (ver. 2.0) was downloaded from the website and used to analyze the data (20).

The scores were analyzed by quartiles and the distribution was graphed using Kernel density estimation.

Ultrasound was used as noninvasive method for detecting the presence of CAP. The following points were required for the characterization of the plaque: 1) abnormal wall thickness (intima-media thickness > 1.5 mm), 2) abnormal structure (protrusion towards the lumen, loss of alignment with the adjacent wall) and 3) abnormal wall echogenicity. Carotid atherosclerotic plaque prevalence was compared between the different risks strata (quartiles) in the different scores used.

Statistical analysis

A receiver operating characteristic (ROC) analysis was carried out to determine the area under the curve, assessing the four scores accuracy to discriminate between subjects with or without CAP. The Youden index [maximum vertical distance between the ROC curve and the line of statistical chance (CJ point)] was used to determine the score OCP. Continuous data were compared between groups using the t test for normal distribution or the Mann-Whitney-Wilcoxon test for non-normal distribution. The analysis of categorical data was performed using the chi-square test. Pearson's test was used to obtain correlation between scores. The concordance between the FSCV, the FSCD, the NS and the UKPDS score for coronary disease was analyzed to classify patients into "high" or "non-high" risk strata (≥ 20% or < 20%), using the Fleiss kappa index. Mild or poor, acceptable or discrete, moderate, significant or almost perfect agreement was defined if the kappa value was < 0.20, between 0.21 and 0.40, 0.41 and 0.60, 0.61 and 0.80 and 0.81 and 1, respectively. Continuous variables were expressed as mean ± standard deviation, and categorical variables as percentages. A two-tailed p value < 0.01 was considered as statistically significant. STATA 11.1 and 3.1 EPIDAT software packages were used for statistical analysis.

Ethics considerations

The study was conducted following the recommendations in medical research suggested by the Declaration of Helsinki, Guidelines for Good Clinical Practice and valid local ethical regulations.

RESULTS

A total of 170 patients (mean age 61.4 ± 11 years, 58.8% men) were included in the study. Average body mass index was 30.6 ± 5 and mean total cholesterol, LDL-C, HDL-C and triglyceride values were 201 ± 36 mg/dL, 121 ± 34 mg/dL, 46 ± 13 mg/dL and 173 ± 101 mg/dL respectively. Mean HbA1c value was 7.0% (53 mmol/mol), 15% received insulin therapy and average duration of diabetes was 7.2 ± 6.5 years. Sixty four percent of patients were receiving antihypertensive treatment, 18.9% was active smokers and only 3.6% have history of atrial fibrillation. The baseline characteristics of the population stratified by sex are described in Table 1.

Average FSCV, FSCD and NS values were 33.6% ± 21%, 20.6% ± 12% and 24.8% ± 18%, respectively. According to the UKPDS score, average risk of coronary disease (fatal and nonfatal), fatal coronary disease, stroke (fatal and non fatal) and fatal stroke were 22.1% ± 16%, 15.1% ± 14%, 14,3% ± 19%, and 2.1% ± 3%, respectively. The Kernel density distributions of the risk scores are showed in Figure 1.

Table 1. Characteristics of the population stratified by sex

Continuous variables, mean (SD)	General population			Population with CAP		
	Women n = 70	Men n = 100	p	Women n = 26	Men n = 60	P
Age, years	61.5 (10.1)	61.0 (11.3)	0.76	68.1 (7.1)	66.8 (8.0)	0.47
BMI, kg/m²	31.6 (6.1)	29.9 (5.3)	0.04	31.5 (6.3)	29.4 (5.0)	0.11
Total cholesterol, mg/dL	197.8 (29.6)	202.7 (40.2)	0.36	202.5 (30.9)	202.3 (39.0)	0.98
LDL-C, mg/dL	113.9 (27.4)	126.3 (37.5)	0.01	118.3 (24.3)	129.8 (38.2)	0.1
HDL-C, mg/dL	51.3 (15.2)	41.8 (10.4)	< 0.001	48.6 (14.3)	42.3 (10.1)	0.05
Triglycerides, mg/dL	155.4 (73.3)	184.3 (115.7)	0.07	165.4 (71.3)	156.9 (67.9)	0.6
HbA1c, %	6.9 (1.4)	7.1 (1.2)	0.33	7.2 (1.4)	7.2 (0.9)	0.81
FSCV, %	20.6 (12.6)	42.4 (21.3)	< 0.001	28.3 (10.5)	51.7 (19.1)	< 0.001
FSCD, %	14.9 (7.2)	24.4 (13.4)	< 0.001	18.5 (6.0)	29.3 (13.2)	< 0.001
NS, %	16.2 (13.7)	30.6 (18.2)	< 0.001	25.3 (12.3)	39.4 (16.3)	< 0.001
UKPDS for CD, %	12.5 (8.6)	28.6 (17.1)	< 0.001	18.6 (9.6)	36.5 (16.7)	< 0.001
UKPDS for stroke, %	8.4 (8.4)	18.3 (22.4)	< 0.001	13.4 (9.8)	26.9 (25.3)	< 0.001
UKPDS for fatal CD, %	8.4 (7.5)	19.6 (15.4)	< 0.001	13.6 (8.8)	26.8 (15.4)	< 0.001
UKPDS for fatal stroke, %	1.3 (1.4)	2.7 (3.3)	< 0.001	1.9 (1.4)	3.9 (3.8)	< 0.001
Categorical variables, %						
Insulin therapy	10.1	18.2	0.15	7.7	21.7	0.14
Antihypertensive treatment	55.7	70.0	0.06	73.1	81.7	0.37
Smoking	10.0	25.0	0.001	15.4	30.0	0.03
Atrial fibrillation	0.0	3.1	0.08	0.0	8.3	0.32
Family history of early CD	10.0	23.0	0.03	7.7	21.7	0.12

SD: standard deviation; BMI: body mass index; FSCV: Framingham score for cardiovascular disease; FSCD: Framingham score for coronary disease; CD: coronary disease; NS: new score proposed by the 2013 ACC/AHA Guideline on the Treatment of Blood Cholesterol.

A significant correlation was found between the estimations of all scores compared, with a range of "r" value between 0.46 and 0.98 (Table 2). However, the agreement (concordance) between the scores in categorizing the population as "high risk" or "no high risk" was moderate (kappa statistic between 0.45-0.59).

Subjects with CAP were older (67.2 ± 7.7 vs. 55.3 ± 10.0 years, p < 0.001) and evidenced higher prevalence of male sex (69.8% vs. 48.2%, p = 0.004), smoking (25.6% vs. 12.1%, p = 0.002) and anti-hypertensive treatment (79.1% vs. 49.4%, p < 0.001) than patients without CAP. The mean duration of diabetes was

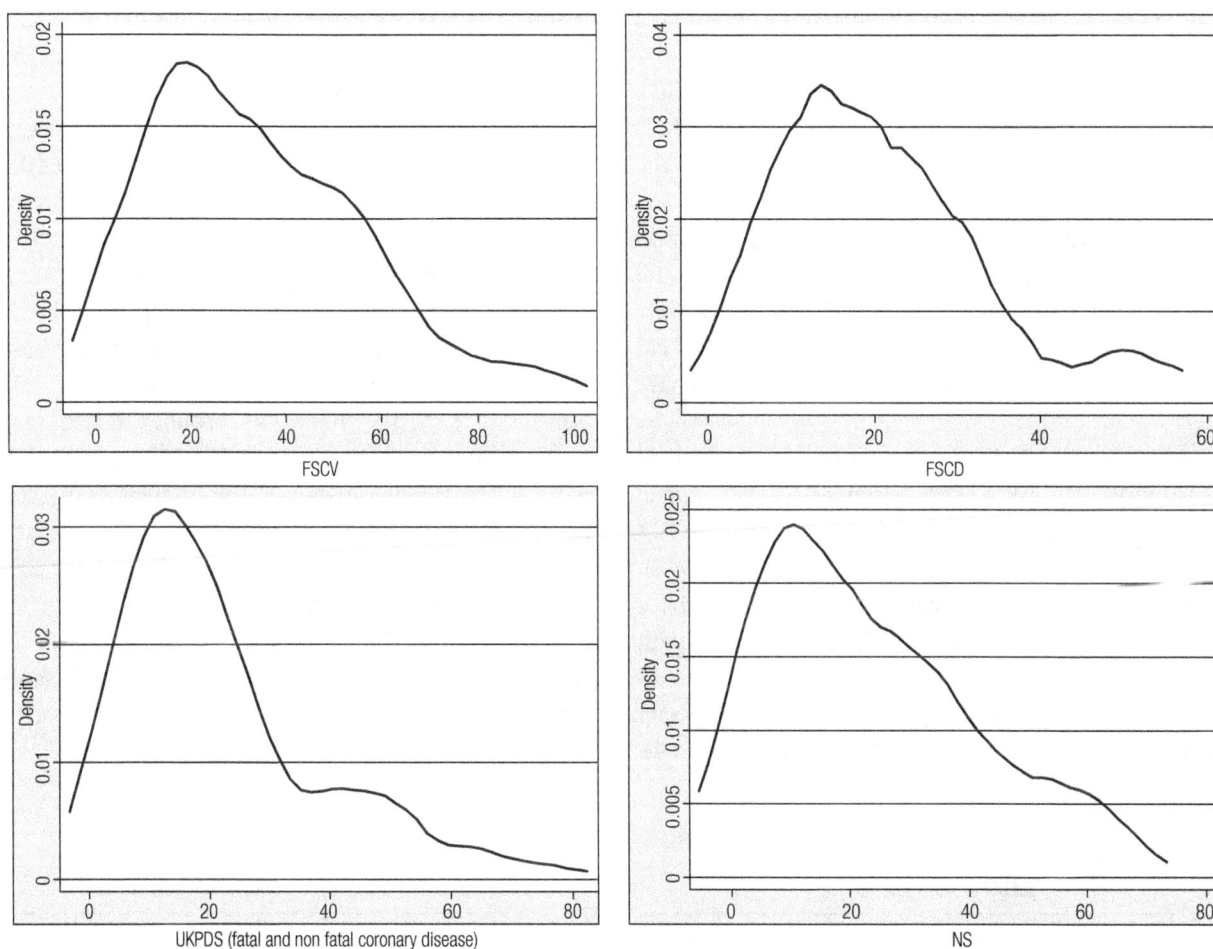

FSCV: Framingham score for cardiovascular disease; FSCD: Framingham score for coronary disease; CD: coronary disease; NS: new score of the 2013 ACC/AHA Guideline; UKPDS: United Kingdom Prospective Diabetes Study.

Figure 1. Kernel density distributions of the risk scores values.

Table 2. Correlations between different risk scores values

	FSCV	FSCD	UKPDS (CD)	UKPDS (fatal CD)	UKPDS (Stroke)	UKPDS (fatal stroke)	NS
FSCV	–	r = 0.89	r = 0.87	r = 0.81	r = 0.58	r = 0.59	r = 0.84
FSCD	r = 0.89	–	r = 0.78	r = 0.71	r = 0.46	r = 0.48	r = 0.72
UKPDS (CD)	r = 0.87	r = 0.78	–	r = 0.98	r = 0.73	r = 0.72	r = 0.86
UKPDS (fatal CD)	r = 0.81	r = 0.71	r = 0.98	–	r = 0.78	r = 0.78	r = 0.86
UKPDS (stroke)	r = 0.58	r = 0.46	r = 0.73	r = 0.78	–	r = 0.98	r = 0.74
UKPDS (fatal stroke)	r = 0.59	r = 0.48	r = 0.72	r = 0.78	r = 0.98	–	r = 0.74
NS	r = 0.84	r = 0.72	r = 0.86	r = 0.86	r = 0.74	r = 0.74	--

FSCV: Framingham score for cardiovascular disease; FSCD: Framingham score for coronary disease; CD: coronary disease; NS: new score proposed by the 2013 ACC/AHA Guideline on the Treatment of Blood Cholesterol.

higher in subjects with CAP in comparison with patients without CAP (9.3 ± 7.6 vs. 4.9 ± 4.3 years, p < 0.001).

Mean scores values were significantly higher in patients with CAP (FSCV: 44.6% ± 20.0% vs. 22.1% ± 15.2%, p < 0.001; FSCD: 26.0% ± 12.5% vs. 14.9% ± 8.6%, p < 0.001; NS: 35.1% ± 16.5% vs. 13.9% ± 11.8%, p < 0.001; UKPDS for coronary disease: 31.1% ± 17.0% vs. 12.6% ± 7.9%, p < 0.001; UKPDS for fatal coronary events: 22.8% ± 15.0% vs. 6.9% ± 5.2%, p < 0.001; UKPDS for stroke: 22.8% ± 22.6% vs. 5.3% ± 4.8%, p < 0.001; UKPDS for fatal stroke: 3.3% ± 3.6% vs. 0.79% ± 0.98%, p < 0.001) compared with the group without CAP.

Overall, the prevalence of CAP was 51% (men: 60%; women 38%), being greater in the higher risk strata (quartiles) in all the scores evaluated (Figure 2). Sixty three percent of diabetic patients with ≥ 7.5% of NS have CAP and only one subject with a NS < 7.5% have CAP.

Applying the NS, 80.4% of the population obtained a cardiovascular risk ≥ 7.5% (men 88.9% vs. women 68.1%, p = 0.001). Thus, considering the 2013 ACC/AHA Guideline on the Treatment of Blood Cholesterol, ≈ 80% of the population had absolute indication for high doses of statin therapy (98.9% in patients with CAP).

ROC analysis showed a good discrimination power between subjects with or without CAP (Figures 3 and 4).

When we analyze the population by sex, the area under the curve showed a good discrimination both in women (SFCV: 0.804, SFCD: 0.738, NS: 0.837, UKPDS score for coronary disease: 0.845, UKPDS for stroke: 0.839, UKPDS for fatal coronary disease: 0.858, UKPDS for fatal stroke: 0.820) and men (SFCV: 0.814, SFCD: 0.769, NS: 0.863, UKPDS score for coronary disease: 0.860, UKPDS for stroke: 0.900, UKPDS for fatal coronary disease: 0.885, UKPDS for fatal stroke: 0.915).

The OCP value of SFCV, SFCD and NS were 25.4% (sensitivity 86%, specificity 69%, Youden 0.547); 16% (sensitivity 79%, specificity 62%, Youden 0.405) and 14.3% (sensitivity 91%, specificity 66%, Youden 0.566) respectively. On the other hand, the OCP value of UKPDS score for coronary disease, fatal coronary disease, stroke and fatal stroke were 17.7% (sensitivity 80%, specificity 79%, Youden 0.592); 8,4% (sensitivity 90%, specificity 69%, Youden 0.587), 7.7% (sensitivity 83%, specificity 79%, Youden 0.616) and 1.1% (sensitivity 84, specificity 77%, Youden 0.603) respectively. When we analyze the population by sex, the OCP values were higher in men in comparison with women (SFCV: 31.0% vs. 15.9%; SFCD: 27% vs. 15.0%; NS: 22.4% vs. 11.8%; UKPDS score for coronary disease: 23.5% vs. 12.0%, UKPDS score for fatal coronary disease 13.1% vs. 7.1%; UKPDS score for stroke: 12.5% vs. 7.3% and UKPDS score for fatal stroke: 1.7% vs. 0.7%).

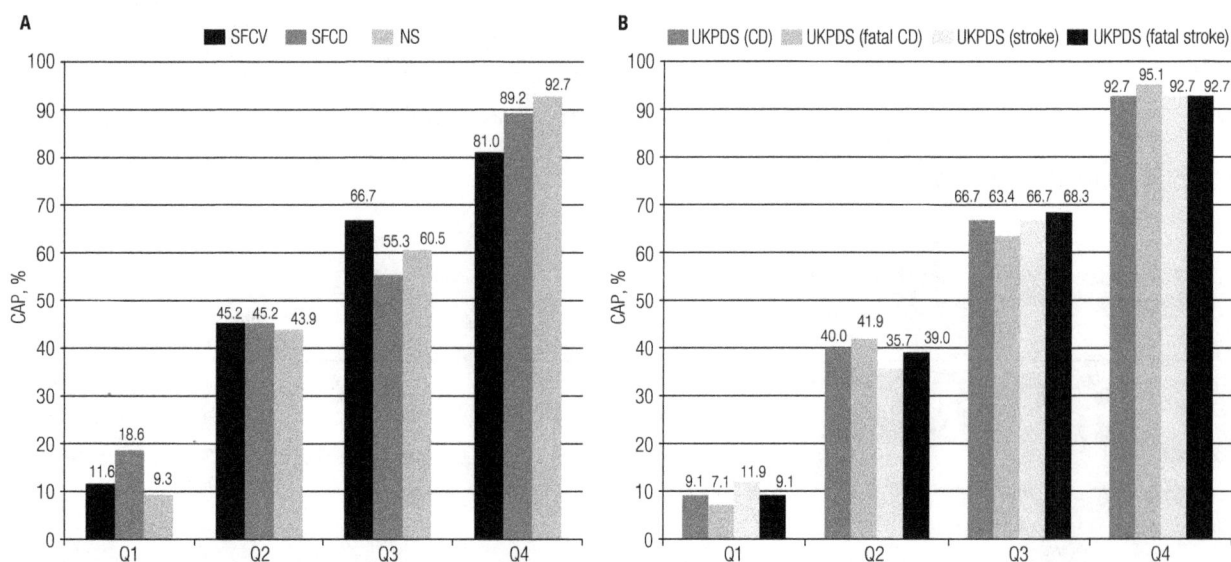

CAP: carotid atherosclerotic plaque; FSCV: Framingham score for cardiovascular disease; FSCD: Framingham score for coronary disease; CD: coronary disease; NS: new score of the 2013 ACC/AHA Guideline; UKPDS: United Kingdom Prospective Diabetes Study; Q: Quartile.

Figure 2. Prevalence of CAP according to different risk scores quartiles. (**A**) FSCV, FSCD and NS. (**B**) UKPDS scores.

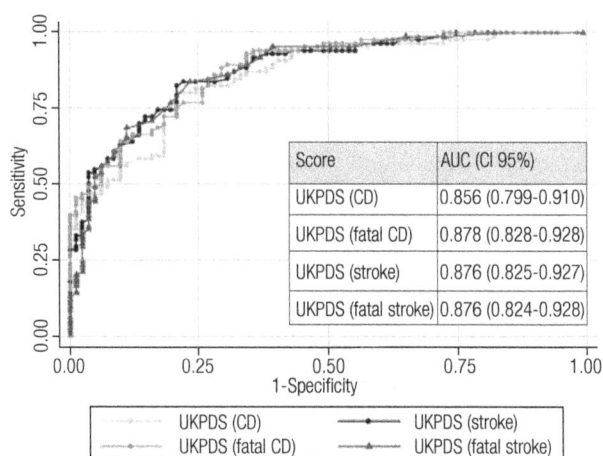

Score	AUC (CI 95%)
UKPDS (CD)	0.856 (0.799-0.910)
UKPDS (fatal CD)	0.878 (0.828-0.928)
UKPDS (stroke)	0.876 (0.825-0.927)
UKPDS (fatal stroke)	0.876 (0.824-0.928)

---- UKPDS (CD)	—•— UKPDS (stroke)
—•— UKPDS (fatal CD)	—▲— UKPDS (fatal stroke)

AUC: area under the curve; CI: interval confidence; CD: coronary disease;
UKPDS: United Kingdom Prospective Diabetes Study.

Figure 3. Discrimination capacity of the UKPDS scores between subjects with or without carotid atherosclerotic plaque (ROC analysis).

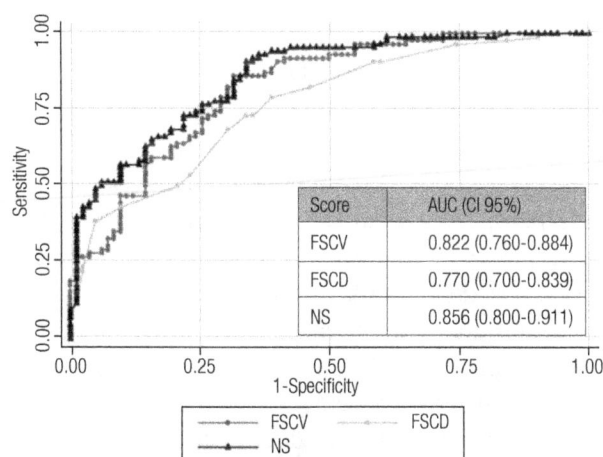

Score	AUC (CI 95%)
FSCV	0.822 (0.760-0.884)
FSCD	0.770 (0.700-0.839)
NS	0.856 (0.800-0.911)

—•— FSCV	----- FSCD
—▲— NS	

AUC: area under the curve; CI: interval confidence; FSCV: Framingham score for cardiovascular disease; FSCD: Framingham score for coronary disease; NS: new score of the 2013 ACC/AHA Guideline.

Figure 4. Discrimination capacity of the FSCV, FSCD and NS between subjects with or without carotid atherosclerotic plaque (ROC analysis).

DISCUSSION

The identification of patients at risk of developing cardiovascular events is one of the most challenging issues in clinical practice. Different risk assessment tools have been proposed to estimate the risk of future events. Although, the Framingham and UKPDS scores are the most frequently used. Recently, a new score has been proposed by the latest ACC/AHA Guideline on the Treatment of Blood Cholesterol. In our study, we compared these predictive scores in a group of patients with diabetes without a history of cardiovascular disease, including the NS, and then we analyzed its relationship with the presence of CAP.

According to what is seen in our results, the estimation of coronary risk at 10 years by using the FSCD and UKPDS score for coronary events is close to the theoretical 20% accepted as "coronary equivalent". Moreover, when scores that predict combined cardiovascular events (FSCV or NS) are used, cardiovascular risk clearly exceeded this threshold. Additionally, stroke risk calculated by the UKPDS score was considerably (14.2%). Our findings were similar to the results of a study conducted in Spain. Using the UKPDS score, the authors found that the risk of coronary events and stroke was 23% and 12% respectively (21).

Although different endpoints were evaluated by each score, the Kernel density distribution on the FSCV, FSCD, NS and UKPDS for coronary events showed similar distributions. This finding is probably related with the good correlation found between different risks estimations. Similarly, a Spanish study showed a significant correlation between the REGICOR equation and UKPDS score in a group of subject with diabetes (22). However, in our study the agreement between the different scores was moderate. Diabetes patients were not classified into the same risk score categories. Therefore, we could not classified into the same categories all diabetes patients using different risk scores.

The prevalence of CAP in our study was 51%. This finding was consistent with previous reports. For example, Ahn and cols. reported a prevalence of 47% in subjects with diabetes in Korea (23) and Catalan and cols. showed a high CAP prevalence (60%) in new-onset diabetes subjects (24). Furthermore, in a group of patients with diabetes but with high cholesterol levels, the prevalence of CAP was even higher (69%) (25).

As expected, patients with CAP had worse clinical risk factors and higher values of all scores than subject without CAP. Our working group had already reported these findings in a cohort that did not include individuals with cardiovascular disease neither people with diabetes (18). Cardoso and cols. showed that in patients with diabetes, older age, male sex, smoking status and the results of ambulatory blood pressure monitoring were the main independent predictors of ultrasonographic carotid atherosclerosis (26).

In our study, the prevalence of CAP was higher in men than in women. This finding could be explained in part by the presence of a worse lipid profile and a higher prevalence of smoking and family history of coronary disease in men.

The prevalence of CAP was elevated in the highest quartiles of all the risk scores. Similarly, in the previously mentioned study, Hong and cols. reported that the prevalence and the number of carotid artery plaques were significantly higher in the high-risk group according to UKPDS risk stratification (25). However, we found that in the lowest quartile of all the scores the prevalence of CAP was between 9 to 19%. Then, a low score does not exclude the possibility of diagnose asymptomatic carotid atherosclerosis. This topic is relevant, especially in women, because the estimated cardiovascular risk for all scores was significantly lower than in men, even analyzing only the population with CAP.

In our investigation, all scores predict CAP with very good accuracy (area under the ROC curves above 0.75). Similarly, a study made in Japan showed area under the ROC curves of 0.76 and 0.79 for FSCV and UKPDS score respectively, for predicting coronary artery stenosis assessment with computed angiography (27).

Applying the NS, only one patient with a score value < 7.5% had CAP. Taking into account these findings, it seems that the recommendation proposed by the 2013 ACC/AHA Guideline on the Treatment of Blood Cholesterol regarding the indication of moderate or intensive doses of statins according to the risk level are appropriate. However, in our study the OCP of NS for the detection of CAP was 14.3%. This cutoff is about twice the one proposed by the NS to stratify patients with diabetes in the highest-risk category and to indicate intensive treatment with statins. This discrepancy might suggest that the cutoff point proposed by the NS in patients with DBT is too low and that the inclusion of the diagnosis of diabetes in the equation probably could increase excessively the impact of the disease on the estimation of risk of events. Something very similar happens in these guides, with the very strong dependence of ageing in the calculation of cardiovascular risk at 10 years. We consider that the equation used by the ACC/AHA Guideline does not capture the heterogeneity of risk present in diabetic patients and the detection of subclinical atherosclerosis could probably improve this limitation.

All other functions evaluated for coronary o cardiovascular events, the OCP was close or over 20%, threshold chosen to classify patients as high risk.

Finally, the OCP values were higher in men compared to women. These findings would suggest that the clinical applicability of the scores would be different in men and women, such as occurs in people without diabetes. However, the low number of individuals analyzed in each group, limiting the conclusions.

This study is associated with several limitations. First, it was cross-sectional with a small number of patients. Second, all participants were enrolled in cardiovascular prevention outpatient clinics of cardiology centers which may have introduced selection bias. Third, in our study, CAP was defined according to the Atherosclerosis Risk in Communities study criteria. Changing the definition of CAP could modify our results. Fourth, the low prevalence of atrial fibrillation in this population may have underestimation the risk of stroke. Finally, this study was not intended to determine whether risk classification was correct. A prospective study should be developed to confirm our findings.

Despite its limitations, our study represents a valuable contribution because we examined patients with diabetes from Argentina, whereas previous reports were limited to other regions of the world.

Several guidelines classify patients with diabetes as high or very high risk regardless of atheroma burden (5,13,28,29). Consequently, the evaluation of atherosclerotic burden by non-invasive imaging has not been definitely incorporated in clinical practice. However, some authors consider that carotid intima-media thickness is a useful marker of the progression of atherosclerosis and is an excellent predictor of cardiovascular events (30). Also, the Brazilian Diabetes Society recommended that patients with diabetes and without a history of cardiovascular disease should be stratified annually by the UKPDS risk-calculator (31). Additionally, through this tool, patients can be distributed between low risk (< 10% in 10 years), intermediate risk (10-20% in 10 years) and high risk (> 20% in 10 years). Furthermore, these recommendations suggest that coronary calcium score should be performed in patients with intermediate risk in order to reclassify their risk. In this context, the search CAP could be suitable for the same purpose, in situations that the computed tomography method is not available.

In conclusion, on average, the cardiovascular risk was elevated for all the scores that were evaluated. However, risk stratification was heterogenic. The prevalence of CAP increased significantly in the higher strata of estimated risk. Understanding the relationship between presence of CAP and scores could improve the estimation of risk in our patients with diabetes.

REFERENCES

1. Seshasai SR, Kaptoge S, Thompson A, Di Angelantonio E, Gao P, Sarwar N, et al. Diabetes mellitus, fasting glucose, and risk of cause-specific death. N Engl J Med. 2011;364:829-41.

2. Haffner SM, Lehto S, Rönnemaa T, Pyörälä K, Laakso M. Mortality from coronary heart disease in subjects with type 2 diabetes and in nondiabetic subjects with and without prior myocardial infarction. N Engl J Med. 1998;339:229-34.

3. Malmberg K, Yusuf S, Gerstein HC, Brown J, Zhao F, Hunt D, et al. Impact of diabetes on long-term prognosis in patients with unstable angina and non-Q-wave myocardial infarction: results of the OASIS (Organization to Assess Strategies for Ischemic Syndromes) Registry. Circulation. 2000;102:1014-9.

4. Juutilainen A, Lehto S, Rönnemaa T, Pyörälä K, Laakso M. Type 2 diabetes as a "coronary heart disease equivalent": an 18-year prospective population-based study in Finnish subjects. Diabetes Care. 2005;28:2901-7.

5. Expert Panel on Detection, Evaluation, and Treatment of High Blood Cholesterol in Adults. Executive Summary of The Third Report of The National Cholesterol Education Program (NCEP) Expert Panel on Detection, Evaluation, And Treatment of High Blood Cholesterol In Adults (Adult Treatment Panel III). JAMA. 2001;285:2486-97.

6. Evans JM, Wang J, Morris AD. Comparison of cardiovascular risk between patients with type 2 diabetes and those who had had a myocardial infarction: cross sectional and cohort studies. BMJ. 2002;324:939-42.

7. Lee CD, Folsom AR, Pankow JS, Brancati FL. Cardiovascular events in diabetic and nondiabetic adults with or without history of myocardial infarction. Circulation. 2004;109:855-60.

8. Bulugahapitiya U, Siyambalapitiya S, Sithole J, Idris I. Is diabetes a coronary risk equivalent? Systematic review and meta-analysis. Diabet Med. 2009;26:142-8.

9. Wilson PWF, D'Agostino RB, Levy D, Belanger A, Silbershatz H, Kannel WB. Prediction of coronary heart disease using risk factor categories. Circulation. 1998;97:1837-47.

10. Conroy RM, Pyorala K, Fitzgerald AP, Sans S, Menotti A, De Backer G, et al. Estimation of ten-year risk of fatal cardiovascular disease in Europe: the SCORE project. Eur Heart J. 2003;24:987-1003.

11. Hippisley-Cox J, Coupland C, Vinogradova Y, Robson J, May M, Brindle P. Derivation and validation of QRISK, a new cardiovascular disease risk score for the United Kingdom: prospective open cohort study. BMJ. 2007;335:136-41.

12. Stevens RJ, Kothari V, Adler AI, Stratton IM. The UKPDS risk engine: a model for the risk of coronary heart disease in Type II diabetes (UKPDS 56). Clin Sci (Lond). 2001;101:671-9.

13. Perk J, De Backer G, Gohlke H, Graham I, Reiner Z, Verschuren M, et al. European Guidelines on cardiovascular disease prevention in clinical practice (version 2012). The Fifth Joint Task Force of the European Society of Cardiology and Other Societies on Cardiovascular Disease Prevention in Clinical Practice (constituted by representatives of nine societies and by invited experts). Eur Heart J. 2012;33:1635-701.

14. Stone NJ, Robinson JG, Lichtenstein AH, Bairey Merz CN, Blum CB, Eckel RH, et al. 2013 ACC/AHA guideline on the treatment of blood cholesterol to reduce atherosclerotic cardiovascular risk in adults: a report of the American College of Cardiology/American Heart Association Task Force on Practice Guidelines. J Am Coll Cardiol. 2014;63:2889-934.

15. Nambi V, Chambless L, Folsom AR, He M, Hu Y, Mosley T, et al. Carotid intima-media thickness and presence or absence of plaque improves prediction of coronary heart disease risk: the ARIC (Atherosclerosis Risk In Communities) study. J Am Coll Cardiol. 2010;55:1600-7.

16. Bernard S, Sérusclat A, Targe F, Charrière S, Roth O, Beaune J, et al. Incremental predictive value of carotid ultrasonography in the assessment of coronary risk in a cohort of asymptomatic type 2 diabetic subjects. Diabetes Care. 2005;28:1158-62.

17. Irie Y, Katakami N, Kaneto H, Kasami R, Sumitsuji S, Yamasaki K et al. Maximum carotid intima-media thickness improves the prediction ability of coronary artery stenosis in type 2 diabetic patients without history of coronary artery disease. Atherosclerosis. 2012;221:438-44.

18. Masson W, Lobo M, Huerín M, Molinero G, Manente D, Pángaro M, et al. Estratificación del riesgo cardiovascular con diferentes puntajes de riesgo en prevención primaria y sus implicaciones en la indicación de estatinas. Rev Argent Cardiol. 2014;82:473-5.

19. D'Agostino RB, Vasan RS, Pencina MJ, Wolf PA, Cobain M, Massaro JM, et al. General cardiovascular risk profile for use in primary care: the Framingham Heart Study. Circulation. 2008;117:743-53.

20. The Oxford Centre for Diabetes, Endocrinology and Metabolism, UKPDS Risk Engine. Oxford: Isis Innovation Ltd; [cited 2009 Apr 10]. Available at: http://www.dtu.ox.ac.uk/riskengine/download.php.

21. Lahoz-Rallo B, Blanco-Gonzalez M, Casas-Ciria I, Marín-Andrade JA, Mendez-Segovia JC, Guillermo Moratalla-Rodriguez G, et al. Cardiovascular disease risk in subjects with type 2 diabetes mellitus in a population in southern Spain. Diabetes Res Clin Pract. 2007;76:436-44.

22. Hernáez R, Choque L, Giménez M, Costa A, Márquez JI, Conget I. Coronary risk assessment in subjects with type 2 diabetes mellitus. General population-based scores or specific scores?. Rev Esp Cardiol. 2004;57:577-80.

23. Ahn HR, Shin MH, Yun WJ, Kim HY, Lee YH, Kweon SS, et al. Comparison of the Framingham risk score, UKPDS risk engine, and SCORE for predicting carotid atherosclerosis and peripheral arterial disease in Korean type 2 diabetic patients. Korean J Fam Med. 2011;32:189-96.

24. Catalan M, Herreras Z, Pinyol M, Sala-Vila A, Amor AJ, de Groot E, et al. Prevalence by sex of preclinical carotid atherosclerosis in newly diagnosed type 2 diabetes. Nutr Metab Cardiovasc Dis. 2015;25:742-8.

25. Hong EG, Ohn JH, Lee SJ, Kwon HS, Kim SG, Kim DJ, et al. Clinical implications of carotid artery intima media thickness assessment on cardiovascular risk stratification in hyperlipidemic Korean adults with diabetes: the ALTO study. BMC. Cardiovasc Disord. 2015;15:114.

26. Cardoso CR, Marques CE, Leite NC, Salles GF. Factors associated with carotid intima-media thickness and carotid plaques in type 2 diabetic patients. J Hypertens. 2012;30:940-7.

27. Fujihara K, Suzuki H, Sato A, Ishizu T, Kodama S, Heianza Y, et al. Comparison of the Framingham risk score, UK Prospective Diabetes Study (UKPDS) Risk Engine, Japanese Atherosclerosis Longitudinal Study-Existing Cohorts Combine (JALS-ECC) and maximum carotid intima-media thickness for predicting coronary artery stenosis in patients with asymptomatic type 2 diabetes. J Atheroscle Thromb. 2014;21:799-815.

28. Standards of medical care in diabetes-2016: Summary of revisions. Diabetes Care. 2016;39 Suppl 1:S4-5.

29. Sociedad Argentina de Cardiología. Área de Normatizaciones y Consensos. Consenso de prevención cardiovascular. Rev Argent Cardiol. 2012;80(Supl 2):1-127.

30. Katakami N, Kaneto H, Shimomura I. Carotid ultrasonography: a potent tool for better clinical practice in diagnosis of atherosclerosis in diabetic patients. J Diabetes Investig. 2014;5:3-13.

31. Bertoluci MC, Pimazoni-Netto A, Pires AC, Pesaro AE, Schaan BD, Caramelli B, et al. Diabetes and cardiovascular disease: from evidence to clinical practice – position statement 2014 of Brazilian Diabetes Society. Diabetol Metab Syndr. 2014;6:58.

26

Leptin as a predictor of metabolic syndrome in prepubertal children

Isabel Madeira[1], Maria Alice Bordallo[2], Nádia Cristina Rodrigues[3], Cecilia Carvalho[4], Fernanda Gazolla[5], Paulo Collett-Solberg[2], Clarice Medeiros[5], Ana Paula Bordallo[5], Marcos Borges[5], Claudia Monteiro[5], Rebeca Ribeiro[6]

[1] Faculdade de Ciências Médicas, Departamento de Pediatria, Universidade do Estado do Rio de Janeiro (UERJ), Rio de Janeiro, RJ, Brasil
[2] Faculdade de Ciências Médicas, Departamento de Medicina Interna, UERJ, Rio de Janeiro, RJ, Brasil
[3] Faculdade de Ciências Médicas, Departamento de Tecnologias da Informação e Educação em Saúde, UERJ, Rio de Janeiro, RJ, Brasil
[4] Instituto de Nutrição, Departamento de Nutrição Aplicada, UERJ, Rio de Janeiro, RJ, Brasil
[5] Hospital Universitário Pedro Ernesto, Unidade Docente Assistencial de Endocrinologia e Metabologia, UERJ, Rio de Janeiro, RJ, Brasil
[6] Faculdade de Ciências Médicas, UERJ, Rio de Janeiro, RJ, Brasil

Correspondence to:
Isabel Madeira
Av. 28 de Setembro, 77
20551-030 – Rio de Janeiro, RJ, Brasil
isamadeira@oi.com.br

ABSTRACT

Objective: Leptin has been suggested as a potential biomarker of cardiovascular risk. This paper aims to ascertain, based on a sample of prepubertal children, which serum leptin value best suited to identify metabolic syndrome (MS). **Subjects and methods:** This observational, cross-sectional study recruited children from the outpatient pediatrics clinic, with the purpose of validating serum leptin level cutoffs to identify MS. All obese and overweight children who met eligibility criteria were included in the study, as was a sample of normal-weight children. The sample underwent clinical assessment and blood fasting glucose, lipid profile, insulin, and leptin were measured. Sensitivity and specificity were estimated for each leptin measurement, using MS as the outcome. These values were used to construct a receiver operating characteristic (ROC) curve. The association between MS and leptin was assessed using logistic models to predict MS. **Results:** A total of 65 normal weight, 46 overweight, and 164 obese children were analyzed (160 boys, 115 girls; age: 93.7 ± 17.8 months). The most appropriate leptin cutoff was 13.4 ng/mL (sensitivity 67.6%; specificity 68.9%; accuracy 72.1%). The logistic model indicated that leptin levels above 13.4 ng/dL were significantly associated with MS and that, for every 1 ng/dL increase in leptin levels, the odds of MS increase by 3% ($p = 0.002$; OR 1.03; 95% CI 1.01-1.05). **Conclusions:** Leptin may be a useful biomarker of cardiovascular risk in prepubertal children, with an optimal cutoff of 13.4 ng/mL. Identification of potential new risk markers for cardiovascular disease in children could contribute to the development of preventive strategies.
Arch Endocrinol Metab. 2017;61(1):7-13

Keywords
Children; ROC curve; leptin; obesity; insulin resistance

INTRODUCTION

Obesity is currently a highly prevalent condition, including in Brazil (1,2). The most significant complication of obesity, atherosclerotic cardiovascular disease, now constitutes the leading cause of death in adults in the western world. The main risk factors for cardiovascular disease are obesity, hypertension, dyslipidemia, and type 2 diabetes mellitus (T2DM), which together compose the so-called metabolic syndrome (MS). In this syndrome, insulin resistance and hyperinsulinemia would explain the core role of obesity and its association with the other abnormal phenomena observed. The effects of these factors appear to begin in childhood (3).

The pathophysiology of obesity involves an imbalance between energy intake and energy expenditure. Several neuroendocrine factors have been implicated in this energy imbalance, such as adipocytokines, proteins produced by adipose tissue. One of the most important adipocytokines is leptin.

This hormone signals, through central pathways, a decrease in food intake and increase in energy expenditure, in addition to having peripheral actions. In muscle, leptin stimulates fatty acid oxidation by activating adenosine monophosphate kinase. It also removes lipids from non-adipose tissue, preventing lipotoxicity, possibly due to its ability to block stearoyl-coenzyme A desaturase, and inhibits hepatic triglyceride buildup by activating phosphatidylinositol 3-kinase (4).

Circulating leptin levels correlate with body adiposity in adults and children (5), and the high leptin levels found in obese individuals are believed to indicate leptin resistance (6). Furthermore, studies in children have shown that high leptin levels correlate with greater fat mass growth over time (7). Although most obese children have high leptin levels, mutations in the leptin receptors are rare. This adipokine is believed to cross the blood–brain barrier by means of a saturable transport system, which would limit its uptake by central receptors (6).

Other aspects related to leptin have been assessed in the pathophysiology of obesity. Leptin may contribute to insulin resistance and its metabolic correlates and appears to have a direct pro-thrombotic effect, in addition to acting synergistically with insulin and free fatty acids to stimulate sympathetic activity and vasoconstriction (8). Hence, leptin and insulin interact to modulate vascular function, and this interaction may have major implications in the vascular dysfunction of MS.

In the pediatric age range, obesity appears to be an important trigger of insulin resistance (3), which makes obese children a high-risk group and has led investigators to search for clinical and laboratory indicators in this population. Nevertheless, there is no consensus definition of MS in children. A review on the topic found 40 different definitions adapted from those proposed for adults (9). In 2007, the International Diabetes Federation (IDF) proposed the latest definition of MS for children over the age of 10 years, based on the presence of increased waist circumference plus two of the following elements: hypertriglyceridemia; low HDL cholesterol; hypertension; and impaired fasting glucose or T2DM (10). A systematic review on MS in children found 26 studies adopting this definition (11).

In a recently published study, our group demonstrated that leptin is positively associated with insulin resistance in prepubertal children after adjusting for sex, age, and body mass index (BMI) Z-score (12). Other authors reported similar results in children (13,14), suggesting a role of leptin as a potential modulator of glucose metabolism and insulin resistance, regardless of obesity. These studies highlight the importance of leptin as a cardiovascular risk marker in this age group.

Identification of potential new risk markers for cardiovascular disease in children could contribute to the development of early intervention strategies, particularly preventive ones. However, no published studies have proposed serum leptin level cutoffs for the pediatric population.

Within this context, the objectives of this study are to ascertain, within a case series of prepubertal children with normal and excess weight, which serum leptin value best suited to identify MS, and to evaluate the association between leptin and MS.

SUBJECTS AND METHODS

This observational, cross-sectional study recruited children from the outpatient general pediatrics clinic of Hospital Universitário Pedro Ernesto da Universidade do Estado do Rio de Janeiro (HUPE-UERJ), a teaching hospital in Rio de Janeiro, Brazil, with the purpose of validating serum leptin level cutoffs to identify MS. All children aged 5–11 years who were prepubertal, overweight or obese, otherwise healthy, and were not taking part in any weight loss program were invited to take part in the study. All eligible children who met these criteria were included. Normal-weight, healthy, prepubertal children, matched by age, from the same Pediatric well-child care clinic were recruited as controls, selected in a first-come first-serve order from May 2008 to December 2011. Study sample size, 275 children, was considered sufficient to achieve statistical power of 80%, with a level of significance set at 5%, for an error of 5%, based on the total population of children seen at the clinic (15).

The children recruited for the study underwent a complete clinical assessment. Weight was measured with the participants barefoot and wearing minimal clothing, on a Filizola scale (Filizola, São Paulo, SP, Brazil) with a resolution of 100 g. Height was measured with a Harpenden-type wall-mounted stadiometer (Tonelli, Criciúma, SC, Brazil) with a resolution of 1 mm. Waist circumference was measured at just above the uppermost lateral border of the right ilium, at the end of a normal expiration, as recommended in the Third National Health and Nutrition Examination Survey (NHANES III) Anthropometry Procedures Manual (16), using a Mabbis® Gulick-type tape measure (Cardiomed, Curitiba, PR, Brazil).

Blood pressure was measured in the right arm using the auscultatory method, with each participant in the sitting position and at rest, using a Tycos® aneroid sphygmomanometer (Welch Allyn Company, Arden, DE, USA) with cuffs of appropriate size.

Blood was collected for laboratory testing after a 12-hour fast. Glucose, total cholesterol, HDL cholesterol, and triglycerides were measured in a Konelab analyzer with the BT 3000 Winer kit, which employs the following assay methods: for glucose, the GOD-PAP (oxidase) enzymatic method; for cholesterol, the CHOP-POD (esterase/oxidase) enzymatic method; for triglycerides, the GPO-PAP (oxidase) enzymatic method; and for HDL cholesterol, the enzymatic colorimetric method (Winterlab, Rosario, Santa Fe, Argentina).

Insulin was measured in a Gamma-C12 counter using the Coat-A-Count solid-phase ^{125}I-labeled radioimmunoassay (DPC, Los Angeles, CA, USA). The intra-assay and inter-assay coefficients of variation were 3.1–9.3% and 4.9–10.0% respectively.

Leptin was also measured in the Gamma-C12 counter, using the double antibody PEG radioimmunoassay method, with a kit that uses ^{125}I-labeled human leptin and human leptin antiserum (Linco Research, St. Charles, MO, USA). The intra-assay and inter-assay coefficients of variation were 3.4–8.3% and 3.0–6.2% respectively.

The HOMA-IR score was calculated by multiplying the fasting blood glucose (in mmol/L) by the fasting insulin level (in μIU/mL) and dividing the product by 22.5, as noted elsewhere (17).

Obesity, overweight, and normal weight were defined using the BMI for sex and age standards proposed by the World Health Organization (WHO). The criteria are as follows: a body mass index (BMI) Z-score greater than +2 denotes obesity; greater than +1 and less than or equal to +2, overweight; and greater than or equal to -2 and less than or equal to +1, normal weight (18).

The definition of MS was adapted from the IDF proposal for children over the age of 10 years (10), and waist circumference was defined as increased when the measurement was within or above the 90th percentile for sex and age in the NHANES III table that combines children of African-American, European-American, and Mexican-American ethnicity (16). Hypertension was defined according to the criteria recommended in the 1st

Brazilian Guideline on the Prevention of Atherosclerosis in Childhood and Adolescence (19). The cutoff points adopted for fasting blood glucose, HDL cholesterol, and triglycerides were those recommended by the same guideline: impaired fasting glucose, values ≥ 5.6 mmol/L (100 mg/dL); low HDL cholesterol, values < 1.16 nmol/L (45 mg/dL); and increased triglycerides, values ≥ 1.46 mmol/L (130 mg/dL) (19).

The collected data were entered into Excel 7 spreadsheets (MapInfo Corporation, Troy, NY, USA) and analyzed in R-Project 3.0.1 (Free Software Foundation, Boston, MA, USA).

Simple and multivariate logistic models, the latter adjusted for sex and age and both having serum leptin levels as the main predictor, were used to predict MS. The results obtained were used to construct two receiver operator characteristic (ROC) curves.

The present study was approved by the HUPE-UERJ Research Ethics Committee with protocol no. 173-CEP/HUPE–CAAE; 0020.0.228.000-07. It is also registered with the Brazilian National Research Ethics Commission under number 127374.

RESULTS

Table 1 describes the clinical and metabolic profile of study participants stratified by nutritional status is provided. A comparison between the MS and no MS groups is shown in Table 2.

Table 1. Profile of study participants stratified by nutritional status

Parameter	Obese children	Overweight children	Normal weight children	P-value
Participants, n (%)	164 (59.6)	46 (16.7)	65 (23.6)	
Age in months	94.68 ± 17.70	92.93 ± 18.68	91.85 ± 17.51	0.52
Sex				
Male	104 (63.4)	21 (45.7)	35 (53.8)	0.07
Female	60 (36.6)	25 (54.3)	30 (46.2)	
Metabolic syndrome	33 (97.1)	1 (2.9)	0 (0)	0.00001
Total cholesterol in mg/dL[‡]	166.43 ± 30.78	166.22 ± 30.36	153.52 ± 33.75	0.02
HDL cholesterol in mg/dL[§]	41.90 ± 9.00	52.48 ± 12.89	49.15 ± 11.70	0.00001
LDL cholesterol in mg/dL[‡]	103.90 ± 28.67	98.22 ± 30.64	89.82 ± 30.17	0.001
Triglycerides in mg/dL[§]	102.96 ± 55.35	77.96 ± 30.08	72.86 ± 28.40	0.00001
HOMA-IR[†]	2.15 ± 1.83	1.67 ± 1.02	0.78 ± 0.67	0.00001
Glucose in mg/dL	86.64 ± 8.72	86.78 ± 7.52	84.45 ± 7.21	0.16
Leptin in ng/mL[*]	18.6 ± 14.47	9.64 ± 9.05	3.29 ± 2.83	0.00001

Data expressed as absolute and relative frequencies (%) or mean ± standard deviation. Tukey test: [*] showed significant difference between all categories (obese, overweight, and normal weight children); [†] showed significant difference between obese and normal weight children and between overweight and normal weight children; [‡] showed significant difference between obese and normal weight children; [§] showed significant difference between obese and normal weight children and between obese and overweight children.

Table 2. Profile of study participants stratified by metabolic syndrome status

Parameter	Metabolic syndrome	No metabolic syndrome	P-value
Participants, n (%)	34 (12.4)	241 (87.6)	
Age in months	103.17 ± 18.6	92.4 ± 17.3	0.0009
Sex			
Male	23 (67.6)	137 (56.8)	0.23
Female	11 (32.4)	104 (43.2)	
BMI z-score[a]	3.54 ± 1.19	1.96 ± 1.77	0.00001
Total cholesterol in mg/dL	175.6 ± 25.1	161.6 ± 32.3	0.02
HDL cholesterol in mg/dL	36.8 ± 4.6	46.6 ± 11.4	0.00001
LDL cholesterol in mg/dL	103.6 ± 24.7	99.1 ± 30.5	0.41
Triglycerides in mg/dL	176.5 ± 62.4	79.7 ± 31.4	0.00001
HOMA-IR	3.3 ± 2.7	1.5 ± 1.2	0.00001
Glucose in mg/dL	88.76 ± 7.89	85.78 ± 8.21	0.046
Leptin in ng/mL	21.2 ± 11.3	12.4 ± 13.5	0.0004

Data expressed as absolute and relative frequencies (%) or mean ± standard deviation.
[a] Z-score for body mass index.

Waist circumference was above the 90th percentile for age in 135 (49.1%) children. Hypertension was detected in 4 (1.45%) children, for a prevalence of 8.82% (n = 3) in the MS group *versus* 0.41% (n = 1) in the no MS group. Impaired fasting glucose was observed in 4 (1.45%) children, all of whom were obese, for a prevalence of 2.94% (n = 3) in the MS group *versus* 1.24% (n = 1) in the no MS group.

Figure 1 shows two ROC curves plotted from the sensitivity and specificity values found for each leptin level measured in the study sample, with MS as the outcome. Curve A represents the simple logistic model for prediction of MS. In this model, a leptin value of 12.3 ng/mL (85% sensibility; 64% specificity) corresponded to the shoulder of the curve and had the best Youden's index. Curve B represents the multiple logistic model, adjusted for sex and age. In this model, a leptin value of 13.4 ng/mL (68% sensibility; 69% specificity) corresponded to the shoulder of the curve and had the best Youden's index.

In the multiple logistic model for prediction of MS, adjusted for sex and age, a leptin level above 13.4 ng/dL was significantly associated with MS (p = 0.002). Figure 2 shows the odds for MS for each leptin value, according to simple and multiple logistic models.

DISCUSSION

The study sample was a very young group of children, and the substantial prevalence of metabolic syndrome according to the adapted IDF criteria is a concerning finding. We decided to use these criteria because they are currently the only standard for diagnosis of the syndrome in children and are recommended by authors who advocate that the use of unified criteria would contribute to the development of studies on the

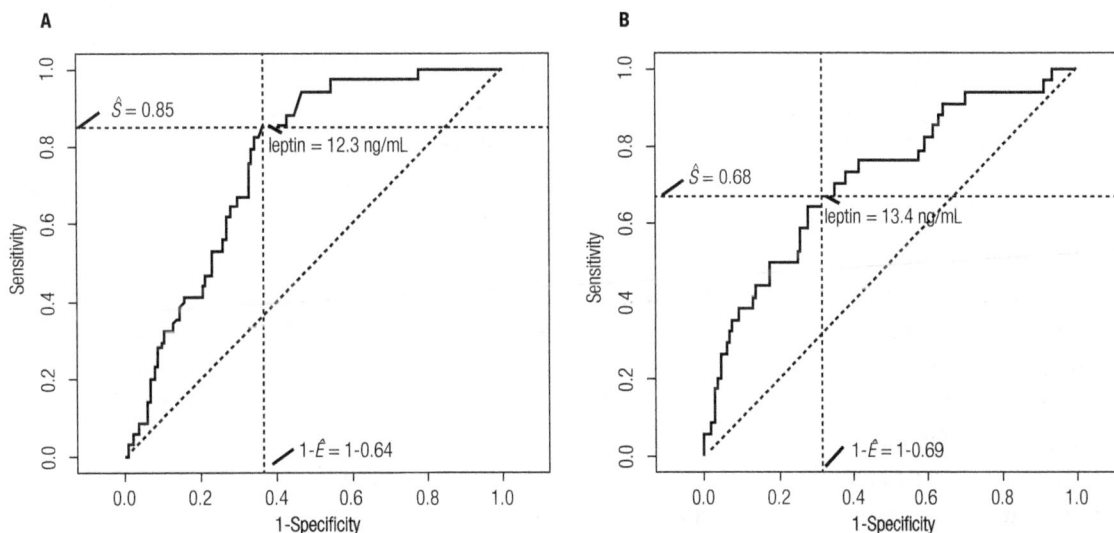

Figure 1. ROC curves of logistic regression prediction models for metabolic syndrome (response variable) in relation to the main predictor (leptin level), based on observations of prepubertal children. (**A**) Crude model: best cutoff point, 12.3 ng/mL; area under the curve, 76.4%; Youden's index, 48.8%. (**B**) Model adjusted for sex and age: best cutoff point, 13.4 ng/mL; area under the curve, 72.1%; Youden's index, 36.5%. On both charts, the best cutoff is denoted by the intersection of the dotted lines. The area under the curve represents the overall accuracy of the test.

A

B

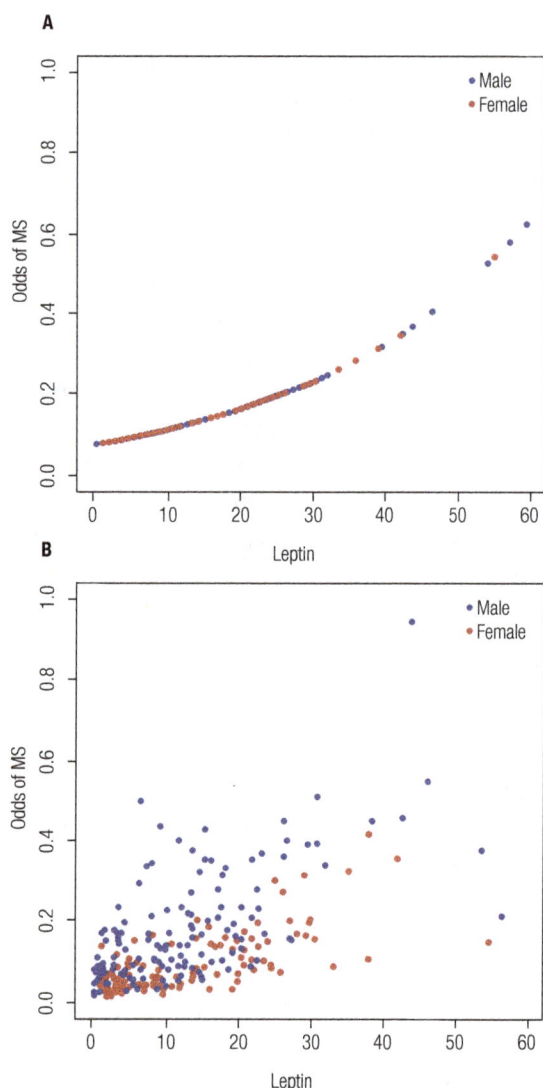

Figure 2. Odds of metabolic syndrome stratified by leptin levels (ng/mL). **(A)** Crude logistic model: odds ratio (95%CI) = 1.04 (1.01-1.06); p < 0.002; equation for the odds of metabolic syndrome = exp (- 2.51 + 0.03 * leptin). **(B)** Model adjusted for sex and age: odds ratio (95%CI) = 1.03 (1.01-1.06); p < 0.002; equation for the odds of metabolic syndrome = exp (-5.19 + 0.03 * leptin – 0,32 * sex + 0.03 * age in months).

topic (11,20). However, in view of the lack of scientific evidence for this classification in under-10 children, these criteria should only be used in clinical practice in patients who are aged 10 years or older (10).

Despite the lack of a consensus definition for MS in children and the fact that the syndrome is not a disease in itself, but rather a constellation of risk factors for cardiovascular disease, its presence in children has been reported and investigated. According to a recent systematic review, the prevalence of MS is nearly 3.3% in the whole pediatric population, 11.9% in the overweight pediatric population, and 29.2% in the obese pediatric

population (11). Longitudinal studies have shown that children with MS components grow into adults with MS, and that adolescents with the syndrome are at greater risk of premature cardiovascular disease in adulthood (21). This evidence justifies the search for new biomarkers of cardiovascular risk in children with excess weight, so as to identify those at the greatest risk, understanding the concept of biomarker as an indicator of pathogenic process (22).

Leptin is one such potential biomarker (23). In children, as in adults, its circulating levels correlate strongly with body fat (5,22), and high leptin levels are associated with greater fat mass growth over time (7) and with difficulty losing weight (24).

In a previous study conducted in the same population of the present study, leptin levels were positively associated with insulin resistance after adjusting for sex, age, and BMI Z-score (12).

Other authors reported similar results in studies of prepubertal children with normal and excess weight (13,14), suggesting a role of leptin as a potential modulator of glucose metabolism and insulin resistance, regardless of obesity.

Knowledge of the role of leptin within this panorama has grown to a point where some authors regard it as a programming factor for future development of obesity and its correlates, possibly via epigenetic mechanisms (25).

Within this perspective, the present study ascertained that, in a sample of prepubertal children with normal and excess weight, a circulating leptin level of 13.4 ng/mL was the optimal cutoff point to identify MS. The sensitivity and specificity of this cutoff were 68% and 69% respectively, which means that its use in prepubertal children will lead to a correct diagnosis of MS in approximately two-thirds of cases and correctly rule out the syndrome in just over two-thirds of children who do not have it.

Use of this cutoff revealed an association between leptin and MS after adjusting for sex and age. The adjusted logistic model showed that, for every 1-ng/dL increase in leptin levels, the odds of MS increase by 3% (p < 0.002).

This association has been described before by other authors, including González and cols., who recruited a randomized sample of 12-to-17-year-olds (26). Papoutsakis and cols., using the IDF definition of MS in a cohort of 1,138 healthy subjects (normal-weight, overweight, and obese) with a mean age of 11.2 years, demonstrated that leptin is a predictor of the number of metabolic syndrome components present (27). Pedrosa and cols., using the definition of MS proposed by the National Cholesterol Education Program Adult Treatment Panel III (NCEP ATP-III), showed that presence of the syndrome was associated with high leptin levels in overweight and obese children aged 7 to 9 years (28).

The novelty of the present study lies in the age range of the recruited participants. Other studies on this topic in young children are scarce, as most authors include adolescents in their series.

In view of their inherent peculiarities, prepubertal children must be studied separately from pubertal and postpubertal subjects, in whom the effects of sex steroids are already present. It has been established that insulin levels and the frequency of insulin resistance increase as puberty progresses (29). The effects of sex steroids are also reflected in leptin levels, which increase during puberty as well (26). Although studies enrolling prepubertal children exclusively are rare, it is known that some risk factors for cardiovascular disease are already present at this age, as shown in our investigation. This justifies further research into potential new biomarkers of cardiovascular risk in childhood, despite the technical difficulties inherent to study of such young subjects.

Now, more than ever, a consensus definition of MS is required (9). Development of such a definition requires proper definition of its components and of cutoffs for better identification of children at increased cardiovascular risk.

The limitations of the present study were mainly those imposed by the young age of the participants, as there is no consensus definition of the MS in this age range. In addition, some cardiovascular risk markers representative of MS, such as hypertension, impaired fasting glucose, and T2DM, are rare in children (23,30), a finding confirmed in the present case series.

Another limitation was the areas under the curves of the ROC curves (Figure 1). Good values are 80-90, while cutoffs 70-80 are considered reasonable (15).

Study of the behavior of potential new biomarkers of cardiovascular risk in childhood may facilitate strategies for prevention and early intervention. Children with high leptin levels constitute a population to which resources and research efforts could be directed. However, due to the dearth of studies in this age group, we must stress that leptin measurement is still not applicable to pediatric clinical practice. Therefore,

caution is warranted when attempting to identify young children at a supposedly increased risk of cardiovascular disease. In this age group, the most suitable approach would be to continue focusing on prophylaxis, i.e., promoting a healthy lifestyle.

REFERENCES

1. Flores LS, Gaya AR, Petersen RDS, Gaya A. Trends of underweight, overweight, and obesity in Brazilian children and adolescents. J Pediatr (Rio J). 2013;89:456-61.

2. Stein AD. Overweight in children: a growing problem. J Pediatr (Rio J). 2014;90:218-20.

3. Steinberger J, Daniels SR. Obesity, insulin resistance, diabetes and cardiovascular risk in children. Circulation. 2003;107:1448-53.

4. Gimeno RE, Klaman LD. Adipose tissue as an active endocrine organ: recent advances. Curr Opin Pharmacol. 2005;5:122-8.

5. Malincikova J, Stejskal D, Hrebicek J. Serun leptin and leptin receptors in healthy pubertal children: relations to insulin resistance and lipid parameters, body mass index, tumor necrosis factor alpha, heart fatty acid binding protein, and IgG anticardiolipin. Acta Univ Palacki Olomuc Fac Med. 2000;143:51-7.

6. Kalra SP. Circumventing leptin resistance for weight control. Proc Natl Acad Sci U S A. 2001;98:4279-81.

7. Fleisch AF, Agarwal N, Roberts MD, Han JC, Theim KR, Vexler A, et al. Influence of serum leptin on weight and body fat growth in children at high risk for adult obesity. J Clin Endocrinol Metab. 2007;92:948-54.

8. Konstantinides K, Schafer K, Neels JG, Dellas C, Loskutoff DJ. Inhibition of endogenous leptin protects mice from arterial and venous thrombosis. Artherioscler Thromb Vasc Biol. 2004;24:2196-201.

9. Ford ES, Li C. Defining the metabolic syndrome in children and adolescents: will the real definition please stand up? J Pediatr. 2008;152:160-4.

10. Zimmet P, Alberti G, Kaufman F, Tajima N, Silink M, Arslanian S, et al. The metabolic syndrome in children and adolescents. Lancet. 2007;369:2059-61.

11. Friend A, Craig L, Turner S. The prevalence of metabolic syndrome in children: a systematic review of the literature. Metab Syndr Relat Dis. 2013;11:71-80.

12. Madeira IR, Bordallo MAN, Carvalho CNM, Gazolla FM, Souza FM, Matos AJ, et al. The role of metabolic syndrome components and adipokines in insulin resistance in prepubertal children. J Pediatr Endocr Metab. 2011;24:289-95.

13. Valle M, Martos R, Gascón F, Cañete R, Zafra MA, Morales R. Low-grade systemic inflammation, hypoadiponectinemia and a high concentration of leptin are present in very young obese children, and correlate with metabolic syndrome. Diabetes Metab. 2005;21:55-62.

14. Slinger JD, Van Breda E, Keizer H, Rump P, Hornstra G, Kuipers H. Insulin resistance, physical fitness, body composition and leptin concentration in 7-8 year old children. J Sci Med Sport. 2008;11:132-8.

15. Fleiss JL, Levin BA, Levin B, Paik MC. Statistical methods for rates and proportions. 3rd ed. Oxford: Wiley InterScience; 2003.

16. Fernández JR, Redden DT, Pietrobelli A, Allison DB. Waist circumference percentiles in nationally representative samples of

African-American, European-American, and Mexican-American children and adolescents. J Pediatr. 2004;145:439-44.

17. Matthews DR, Hosker JP, Rudenski AS, Naylor BA, Treacher DF, Turner RC. Homeostasis model assessment: insulin resistance and beta-cell function from fasting plasma glucose and insulin concentrations in man. Diabetologia. 1985;28:412-9.

18. de Onis M, Onyango AW, Borghi E, Siyam A, Nishida C, Siekmann J. Development of a WHO growth reference for school-aged children and adolescents. Bull World Health Organ. 2007;85:660-7.

19. Giuliano ICB, Caramelli B, Pellanda L, Duncan B, Mattos S, Fonseca FH. Sociedade Brasileira de Cardiologia. I Diretriz de Prevenção da Aterosclerose na Infância e na Adolescência. Arq Bras Cardiol. 2005;85(supl VI):1-36.

20. D'Adamo E, Santoro N, Caprio S. Metabolic syndrome in pediatrics: old concepts revised, new concepts discussed. Curr Probl Pediatr Adolesc Health Care. 2013;43:114-23.

21. Morrison JA, Friedman LA, Wang P, Gluec CJ. Metabolic syndrome in childhood predicts adult metabolic syndrome and type 2 diabetes mellitus 25 to 30 years later. J Pediatr. 2008;152:201-6.

22. Leoni MC, Valsecchi C, Mantelli M, Marastoni L, Tinelli C, Marchi A, et al. Impact of child obesity on adipose tissue physiology: assessment of adipocytokines and inflammatory cytokines as biomarkers of obesity. Pediatr Rep. 2010;2:e19.

23. Poyrazoglu S, Bas F, Darendeliler F. Metabolic syndrome in young people. Curr Opin Endcrinol Diabetes Obes. 2014;21:56-63.

24. Reinehr T, Kleber M, de Sousa G, Andler W. Leptin concentrations are a predictor of overweight reduction in a lifestyle intervention. Int J Pediatr Obes. 2009;4:215-23.

25. Vickers MH, Sloboda DM. Leptin as mediator of the effects of developmental programming. Best Pract Res Clin Endocrinol Metab. 2012;26:677-87.

26. González M, del Mar Bibiloni M, Pons A, Llompart I, Tur JA. Inflammatory markers and metabolic syndrome among adolescents. Eur J Clin Nutr. 2012;66:1141-5.

27. Papoutsakis C, Yannakoulia M, Ntalla I, Dedoussis GV. Metabolic syndrome in a Mediterranean pediatric cohort: prevalence using International Diabetes Federation-derived criteria and associations with adiponectin and leptin. Metabolism. 2012;61:140-5.

28. Pedrosa C, Oliveira BM, Albuquerque I, Simões-Pereira C, Vaz-de-Almeida MD, Correia F. Obesity and metabolic syndrome in 7-9 years-old Portuguese schoolchildren. Diabetol Metab Syndr. 2010;2:40.

29. Druet C, Dabbas B, Baltakse V, Payen C, Jouret B, Baud C, et al. Insulin resistance and the metabolic syndrome in obese French children. Clin Endocrinol (Oxf). 2006;64:672-8.

30. Sinayko AR. Metabolic Syndrome in children. J Pediatr (Rio J). 2012;88:286-8.

27

Thyroid cancer burden and economic impact on the Brazilian public health system

Carolina Castro Porto Silva Janovsky[1,2], Marcio Sommer Bittencourt[2,3],
Maykon Anderson Pires de Novais[4], Rui M. B. Maciel[1],
Rosa Paula M. Biscolla[1], Paola Zucchi[4]

ABSTRACT

Objective: Recent data indicates an increasing incidence of thyroid cancer not accompanied by a proportional increase in mortality, suggesting *overdiagnosis*, which may represent a big public health problem, particularly where resources are scarce. This article aims to describe and evaluate the procedures related to investigation of thyroid nodules and treatment and follow-up of thyroid cancer and the costs for the Brazilian public health system between 2008 and 2015. **Materials and methods:** Data on procedures related to investigation of thyroid nodules and treatment/follow-up of thyroid cancer between 2008 and 2015 in Brazil were collected from the Department of Informatics of the Brazilian Unified Health System (Datasus) website. **Results:** A statistically significant increase in the use of procedures related to thyroid nodules investigation and thyroid cancer treatment and follow-up was observed in Brazil, though a reduction was noted for procedures related to the treatment of more aggressive thyroid cancer, such as total thyroidectomy with neck dissection and higher radioiodine activities such as 200 and 250 milicuries (mCi). The procedures related to thyroid nodules investigation costs increased by 91% for thyroid ultrasound (p = 0.0003) and 128% in thyroid nodule biopsy (p < 0.001). Costs related to treatment and follow-up related-procedures increased by 120%. **Conclusion:** The increase in the incidence of thyroid cancer in Brazil is directly associated with an increased use of diagnostic tools for thyroid nodules, which leads to an upsurge in thyroid cancer treatment and follow-up-related procedures. These data suggest that substantial resources are being used for diagnosis, treatment and follow-up of a potentially indolent condition. Arch Endocrinol Metab. 2018;62(5):537-44

[1] Centro de Doenças da Tireoide e Laboratório de Endocrinologia Molecular e Translacional, Divisão de Endocrinologia, Departamento de Medicina, Escola Paulista de Medicina, Universidade Federal de São Paulo (EPM-Unifesp), São Paulo, SP, Brasil
[2] Centro de Medicina Preventiva, Hospital Israelita Albert Einstein, São Paulo, SP, Brasil
[3] Núcleo de Pesquisa Clínica e Epidemiológica, Hospital das Clínicas da Faculdade de Medicina da Universidade de São Paulo (HCFMUSP), São Paulo, SP, Brasil
[4] Divisão de Economia da Saúde, Departamento de Medicina, Escola Paulista de Medicina, Universidade Federal de São Paulo, São Paulo, SP, Brasil

Correspondence to:
Rosa Paula Mello Biscolla
Rua Pedro de Toledo, 669, 11th floor
04039-032 – São Paulo, SP, Brasil
rosapaula.biscolla@grupofleury.com.br

Keywords
Thyroid cancer; economic impact; Brazilian public health system; costs; overdiagnosis

INTRODUCTION

Thyroid nodules are a very common condition, found by palpation in 4-7% of the adult population and in more than 50% if an image exam is used (1-4). Despite the general knowledge that thyroid nodules are seldom malignant, about 5%, some studies with necropsies have shown that thyroid cancer may be present in up to 36% of individuals who died from other causes not thyroid-related (5-9).

Indeed, thyroid cancer is the most common endocrine cancer, with an incidence rate of 7.57 per 100,000 women and 1.49 per 100,000 men in Brazil (10), though recent data indicate an increase in incidence worldwide (2,11-14). Interestingly, this increase is not accompanied by a proportional increase in mortality, suggesting the potential diagnosis of early-stage cancer associated with a lower risk of recurrence or the potential occurrence of *overdiagnosis*, which means diagnosing a disease that would never cause symptoms or death during a patient's expected life span (2,15-18).

This phenomenon has been documented in a recent South Korean study, which reported a dramatic rise in the diagnosis of thyroid cancer, reaching epidemic levels, due to the incorporation of a neck ultrasound as part of a routine screening check-up (11). In addition, data from the United States suggest that despite an overall increase in the incidence of thyroid cancers, this phenomenon was more prominent in regions with widely available health care access (15,19,20). Interestingly, such findings seem to be occurring worldwide, leading to increased concern over its public health impact (20).

Recent Brazilian data from the population-based cancer registry (RCBP) has demonstrated a significant increase in the incidence of thyroid cancer in the city of São Paulo from 2008 to 2012 (21). Although this seems to occur throughout the country, the results are more impressive in the southern, southeastern and northeastern regions, where diagnostic tools are more widely available (10,15,22-25).

Since *overdiagnosis* may represent an outsize problem for public health services, it is fundamental to evaluate this phenomenon especially in developing countries, where resources are scarce (22). However, no data on the quantity of procedures performed to investigate a thyroid nodule, treat and follow thyroid cancer patients, as well as its costs for the Brazilian public health system (SUS) are currently available. Therefore, the aim of this study is to describe and discuss the procedures related to investigation of thyroid nodules, treatment and follow-up of thyroid cancer and the direct costs for the Brazilian public health system between 2008 and 2015.

MATERIALS AND METHODS

A retrospective study was performed using the Department of Informatics of the Unified Health System (Datasus) database (datasus.saude.gov.br) as the main source of information, accessed during the month of December 2016.

We considered all the procedures present in the algorithm proposed by the national endocrine society for the investigation and management of thyroid nodules (Figure 1 – supplementary material) (26). As thyroid-stimulating hormone TSH measurements are used to investigate thyroid disfunctions and there is not a specific Datasus code for TSH dosage requested for thyroid nodule evaluation, data about TSH measurements were not included.

The quantity and tariffs of the procedures between 2008 and 2015 were accessed through the TABNET link on the Datasus homepage. The data were organized according to the place where the procedure was performed, not by the patient's birthplace. We analyzed data from the entire country, stratified by the five Brazilian regions (south, southeast, northeast, north, and central-west). It was considered only the treatment related-procedures restricted to the 10th edition International Classification of disease code C-73 ('Thyroid Cancer') (27).

The tariffs were described in the Brazilian local currency, i.e. *reais*. Considering that the tariff (direct cost) of each procedure for our Public Health System, collected from the SIGTAP (sigtap.datasus.saude.gov. br), hasn't changed since 2008, there was no need for adjusting to the inflation rate.

The thyroid nodule investigation and treatment/ follow-up-related procedures analyzed, as well as each tariff are described in Tables 1 and 2.

Brazilian population estimates were obtained from the Brazilian Institute of Geography and Statistics (IBGE) website to adjust the quantity of procedures per 100,000 people in each region. The incidence and mortality rate of thyroid cancer was obtained from the latest version of the National Cancer Institute/ Population-based Cancer Registry (INCA/RCBP) database, using the tenth edition of the International Classification of Disease (ICD-10) code "C73" (27).

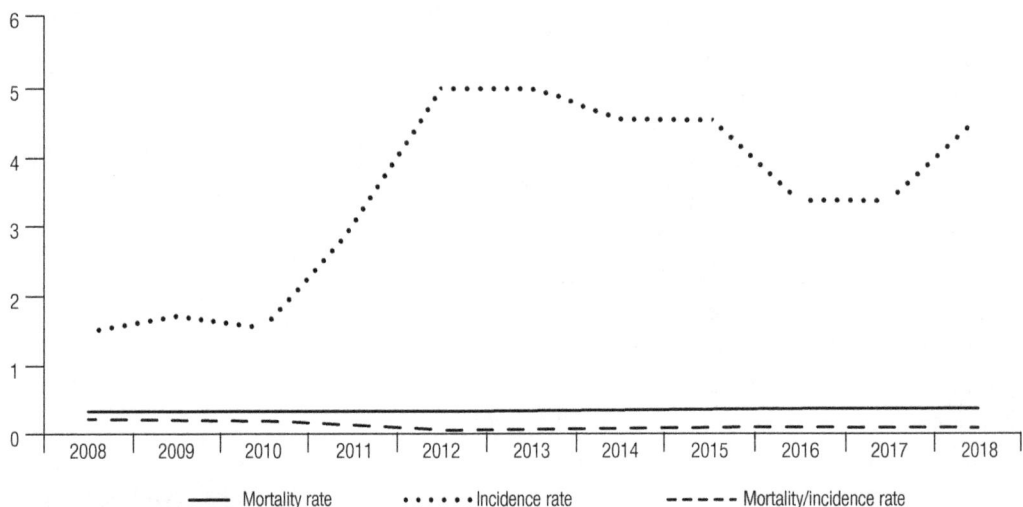

Figure 1. Incidence versus Mortality of Thyroid Cancer (ICD-10: C73) between 2008 and 2018 in Brazil (rate per 100,000 people). Source: Data obtained from the National Cancer Institute (INCA).

The statistical analysis was performed with Stata 13.0 (28). To verify the trend of each variable during the period of the study, a Spearman correlation was used. The significance level adopted was 5%.

Table 1. Thyroid Cancer Diagnosis-related Procedures Available at Datasus in December 2016 (sigtap.datasus.saude.gov.br)

Procedure name	Datasus code	Tariff (R$)
Thyroid ultrasound	02.05.02.012-7	24.20
Thyroid FNAB	02.01.01.047-0	23.73
Thyroid scintigraphy	02.08.03.002-6	77.28
Thyroid scintigraphy with suppression and/or stimulus*	02.08.03.003-4	107.30

* Suppression with T3 or T4/stimulus with recombinant human TSH (thyroid-stimulating hormone).
FNAB: fine-needle aspiration biopsy.

Table 2. Thyroid Cancer Treatment-related Procedures Available at Datasus in December 2016 (sigtap.datasus.saude.gov.br)

Procedure name	Datasus code	Tariff (R$)
Oncologic total thyroidectomy	04.16.03.027-0	2836.30
Total thyroidectomy with neck dissection	04.02.01.005-1	767.77
Total thyroidectomy with neck dissection in oncology	04.16.03.012-2#	1606.86
Trans sternal resection of thyroid cancer	04.16.03.036-0	4186.64
Trans sternal resection of goiter in oncology	04.16.03.005-0*	2618.25
RAI 30 mCi	03.04.09.005-0	443.70
RAI 50 mCi	03.04.09.006-9	614.70
RAI 100 mCi	03.04.09.002-6	1071.90
RAI 150 mCi	03.04.09.001-8	1289.90
RAI 200 mCi	03.04.03.003-4	1471.32
RAI 250 mCi	03.04.09.004-2 03.03.12.001-0	1810.32
WBS	02.08.03.004-2	338.70
Serum thyroglobulin	02.02.06.036-5	15.35

Code 04.16.03.012-2 was revoked in January 2013. Afterwards, codes 04.16.02.018-6 (unilateral neck dissection in oncology) and 04.16.03.027-0 (total thyroidectomy in oncology) were used to describe this procedure.
* Code 04.16.03.005-0 was revoked in January 2013. Afterwards, code 04.16.03.036-0 (trans sternal resection of thyroid cancer) was used to describe this procedure.
RAI: radioiodine treatment; WBS: whole body scan.

RESULTS

In 2008, thyroid cancer incidence rate was 1.51 per 100,000 individuals, rising progressively to 4.57 per 100,000 individuals in 2018 (p = 0.06). The mortality rate rose from 0.30 in 2008 to 0.36 in 2018 (p = 0.004). However, comparing the mortality rate to the incidence rate (mortality rate/incidence rate) there was a negative trend (p = 0.07, rho -0.0674, Figure 1).

Contributing to this incidence's upsurge, it was observed a statistically significant increase in the number of thyroid nodule investigation tools (thyroid ultrasound and fine-needle aspiration biopsy – FNAB), and treatment/follow-up-related procedures (oncologic total thyroidectomy and radioiodine treatment 100 mCi and 150 mCi) between 2008 and 2015 in Brazil and in all geographic regions (Tables 3, 4 and Figure 2). Data on the increase in treatment-related procedures per geographic region are described in the supplementary material.

The use of thyroid scintigraphy with or without stimulus and/or suppression has reduced during the analyzed period (Table 3).

However, the procedures related to more aggressive thyroid cancer treatment reduced significantly during the same period. For example, total thyroidectomy with neck dissection decreased from 0.21 per 100,000 people in 2008 to 0.12 per 100,000 people in 2015 (p = 0.03), while the number of higher radioiodine activities, such as 200 mCi and 250 mCi, both decreased from 0.33 and 0.32 per 100,000 people in 2008, to 0.26 and 0.19 per 100,000 people in 2015, respectively (p = 0.0991 and p < 0.0001). The comparison among levels of radioiodine used for thyroid cancer ablation is shown in Figure 3.

Considering treatment for low-risk patients, an increase in the use of lower doses of RAI (30-50 mCi) for thyroid cancer treatment was noted, although this data is only available since 2014.

Table 3. Number of Thyroid Cancer Diagnosis-related Procedures per 100,000 People, between 2008 and 2015 in the Brazilian Public Health System (SUS)

	2008	2009	2010	2011	2012	2013	2014	2015	p
Thyroid ultrasound	154.5	173.2	196.7	173.5	196.1	207.7	232.8	229.6	< 0.001
Thyroid FNAB	10.3	10.1	10.4	11.2	13.5	14.6	15.6	16.9	< 0.001
Thyroid scintigraphy	6.2	5.5	5.6	5.6	5.4	5.5	5.3	4.8	0.001
Thyroid scintigraphy with suppression/stimulus*	0.09	0.06	0.06	0.04	0.04	0.05	0.07	0.08	0.795

* Suppression with T3 or T4/stimulus with recombinant human TSH (thyroid-stimulating hormone).
FNAB: fine-needle aspiration biopsy.
Source: datasus.saude.gov.br.

Table 4. Number of Thyroid Cancer Treatment and Follow-up-related Procedures per 100,000 People, between 2008 and 2015 in the Brazilian Public Health System (SUS)

	2008	2009	2010	2011	2012	2013	2014	2015	p
Oncologic TT	0.8	0.9	1.0	1.1	1.2	1.7	1.8	1.9	< 0.001
TT with neck dissection	0.2	0.2	0.2	0.2	0.2	0.2	0.2	0.1	0.027
TT with neck dissection in oncology	0.48	0.56	0.65	0.73	0.84	-	-	-	< 0.001
Trans sternal resection of thyroid cancer*	0.03	0.04	0.03	0.04	0.02	0.02	0.02	0.03	0.046
RAI 30 mCi**	-	-	-	-	-	-	0.06	0.07	< 0.001
RAI 50 mCi**	-	-	-	-	-	-	0.04	0.07	< 0.001
RAI 100 mCi	0.4	0.5	0.7	0.7	0.8	0.9	0.9	0.9	0.027
RAI 150 mCi	0.4	0.5	0.7	0.7	0.8	0.9	0.8	0.8	0.055
RAI 200 mCi	0.3	0.3	0.3	0.3	0.3	0.3	0.3	0.3	0.127
RAI 250 mCi	0.3	0.3	0.3	0.2	0.2	0.2	0.2	0.2	0.007
WBS	3.8	3.7	4.2	4.6	4.4	5.1	4.9	4.9	0.008
Serum thyroglobulin	23.3	27.3	37.3	39.4	38.7	39.8	44.9	48.5	< 0.001

* Data includes codes 04.16.03.005-0 (from 2008 to 2013) and 04.16.03.036-0 (from 2013 to 2016).
** Data available since 2014.
RAI: radioiodine treatment; TT: total thyroidectomy; WBS: whole body scan.
Only the procedures restricted to the IDC: C73 were considered.
Source: Data obtained from datasus.saude.gov.br

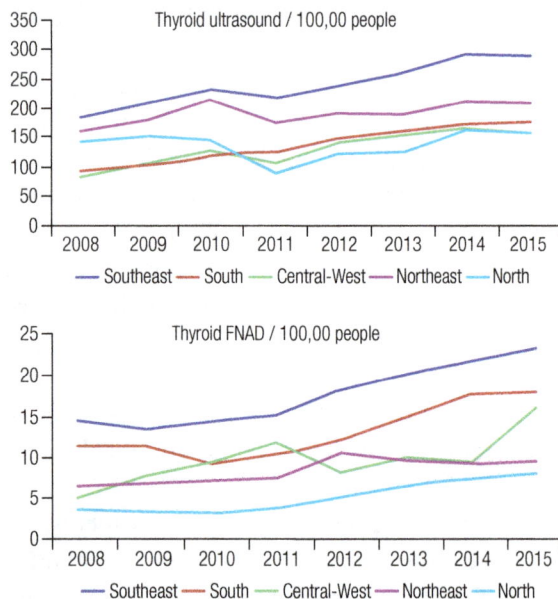

Figure 2. Increase in Numbers of Procedures Related to Thyroid Nodule Investigation between 2008 and 2015 in the Brazilian Public Health System (SUS) by Regions.

FNAB: fine-needle aspiration biopsy.

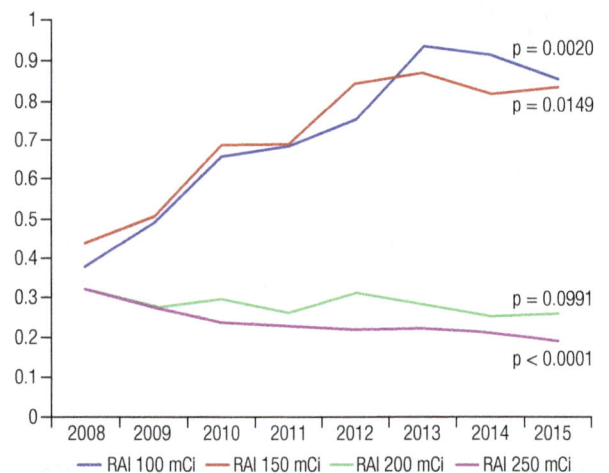

Figure 3. Radioactive Iodine Use per 100,000 People During 2008–2015 in the Brazilian Public Health System (SUS).

RAI: radioiodine treatment.

Regarding direct costs to the Brazilian public health system, a 84% increase in procedures related to thyroid nodule investigation costs was noted in this period. Thyroid ultrasound costs increased by 91% (p = 0.0003), and thyroid nodule biopsy (fine-needle aspiration biopsy) costs increased by 128% (p < 0.001)

from 2008 to 2015 (Figure 4A). Similarly, there was a 120% increase in the total costs of treatment-related procedures performed during the same period, mainly due to the increase in the use of oncologic total thyroidectomy, radioiodine activities of 100 and 150 mCi RAI and follow-up procedures (Figure 4B). These procedures (diagnostic and therapeutic) altogether represented an expense of almost 230 million *reais* for the unified health system (SUS) in this 8-year period.

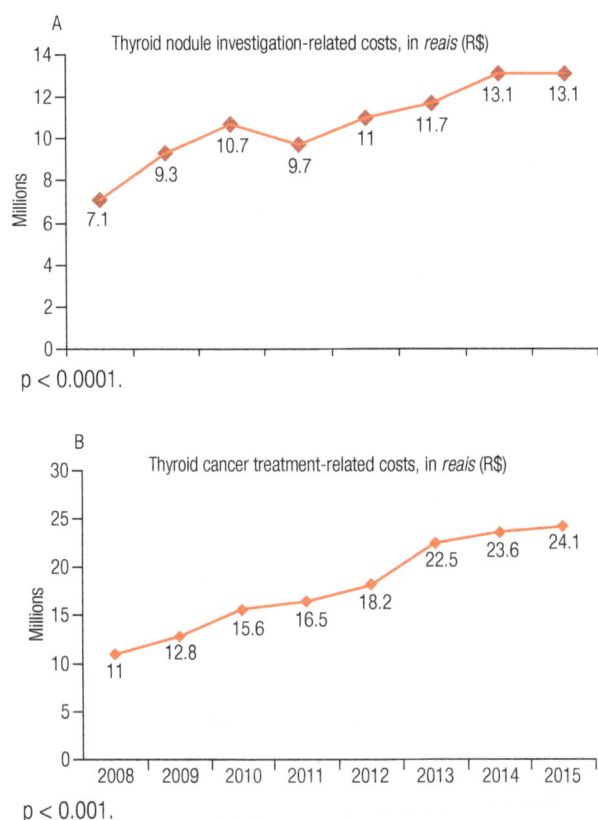

Figure 4. Increase in Costs Related to Thyroid Cancer Diagnosis (**A**) and Treatment (**B**) between 2008 and 2015 in the Brazilian Public Health System.

DISCUSSION

Our study demonstrates an important upsurge in the use of procedures related to thyroid nodule investigation and thyroid cancer treatment and follow-up in Brazil from 2008 to 2015. This overuse of resources has increased the costs of the disease for the Brazilian public health system.

Interestingly, this increase seems to be mostly driven by procedures related to early-stage cancer, as the use of more aggressive surgery and higher-dose radiation therapy has decreased over time. Although this trend might be interpreted as earlier diagnosis due to more intensive use of screening strategies, one would expect a reduction in mortality if this were true. Collectively, this evidence can be interpreted as a potential *overdiagnosis* of cases, which are unlikely to progress to overt or aggressive forms of cancer.

The clinical relevance of a nodule incidentally found by ultrasound is unclear because it probably will not prompt symptoms or neoplastic dissemination (29-31). Indeed, studies have shown that 19% to 68% of the population presents with a thyroid nodule on a neck ultrasound (32,33). In these cases, an early thyroid cancer diagnosis would not improve prognosis, but it may increase the risks related to unnecessary aggressive treatment (31).

To avoid *overdiagnosis* and overuse of resources, health systems in different countries are reconsidering the usefulness of neck ultrasound to screen for thyroid cancer in asymptomatic individuals. In the United Kingdom, only a thyroid specialist is allowed to order neck ultrasounds for patients with thyroid nodules (34). Along the same lines, the American Preventive Service Task Force (USPSTF) recently released its guidelines, in which it strongly recommends against using neck ultrasounds for thyroid cancer screening in asymptomatic people (35). Restricting the use of neck ultrasounds to cases in which palpable nodules are detected by a specialist could be an option for reducing healthcare resource utilization in the Brazilian public health system.

Despite the increase in total thyroidectomies performed during the period of this study, a significant reduction in the use of more complex surgeries, such as total thyroidectomies with neck dissection, was noted. This finding suggests that smaller tumours are being resected, without lymph node metastasis and probably with no important clinical repercussion, which corroborates the hypothesis of *overdiagnosis* (36-38). This concept is reinforced by recent data showing a similar effect with *watchful waiting* compared with surgery when a thyroid nodule is diagnosed as cancer (39,40).

Our results have also documented a significant increase in radioiodine treatment with 100 and 150 mCi, the most common activities prescribed for thyroid cancer patients with intermediate or high risk of recurrence. Lately, national and international guidelines on thyroid cancer management have recommended against the use of radioiodine in low risk of recurrence cases (26,41). Even so, Roman and cols. (42) observed that 30% of the patients with tumours < 1 cm still receive radioiodine activities despite recent guidelines against it (42). In our study, it is not clear if the rise observed in the use of RAI is associated with diagnosis of higher-risk tumours or if clinicians continue to prescribe RAI due to a lack of knowledge or for thyroid remnant ablation. In these cases, the use of RAI could facilitate the use of serum thyroglobulin measurements in the thyroid cancer follow-up (43). Nevertheless, the reduction in prescribing higher RAI activities (200 and

250 mCi) implies that less aggressive cases are being diagnosed.

There was a numerical increase in the use of low radioiodine activities (30-50 mCi), despite the small absolute number of those procedures, as they were only included in the list of authorized procedures by the Brazilian Public Health System in 2014. Recent studies have shown that the benefits of lower RAI doses equal higher doses, such as 100 mCi for low- to intermediate-risk patients, with fewer side effects and reduced costs (44,45). This may be a tendency as low-risk cases are being dignosed. However, the low request for these procedures may indicate that low-risk patients have not received any RAI treatment, which is the most recent standard of care expected for low-risk cases (46,47), or they have received 100 mCi despite the recent literature recommendations (46-49).

The southeastern region of Brazil had the highest increase in number of procedures as well as expenditures related to thyroid cancer diagnosis and treatment. This may have occurred due to the choice of using the Datasus search filter of patients' treatment place and not their birthplace. It is known that the southeastern region is the richest region and has the largest cancer centres in Brazil, which are referred centres for people from other regions. So the expectation on overuse of resources is higher. Nonetheless, this important upsurge in diagnostic and treatment-related procedures seems to be spread throughout the country, irrespective of region.

From 2010 to 2015, there was a 66% increase in costs related to cancer in Brazil, from 2.1 billion *reais* to 3.5 billion *reais*, according to the National Cancer Institute (INCA). During the 8-year study period, there was also a significant increase in the cost of thyroid nodule investigation and thyroid cancer treatment and follow-up in all Brazilian regions, proportionally higher than what was observed for other types of cancer (106% for thyroid cancer vs 66% for all types of cancer). This excessive expenditure for a potentially indolent disease adds on to the hypothesis of *overdiagnosis*.

Our study, however, must be read within the context of its design. The completeness of the INCA/RCBP database is questionable in some regions. Therefore, the inputs on thyroid cancer incidence may be underestimated. Also, the Datasus database depends on the registry of the procedures performed in each hospital or healthcare service across the country, thus it does not warrant a completely reliable source of information.

Additionally, there are different codes to describe the same procedure, for example, "total thyroidectomy" *versus* "total thyroidectomy in oncology". This study considered only the code for total thyroidectomy in oncology, which excludes thyroid surgeries for benign diseases. However, the figures may be underestimated, as it is possible that the code for total thyroidectomy (not oncologic) also might have been used to describe surgeries for cancer. Another coding problem is that the code used to describe thyroid FNAB because it is used to describe thyroid as well as parathyroid FNAB. It is known that thyroid tumors are 16 times more common than parathyroid tumors (50). We therefore assumed all FNAB were related to thyroid cancer. Although this may result in a small overestimation of its use, there has been no change in the incidence of parathyroid tumors, and the documented increase over the last eight years is unlikely to have changed if the cases used for parathyroid disease were excluded. Finally, the treatment related-procedure codes that referred to other diseases despite thyroid cancer were disregarded as they might have overestimated the results.

In conclusion, the increasing incidence of thyroid cancer in Brazil seems to be directly associated with the performance of diagnostic procedures, as well as an increase in treatment-related procedures. These data suggest that large resources are allocated for diagnosis and treatment of a potentially indolent condition, which could remain unnoticed throughout one's lifetime. Therefore, it is important that thyroid cancer care be reexamined with a cost-conscious view, providing the best outcome that matters to the patient, relative to the cost of delivering it, especially in developing countries where healthcare resources are scarce.

Ethics approval and consent to participate: the study was approved by the Ethics Committee on Research from Federal University of Sao Paulo (Unifesp) under the National Research Database (Plataforma Brasil). The committee's reference number (CAAE) is: 58914516.8.0000.5505.

Availability of data and material: all data is available publicly at www.datasus.gov.br. The raw data on the statistical analysis is available from the corresponding author upon reasonable request.

Authors' contributions: Carolina Castro Porto Silva Janovsky designed the study, collected the data, conducted the statistical analysis and wrote the manuscript. Marcio Sommer Bittencourt contributed to the statistical analysis, contributed to the discussion and reviewed the manuscript. Maykon Anderson Pires de Novais contributed to the study design and reviewed the manuscript. Rui Monteiro de Barros Maciel contributed to the discussion and reviewed the manuscript. Rosa Paula de Mello Biscolla designed the study, contributed to the discussion and reviewed the manuscript. Paola Zucchi designed the study, contributed to the discussion and reviewed the manuscript. All authors read and approved the final version.

Acknowledgements: the authors would like to acknowledge the Department of Informatics of the Brazilian Unified Health System (DATASUS) for the availability of the material and technical support when needed.

Funding: none.

REFERENCES

1. Ezzat S, Sarti DA, Cain DR, Braunstein GD. Thyroid incidentalomas. Prevalence by palpation and ultrasonography. Arch Intern Med. 1994;154(16):1838-40.

2. Leenhardt L, Bernier MO, Boin-Pineau MH, Conte Devolx B, Maréchaud R, Niccoli-Sire P, et al. Advances in diagnostic practices affect thyroid cancer incidence in France. Eur J Endocrinol. 2004;150(2):133-9.

3. Udelsman R, Zhang Y. The epidemic of thyroid cancer in the United States: the role of endocrinologists and ultrasounds. Thyroid. 2014;24(3):472-9.

4. Guth S, Theune U, Aberle J, Galach A, Bamberger CM. Very high prevalence of thyroid nodules detected by high frequency (13 MHz) ultrasound examination. Eur J Clin Invest. 2009;39(8):699-706.

5. Wartofsky L. The thyroid nodule: evaluation, risk of malignancy, and management. in: thyroid cancer. 2nd ed. New York, NY: Springer New York; 2016. p. 257-75.

6. de Matos PS, Ferreira APC, Ward LS. Prevalence of papillary microcarcinoma of the thyroid in Brazilian autopsy and surgical series. Endocr Pathol. 2006;17(2):165-73.

7. Yamamoto Y, Maeda T, Izumi K, Otsuka H. Occult papillary carcinoma of the thyroid. A study of 408 autopsy cases. Cancer. 1990;65(5):1173-9.

8. Franssila KO, Rubén Harach H. Occult papillary carcinoma of the thyroid in children and young adults: a systemic autopsy study in Finland. Cancer. 1986;58(3):715-9.

9. Ottino A, Pianzola HM, Castelletto RH. Occult papillary thyroid carcinoma at autopsy in La Plata, Argentina. Cancer. 1989;64(2):547-51.

10. Brasil. Instituto Nacional do Câncer (Inca). Estimativa da incidência de câncer no Brasil em 2018. Brasília, DF. Ministério da Saúde; 2018.

11. Ahn HS, Kim HJ, Welch G. Korea's Thyroid-Cancer "Epidemic" – Screening and Overdiagnosis. N Engl J Med. 2014; 371(19):1765-7.

12. Veiga LH, Neta G, Aschebrook-Kilfoy B, Ron E, Devesa SS. Thyroid cancer incidence patterns in Sao Paulo, Brazil, and the U.S. SEER program, 1997-2008. Thyroid. 2013;23(6):748-57.

13. Davies L, Welch HG. Increasing incidence of thyroid cancer in the United States, 1973-2002. JAMA. 2006;295(18):2164-7.

14. Ito Y, Nikiforov YE, Schlumberger M, Vigneri R. Increasing incidence of thyroid cancer: controversies explored. Nat Rev Endocrinol. 2013;9(3):178-84.

15. Ward L, Graf H. Câncer da tiroide: aumento na ocorrência da doença ou simplesmente na sua detecção? Arq Bras Endocrinol Metabol. 2009;52(9):1-2.

16. International Atomic Energy Agency (IAEA). Investigation of excess thyroid cancer incidence in Los Alamos County (DOE/AL/75237--T1). United States. Available from: https://inis.iaea.org/search/citationdownload.aspx.

17. Brito JP, Al Nofal A, Montori VM, Hay ID, Morris JC. The Impact of Subclinical Disease and Mechanism of Detection on the Rise in Thyroid Cancer Incidence: A Population-Based Study in Olmsted County, Minnesota During 1935 Through 2012. Thyroid. 2015;25(9):999-1007.

18. Welch HG, Black WC. Overdiagnosis in cancer. J Natl Cancer Inst. 2010;102(9):605-13.

19. Sprague BL, Warren Andersen S, Trentham-Dietz A. Thyroid cancer incidence and socioeconomic indicators of health care access. Cancer Causes Control. 2008;19(6):585-93.

20. Vaccarella S, Franceschi S, Bray F, Wild CP, Plummer M, Dal Maso L. Worldwide thyroid-cancer epidemic? the increasing impact of overdiagnosis. N Engl J Med. 2016;375(7):614-7.

21. Registro de Câncer de Base Populacional. Câncer em São Paulo (RCBP-SP) 2008-2012.

22. Ward LS. Epidemiologia do câncer da tiroide no Brasil: apontando direções na política de saúde do país. Arq Bras Endocrinol Metabol. 2005;49(4):474-6.

23. Coeli CM, Brito AS, Barbosa FS, Ribeiro MG, Sieiro APAV, Vaisman M. Incidência e mortalidade por câncer de tireoide no Brasil. Arq Bras Endocrinol Metabol. 2005;49(4):503-9.

24. Brasil. Estimativa da incidência de câncer no Brasil em 2012. Instituto Nacional do Câncer (Inca). Brasília. DF: Ministério da Saúde; 2012.

25. Cordioli MICV, Canalli MHBS, Coral MHC. Increase incidence of thyroid cancer in Florianopolis, Brazil: comparative study of diagnosed cases in 2000 and 2005. 2009;53(4):453-60.

26. Rosario PW, Ward LS, Carvalho GA, Graf H, Maciel RMB, Maciel LMZ, et al. Thyroid nodules and differentiated thyroid cancer: update on the Brazilian consensus. Arq Bras Endocrinol Metabol. 2013;57:240-64.

27. Sinha P, Sunder G, Bendale P, Mantri M, Dande A. Coding System for Classification of Diseases and Related Health Problems. In: Sinha P, Sunder G, Bendale P, Mantri M, Dande A. Electronic Health Record. Hoboken, NJ, USA: John Wiley & Sons, Inc; 2012. p. 111-7.

28. Stata 13.0. Disponível em: https://www.stata.com.

29. Sugitani I, Fujimoto Y. Management of low-risk papillary thyroid carcinoma: Unique conventional policy in Japan and our efforts to improve the level of evidence. Surgery Today. Springer Japan. 2010;40(3):199-215.

30. Penna GC, Mendes HG. Thyroid nodule < 1 cm and low-risk papillary thyroid microcarcinoma: what are today's management options? Endocrinol Metab Int J. 2016;3(4):1-3.

31. Oda H, Miyauchi A, Ito Y, Sasai H, Masuoka H, Yabuta T, et al. Comparison of the costs of active surveillance and immediate surgery in the management of low-risk papillary microcarcinoma of the thyroid. Endocr J. 2017;64(1):59-64.

32. Tan GH. Thyroid incidentalomas: management approaches to nonpalpable nodules discovered incidentally on thyroid imaging. Ann Intern Med. 1997;126(3):226-31.

33. Guth S, Theune U, Aberle J, Galach A, Bamberger CM. Very high prevalence of thyroid nodules detected by high frequency (13 MHz) ultrasound examination. Eur J Clin Invest. 2009;39(8):699-706.

34. Perros P, Boelaert K, Colley S, Evans C, Evans RM, Gerrard Ba G, et al.; British Thyroid Association. Guidelines for the management of thyroid cancer. Clin Endocrinol (Oxf). 2014 Jul;81 Suppl 1:1-122.

35. Jin J. The US Preventive Services Task Force. JAMA. 2016;315(16):1804.

36. Park S, Oh CM, Cho H, Lee JY, Jung KW, Jun JK, et al. Association between screening and the thyroid cancer "epidemic" in South Korea: evidence from a nationwide study. BMJ. 2016;355:i5745.

37. Tan GH, Gharib H. Thyroid incidentalomas: management approaches to nonpalpable nodules discovered incidentally on thyroid imaging. Ann Intern Med. 1997;126(3):226-31.

38. Ukrainski MB, Pribitkin EA, Miller JL. Increasing incidence of thyroid nodules and thyroid cancer: does increased detection of a subclinical reservoir justify the associated anxiety and treatment? Clin Ther. 2016;38(4):976-85.

39. Ito Y, Miyauchi A, Inoue H, Fukushima M, Kihara M, Higashiyama T, et al. An observational trial for papillary thyroid microcarcinoma in Japanese patients. World J Surg. 2010;34(1):28-35.

40. Ito Y, Miyauchi A. Is surgery necessary for papillary thyroid microcarcinomas? Nat Rev Endocrinol. 2011;8(1):1-1.

41. Haugen BR. 2015 American Thyroid Association Management Guidelines for Adult Patients with Thyroid Nodules and Differentiated Thyroid Cancer: What is new and what has changed? Cancer. 2016;123(3):372-81.

42. Roman BR, Feingold JH, Patel SG, Shaha AR, Shah JP, Tuttle RM, et al. The 2009 American Thyroid Association Guidelines modestly reduced radioactive iodine use for thyroid cancers less than 1 cm. Thyroid. 2014;24(10):1549-50.

43. Cabana MD, Rand CS, Powe NR, Wu AW, Wilson MH, Abboud PAC, et al. Why don't physicians follow clinical practice guidelines? JAMA. 1999;282:1458-65.

44. Schlumberger M, Catargi B, Borget I, Deandreis D, Zerdoud S, Bridji B, et al. Strategies of radioiodine ablation in patients with low-risk thyroid cancer. N Engl J Med. 2012;366(18):1663-73.

45. Yamazaki CA, Padovani RP, Biscolla RPM, Ikejiri ES, Marchetti RR, Castiglioni MLV, et al. Lithium as an adjuvant in the postoperative ablation of remnant tissue in low-risk thyroid carcinoma. Thyroid. 2012;22(10):1002-6.

46. Janovsky CCPS, Maciel RMB, Camacho CP, Padovani RP, Nakabashi CC, Yang JH, et al. A prospective study showing an excellent response of patients with low-risk differentiated thyroid cancer who did not undergo radioiodine remnant ablation after total thyroidectomy. Eur Thyroid J. 2016;5(1):44-9.

47. Durante C, Montesano T, Attard M, Torlontano M, Monzani F, Costante G, et al. Long-term surveillance of papillary thyroid cancer patients who do not undergo postoperative radioiodine remnant ablation: is there a role for serum thyroglobulin measurement? J Clin Endocrinol Metab. 2012;97(8):2748-53.

48. Durante C, Attard M, Torlontano M, Ronga G, Monzani F, Costante G, et al. Identification and optimal postsurgical follow-up of patients with very low-risk papillary thyroid microcarcinomas. J Clin Endocrinol Metab. 2010;95(11):4882-8.

49. Lamartina L, Durante C, Filetti S, Cooper DS. Low-risk differentiated thyroid cancer and radioiodine remnant ablation: a systematic review of the literature. J Clin Endocrinol Metab. 2015;100(5):1748-61.

50. James BC, Aschebrook-Kilfoy B, Cipriani N, Kaplan EL, Angelos P, Grogan RH. The Incidence and survival of rare cancers of the thyroid, parathyroid, adrenal, and pancreas. Ann Surg Oncol. 2016;23(2):424-33.

28

Clinical impact of thyroglobulin (Tg) and Tg autoantibody (TgAb) measurements in needle washouts of neck lymph node biopsies in the management of patients with papillary thyroid carcinoma

M. Cecilia Martins-Costa[1,2], Rui M. B. Maciel[1,3,4], Teresa S. Kasamatsu[1],
Claudia C. D. Nakabashi[1,3,4], Cleber P. Camacho[1,3],
Felipe Crispim[1], Elza S. Ikejiri[1,3], M. Conceição O. Mamone[1,3],
Danielle M. Andreoni[1,3], Rosa Paula M. Biscolla[1,3,4]

ABSTRACT

Objectives: The presence of thyroglobulin (Tg) in needle washouts of fine needle aspiration biopsy (Tg-FNAB) in neck lymph nodes (LNs) suspected of metastasis has become a cornerstone in the follow-up of patients with papillary thyroid carcinoma (PTC). However, there are limited data regarding the measurement of anti-Tg antibodies in these washouts (TgAb-FNAB), and it is not clear whether these antibodies interfere with the assessment of Tg-FNAB or whether there are other factors that would more consistently justify the finding of low Tg-FNAB in metastatic LNs. **Materials and methods:** We investigated 232 FNAB samples obtained from suspicious neck LNs of 144 PTC patients. These samples were divided according to the patient's serum TgAb status: sTgAb- (n = 203 samples) and sTgAb+ (n = 29). The TgAb-FNAB levels were measured using two different assays. Tg-FNAB was also measured using two assays when low levels (< 10 ng/mL) were identified in the first assay of the metastatic LNs from the sTgAb+ samples. **Results:** The TgAb-FNAB results were negative in both assays in all samples. Low levels of Tg-FNAB were identified in 11/16 of the metastatic LNs of the sTgAb+ patients and 16/63 of the sTgAb- patients (p < 0.05) using assay 1. The measurement of the Tg-FNAB levels using assay 2 indicated additional metastases in 5 LNs of the sTgAb+ patients. **Conclusions:** Factors other than the presence of TgAb-FNAB may contribute to the higher number of metastatic LNs with undetectable Tg-FNAB in the sTgAb+ group. In addition, the measurement of Tg-FNAB using different assays was useful to enhance the diagnosis of metastatic LNs, particularly when cytological and Tg-FNAB results are discordant. Arch Endocrinol Metab. 2017;61(2):108-14

Keywords
Fine needle aspiration biopsy; anti-thyroglobulin antibody; thyroglobulin; papillary thyroid cancer; neck lymph nodes

[1] Centro de Doenças da Tireoide e Laboratório de Endocrinologia Molecular e Translacional, Divisão de Endocrinologia, Departamento de Medicina, Escola Paulista de Medicina da Universidade Federal de São Paulo (EPM--Unifesp), São Paulo, SP, Brasil
[2] Departamento de Medicina, Universidade de Fortaleza (Unifor), Fortaleza, CE, Brasil
[3] Centro de Doenças da Tireoide, Instituto Israelita de Ensino e Pesquisa Albert Einstein (IIEPAE), São Paulo, SP, Brasil
[4] Fleury Medicina e Saúde, São Paulo, SP, Brasil

Correspondence to:
Rui M. B. Maciel
Laboratório de Endocrinologia
Molecular e Translacional,
Disciplina de Endocrinologia,
Departamento de Medicina,
Escola Paulista de Medicina,
Universidade Federal de São Paulo
Rua Pedro de Toledo, 669, 11° andar
04039-32 – São Paulo, SP, Brasil
rui.maciel@unifesp.br

INTRODUCTION

Papillary thyroid carcinoma (PTC) is the most common endocrine malignancy, with a propensity for cervical lymphatic spread, which occurs in 20% to 50% of patients based on reports of surgical pathological specimens using standard methods of description; however, the prevalence may reach 90% of patients when the surgical sample is scrutinized in detail for micrometastases (1,2).

The confirmation of malignancy in lymph nodes (LNs) with a suspicious ultrasonographic (US) appearance is achieved by US-guided fine needle aspiration biopsy (FNAB) for cytological study (cyto-FNAB) and the measurement of thyroglobulin levels (Tg) in needle washouts (Tg-FNAB) (3-8).

Considering only the data from cyto-FNAB, approximately 6% to 8% of metastases are misdiagnosed as a result of false-negative results (9,10). These results may occur in cases of small or cystic LN metastases, which reflect a lack of tumor cells detected during the FNAB procedure (11). Nevertheless, the use of Tg-FNAB alone has several limitations, and despite being well established as an important tool in the investigation of suspicious LN metastases, Tg-FNAB presents variable results between metastatic and non-metastatic LNs (3,4,11-23). This subject has been the topic of recent reviews and meta-analysis studies (12,13).

Another aspect for consideration during the follow-up of patients with PTC is the interpretation of serum Tg (sTg) values in the presence of serum anti-Tg antibodies (sTgAb), which occurs in approximately 25% of patients with PTC; these antibodies may interfere with the measurement of sTg, which compromises the use of this tumor marker in the follow-up of patients with PTC (24). It remains controversial whether these antibodies also interfere with the assessment of TgAb-FNAB. Previous studies on this topic have included a limited number of patients with positive serum anti-Tg antibodies (sTgAb+) (25-27) and limited direct measurements of TgAb-FNAB (16,18,20,25,26).

Therefore, the objectives of the present study were to: 1) assess the presence of TgAb in a substantial amount of washout fluid samples (TgAb-FNAB) of cervical LNs suspicious for PTC metastases; 2) analyze whether the presence of serum sTgAb+ interfered with the assessment of Tg-FNAB for the management of neck lymphadenopathy in PTC patients; and 3) compare the TgAb values of the serum and FNAB washout.

MATERIALS AND METHODS

Patients

We assessed 144 patients who presented suspicious LNs via US assessment during follow-up for PTC. These patients were followed by a single team of physicians at associated Thyroid Disease Centers at the Division of Endocrinology, Department of Medicine, *Escola Paulista de Medicina, Universidade Federal de Sao Paulo* and the *Instituto Israelita de Ensino e Pesquisa Albert Einstein*, both in Sao Paulo, Brazil.

Suspicious LNs were submitted to FNAB guided by neck US assessment. The minimum follow-up period was 4 years after the last FNAB. Some patients had more than one FNAB performed when multiple suspicious LNs appeared during the follow-up or the FNAB had to be repeated because of inadequate or non-diagnostic

cyto-FNAB results with undetectable Tg-FNAB values. Two hundred eighty-six FNABs were performed, and 232 FNAB samples were analyzed. Fifty-four FNAB samples were excluded because the patients were lost during follow-up (n = 32) or the diagnosis of lymphadenopathy could not be confirmed (n = 22), as cytopathology indicated that these samples were obtained from other cervical lesions rather than LNs.

The confirmation of LN metastases was obtained via histopathological examination after surgery or the ^{131}I uptake after radioiodine treatment. In two particular situations, LNs that initially fulfilled suspicious criteria via US assessment were considered reactive over time: 1) LNs that spontaneously disappeared at the subsequent US assessment performed during follow-up; and 2) LNs that initially had inadequate or non-diagnostic cytology results on the first FNAB attempt and presented a reactive cytology with Tg-FNAB < 10 ng/mL after a second FNAB.

All diagnostic procedures were performed in accordance with the regulations of the local ethics committee. Written informed consent was obtained from each patient.

Assays

Tg-FNAB was measured with a commercial immunofluorometric assay using monoclonal antibodies (DELFIA®, PerkinElmer, Turku, Finland), with a functional sensitivity of 1.0 ng/mL (assay 1). A second immunofluorometric Tg assay (assay 2), using mono and polyclonal antibodies, was performed on the washout fluids of sTgAb+ patients with a Tg-FNAB value < 10 ng/mL in assay 1 to determine whether low Tg-FNAB persisted using a different method. Assay 2 has a functional sensitivity of 0.3 ng/mL (28). The Tg assay 2 was assessed only in this specific group of patients for whom the TgAb-FNAB results, in the case of positivity by contamination with sTgAb, could interfere with the Tg-FNAB levels. We verified whether these lower Tg-FNAB levels would be maintained when examined using another assay.

The Tg-FNAB cutoff point for the diagnosis of malignancy has not been unanimously established in the literature (12,13). We used the value of 10 ng/mL, which is consistent with the majority of published reports (11,14,20-22).

TgAb was measured using an in house immunofluorometric assay in both serum and FNAB washout samples, and negative values for TgAb were considered < 40 IU/mL (29). In addition, we also measured TgAb in FNAB washout samples using a chemiluminescence immunoassay (ECLIA Roche, Mannheim, Germany). The cutoff value for positive TgAb was 115 IU/mL.

Ultrasonography

A cervical US assessment was performed using a linear, multi-frequency, 7.5-10-MHz transducer and integrated using color-Doppler examination by the same radiologist. The images were obtained in transversal and longitudinal planes by scanning the hyperextended neck, which enabled the visualization of the central compartment. All cervical LNs were identified, localized, and measured. LNs with 1 or more suspicious features indicative of PTC neck metastasis, i.e., round shape, hypoechogenic aspect, absence of hilum, non-homogeneous pattern, including fluid areas, and intralesional punctate calcifications, were submitted to FNAB.

Cyto-FNAB and Tg-FNAB

US-guided FNAB was performed using a 22-25-gauge needle attached to a 10-mL syringe inserted into the LN under US visual control. The needle was repeatedly moved inside each LN until the needle hub was filled with material. The smears (4-8 per LN) were immediately fixed and stained with panoptic dye. All cytological examinations were performed by the same cytopathologist.

The cyto-FNAB results were classified into 3 distinct diagnostic categories: 1) reactive: presence of lymphocytes and occasional plasma cells without malignant epithelial cells; 2) inadequate or non-diagnostic: presence of blood cells and absence of inflammatory and epithelial cells; and 3) positive for PTC metastases: presence of epithelial cells with malignant cytological characteristics (e.g., abnormal nuclear shape, nuclear enlargement and nuclear polymorphisms, presence of papillae, and/or characteristic nuclear changes, such as grooves and pseudo-inclusions).

Following the smear preparation, the needle was washed with 1 mL of saline, and the solution was processed for Tg-FNAB measurement and subsequently stored at -20°C. The same samples were used to measure the TgAb-FNAB levels.

Statistical analysis

The number of metastatic LNs in Group 1 (sTgAb-) and Group 2 (sTgAb+), as well as their Tg-FNAB levels (assay 1) and cyto-FNAB results were compared using Fisher's Exact Tests and χ^2 tests as appropriate, with a two-tailed $p < 0.05$ considered statistically significant. The sensitivity, specificity, positive predictive value and negative predictive value of a positive Tg-FNAB were calculated using assay 1 (Tg-FNAB $\geq$ 10 ng/mL). All analyses were performed using the Statistical Package for Social Science professional software version 15.0 (SPSS, Chicago, IL, USA).

RESULTS

A general overview of the present study that indicates the results of 232 FNABs in 144 patients is presented in Figure 1. The patients were divided into 2 groups: Group 1, which included patients who presented negative sTgAb values (sTgAb-) (203 FNABs), and Group 2, which included patients who presented positive sTgAb values (sTgAb+) (29 FNABs). These groups were subsequently subdivided according to the Tg-FNAB levels (Tg-FNAB $\geq$ 10 ng/mL and Tg-FNAB < 10 ng/mL) and the cyto-FNAB results (reactive, inadequate/non-diagnostic or positive for PTC metastasis) (Figure 1).

We identified metastases in 63 (31%) LNs in Group 1 (sTgAb-) and 16 (55%) LNs in Group 2 (sTgAb+). This difference was statistically significant ($p < 0.05$, Fisher's Exact test) (Table 1). All metastatic LNs presented classical and follicular PTC histological variants.

Sixteen of the 63 metastatic LNs in Group 1 and 11 of the 16 metastatic LNs in Group 2 had Tg-FNAB levels < 10 ng/dL. Therefore, Group 2 (sTgAb+) had a higher number of metastatic LNs with Tg-FNAB values < 10 ng/dL than Group 1 (68.8% in Group 2 vs. 25.4% in Group 1; $p < 0.05$, χ^2 test) (Table 1). Consistent with the serum results, this finding suggests that the presence of sTgAb may underestimate the measurement of Tg-FNAB.

The cutoff of Tg-FNAB of 10 ng/mL (assay 1) for the diagnosis of metastatic PTC in cervical LNs in Group 1 (sTgAb-) exhibited a sensitivity of 74.6%, with a specificity of 100%, a positive predictive value of 100% and a negative predictive value of 89.7%; Group 2 (sTgAb+) exhibited a sensitivity of 31.2%, with a specificity of 100%, a positive predictive value of 100% and a negative predictive value of 54.2%. Notably, it was not possible to perform the same analysis for Tg-FNAB using assay 2 because it was only tested in the washout fluids of the sTgAb+ patients with Tg-FNAB levels < 10 ng/mL in assay 1.

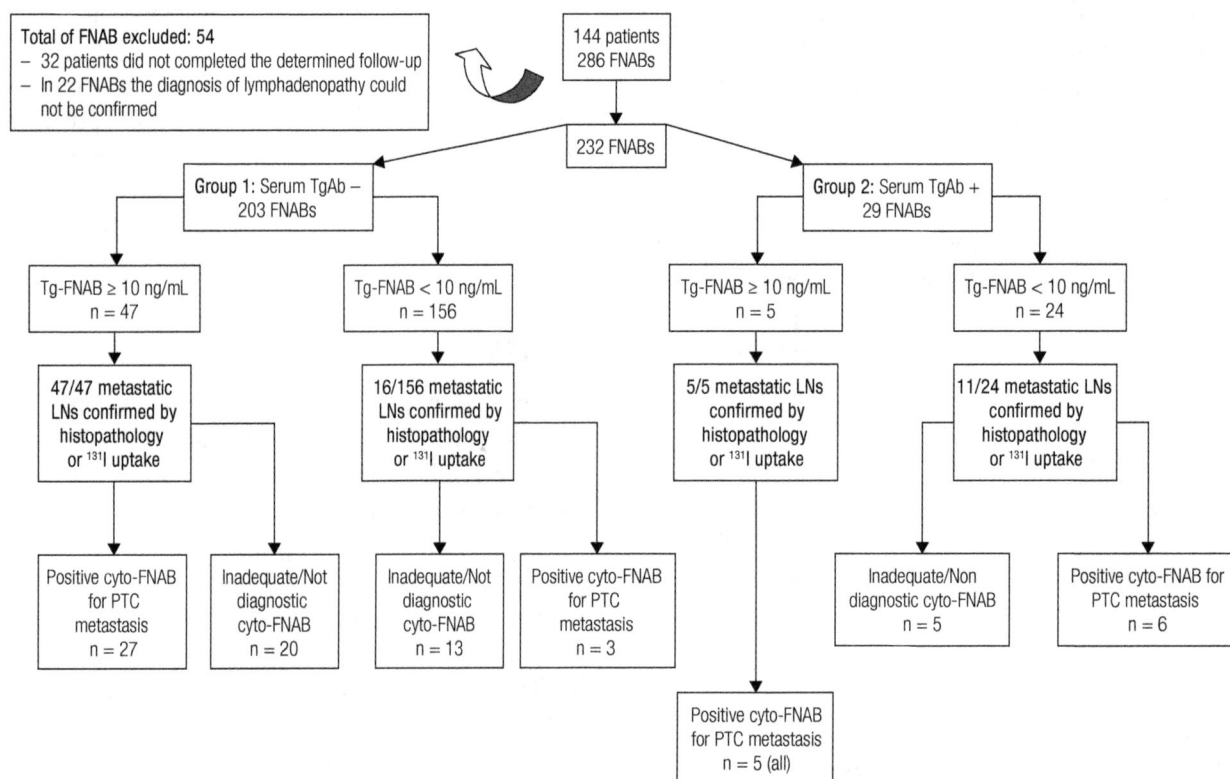

Figure 1. General overview of the study with detailing of Tg-FNAB (by assay 1-(immunofluorometric, with monoclonal antibodies) and cyto-FNAB results of Group 1 (sTgAb–) and Group 2 (sTgAb+).

Table 1. Comparison of Tg-FNAB levels (assay 1) and cyto-FNAB results of metastatic lymph nodes from Group 1 (sTgAb-) and Group 2 (sTgAb+)

	GROUP 1 sTgAb-Metastatic/TOTAL (%) 63 / 203 (31%)[a]		GROUP 2 sTgAb+Metastatic/TOTAL (%) 16 / 29 (55%)[a]	
	Tg-FNAB < 10 ng/mL	Tg-FNAB ≥ 10 ng/mL	Tg-FNAB < 10 ng/mL	Tg-FNAB ≥ 10 ng/mL
	n	n	n	n
Inadequate/not diagnostic cyto-FNAB	13	20	5	0
Positive for metastasis cyto-FNAB	3	27	6	5
TOTAL	16 (25.4%)[b]	47 (74.6%)[c]	11 (68.8%)[b]	5 (31.3%)[c]

[a] Statistical difference between groups (p < 0.05) using Fisher's Exact Test 2 test.
[b,c] Statistical difference between groups (p < 0.05) using χ^2 test.

To evaluate the potential differences in the performance of Tg assay 1 in the sTgAb+ patients (Group 2), we performed a different Tg-FNAB assay (using mono and polyclonal antibodies, Tg assay 2) in all washout fluid samples of metastatic LNs with Tg-FNAB levels < 10 ng/mL using assay 1 (using monoclonal antibodies). We obtained different results between both assays in 4 patients whose cyto-FNABs were positive for PTC metastases and the levels of Tg-FNAB were low (< 10 ng/mL) according to assay 1 and high (≥ 10 ng/mL) according to assay 2 (Table 2). In these

patients, the measurements of Tg-FNAB using assay 2 were consistent with the cyto-FNAB measurements. These findings also indicated that the presence of sTgAb could interfere with the interpretation of Tg-FNAB measurements. Furthermore, these findings suggest methods that employ polyclonal antibodies, such as radioimmunoassays and assay 2, appeared more resistant to TgAb interference (24). Moreover, in one patient, a suspicious LN based on US assessment presented inadequate/non-diagnostic cyto-FNAB, and the level of Tg-FNAB was 8.7 ng/mL according to assay 1 and 142 ng/mL according to assay 2. This patient underwent ^{131}I treatment, and the subsequent scintigraphy indicated substantial ^{131}I uptake in the area of the corresponding LN. Consequently, in this patient, the measurement of Tg-FNAB using assay 2 was important for the diagnosis of metastasis.

However, the direct measurement of TgAb-FNAB based on immunofluorometric assays was negative in all 232 samples of both groups, including the FNAB washouts of the sTgAb+ patients. Using a second assay (electrochemiluminescence assay, ECLIA, Roche), we identified 7 samples with positive TgAb-FNAB values, all of which were obtained from Group 1 (sTgAb-) patients, with high levels of Tg-FNAB, which likely lead to false elevations of TgAb-FNAB. Moreover, this artifact represents an established competitive effect that occurs when the Tg levels are > 2000 ng/mL, and these values must be considered false-positive results, as described by the manufacturer.

Table 2. Comparison of Tg-FNAB by assay 1 (immunofluorometric, with monoclonal antibodies) and assay 2 (immunofluorometric with mono and polyclonal antibodies) and cytological results of metastatic lymph nodes (LNs) of Group 1 (sTgAb-) and Group 2 (sTgAb+) with Tg-FNAB levels < 10 ng/mL by assay 1

	Tg-FNAB Assay 1	Tg-FNAB Assay 2
Reactive cyto-FNAB	–	–
Inadequate/not diagnostic cyto-FNAB	8.7	142
	< 1.0	1.6
	< 1.0	0.5
	< 1.0	0.9
	< 1.0	0.6
Positive for metastasis cyto-FNAB	< 1.0	28.6
	5.9	42.7
	< 1.0	142
	< 1.0	1.4
	2.1	101
	< 1.0	1.1

DISCUSSION

The evaluation of cervical LNs is difficult during the follow-up of PTC patients because inflammatory LNs are frequently present. The use of Tg-FNAB is well recognized as a valuable instrument in the examination of suspicious LN metastases (3,4,11-23). However, there are limited data regarding factors that may interfere with the diagnostic sensitivity of Tg-FNAB, such as the presence of TgAb in washout fluid samples.

The presence of TgAb in FNAB washout fluids may reflect the active LN synthesis of TgAb (30) or the contamination of the washout fluids with blood; thus, we measured the TgAb-FNAB levels in both positive and negative sTgAb patients (n = 232). The results indicated that all washout fluid samples obtained from the patients in both groups were negative for TgAb-FNAB based on immunofluorometric assays. Notably, when we retested the TgAb-FNAB levels using a chemiluminescence immunoassay, we identified 7 samples in Group 1 (sTgAb-) patients with positive TgAb-FNAB values. However, as previously described, these patients had extremely high levels of Tg-FNAB, and according to the manufacturer's description, these results must be interpreted as false-positive because of the high titers of Tg-FNAB. We thus considered that all washout fluid samples of Groups 1 and 2 were negative for TgAb-FNAB in both assays performed. However, we raised several speculations to justify the negative results of TgAb-FNAB in all samples in the present study, including the samples obtained from sTgAb+ patients: 1) active LN synthesis of TgAb, which may eventually occur, was scarce in the samples, and consequently, there was no detection of TgAb in the washouts; 2) there was no contamination of the washout fluid with blood during the FNAB procedure in the sTgAb+ patients; and 3) the washouts of LNs perfused with blood that contain TgAb may have a low concentration of these antibodies; however, it is insufficient to measure.

Other studies have presented similar results. Following the inclusion of a limited number of TgAb-FNAB measurements of LN washout in sTgAb+ patients, the authors did not detect TgAb via direct measurement in the washout fluids of LNs, which suggests that sTgAb do not interfere with the detection of Tg-FNAB levels (16,18,20,26).

Boi and cols. evaluated washout fluid samples from 8 sTgAb+ patients and suggested that the presence of TgAb-FNAB may interfere with the interpretation of Tg-FNAB results because lower levels of Tg-FNAB were detected in 2 metastatic LNs with positive TgAb-FNAB levels compared with metastatic LNs with negative TgAb-FNAB levels (25). These authors proposed that this interference is minimized by the high Tg concentrations in the FNAB washouts of metastatic LNs, which saturate TgAb binding sites and therefore do not compromise the value of Tg-FNAB in the diagnosis of metastases. The results of the present study, which included a larger number of patients (11/24 patients sTgAb+ and Tg-FNAB < 10 ng/mL, Group 2, Figure 1), confirm this finding.

TgAb-FNAB was negative in all samples examined in the present study; thus, further comparisons between the TgAb values in the serum and FNAB washout would not be plausible. Instead, we considered other potential reasons why low levels of Tg-FNAB were present in the metastatic LNs of patients with PTC, including difficulties in sampling a representative area of neoplasia during the FNAB procedure, heterogenic Tg production by metastatic cells and differences in Tg assay performance.

Regarding the difficulties in sampling a representative area of neoplasia during FNAB, we identified metastatic LNs with Tg-FNAB < 10 ng/mL in both Group 1 (n = 16) and Group 2 (n = 11). We proposed that this Tg-FNAB value represented a true negative result in most cases based on the finding that the majority of these LNs also exhibited inadequate/non-diagnostic cyto-FNAB results (Group 1: n = 13/16 and Group 2: n = 5/11) (Table 1). However, this result may also reflect the non-homogeneous patterns and fluid areas that occur in some metastatic LNs.

In the present study, we did not identify undifferentiated variants of PTC carcinoma in metastatic LNs with low Tg-FNAB levels (< 10 ng/mL). In both Groups 1 and 2, all metastatic LNs with low Tg-FNAB values presented classical and follicular PTC histological variants. However, variable levels of Tg-FNAB have been described, even in samples with the same variant, which reflects heterogenic Tg production by differentiated metastatic cells (24).

Differences in Tg assays were also identified in the present study. The finding of negative TgAb-FNAB in all samples and a higher percentage of metastatic LNs with Tg-FNAB < 10 ng/dL in the sTgAb+ patients than the sTgAb- patients (68.75% vs. 25.4%, respectively, $p < 0.05$) prompted us to perform a second Tg assay in the washout fluids of all proven metastatic LNs of the sTgAb+ patients with Tg-FNAB < 10 ng/dL (Table 2). In some patients, we obtained different results between both assays. The Tg-FNAB levels according to assay 2 were consistent with the cytological results in 4 LNs with positive cyto-FNAB for PTC metastasis with undetectable Tg-FNAB based on assay 1, and these LNs were metastatic. The Tg-FNAB level of 142 ng/mL detected using assay 2 also clarified the diagnosis of a metastatic LN with inadequate/non-diagnostic cyto-

FNAB and a Tg-FNAB level of 8.7 ng/mL according to assay 1 (Table 2).

Similar to the results obtained in the present study, Jeon and cols. (27) and Jo and cols. (31) also identified a higher percentage of LNs with low levels of Tg-FNAB in sTgAb+ patients than sTgAb- patients. These authors concluded that the presence of sTgAb interfered with the Tg-FNAB levels; however, these researchers did not measure TgAb in FNAB washout fluid samples (27,31).

In conclusion, we propose that other factors, rather than the presence of TgAb, may contribute to the higher number of metastatic LNs with undetectable Tg-FNAB identified in the sTgAb+ group because TgAb-FNAB was negative in all samples according to 2 different assays. Furthermore, for the analysis of Tg-FNAB in the sTgAb+ patients, assay 2 (mono/polyclonal) had a better performance in the detection of metastatic LNs than the monoclonal assay; however, it exhibited limitations in the identification of some LN metastases. Nevertheless, this analysis was useful in some cases in which there was no concordance between the cyto-FNAB and Tg-FNAB results or when the cyto-FNAB was inadequate/non-diagnostic and the Tg-FNAB levels were low based on the monoclonal assay. Therefore, we proposed that the measurement of Tg using another assay would be helpful in LNs with a positive cytology for PTC and low levels of Tg-FNAB using the first assay and in cases of inadequate/non-diagnostic cytology and low Tg-FNAB levels. However, in this latter situation, we emphasize that the low value of Tg-FNAB may persist in every additional assay assessed, as a matter of material scarcity. When employed alone, cyto-FNAB or Tg-FNAB (independent of the tested assay) did not provide a guarantee of establishing the diagnosis of cervical lymphadenopathy in patients.

In addition, false-positive and false-negative results may occur, which reinforce the recommendations that these LNs require monitoring and physicians must interpret clinical, laboratory, cytology, and ultrasound data together to achieve successful management in the follow-up of patients with PTC.

Acknowledgements: this work was supported by grants from the São Paulo State Research Foundation (Fapesp-09/50573-1) and from the Brazilian Ministry of Health (25000.168513/2008-11) to R.M.B.M. and R.P.M.B are investigators of the Fleury Group.

REFERENCES

1. Arturi F, Russo D, Giuffrida D, Ippolito A, Perrotti N, Vigneri R, et al. Early diagnosis by genetic analysis of differentiated thyroid cancer metastases in small lymph nodes. J Clin Endocrinol Metab. 1997;82:1638-41.

2. Hughes DT, Doherty GM. Central neck dissection for papillary thyroid cancer. Cancer Control. 2011;18:83-8.

3. Frasoldati A, Toschi E, Zini M, Flora M, Caroggio A, Dotti C, et al. Role of thyroglobulin measurement in fine-needle aspiration biopsies of cervical lymph nodes in patients with differentiated thyroid cancer. Thyroid. 1999;9:105-11.

4. Pacini F, Fugazzola L, Lippi F, Ceccarelli C, Centoni R, Miccoli P, et al. Detection of thyroglobulin in fine needle aspirates of nonthyroidal neck masses: a clue to the diagnosis of metastatic differentiated thyroid cancer. J Clin Endocrinol Metab. 1992;74:1401-4.

5. Cooper DS, Doherty GM, Haugen BR, Kloos RT, Lee SL, Mandel SJ, et al. Revised American Thyroid Association management guidelines for patients with thyroid nodules and differentiated thyroid cancer. Thyroid. 2009;19:1167-214.

6. Stak BC Jr, Ferris RL, Goldenberg D, Haymart M, Shaha A, Sheth S, et al. American Thyroid Association consensus review and statement regarding the anatomy, terminology, and rationale for lateral neck dissection in differentiated thyroid cancer. Thyroid. 2012;22:501-8.

7. Rosário PW, Ward LS, Carvalho GA, Graf H, Maciel RMB, Maciel LMZ, et al. Thyroid Nodule and Differentiated Thyroid Cancer: Update on the Brazilian Consensus. Arq Brasil Endocrinol Metab. 2013;57:240-67.

8. Leehardt L, Erdogan MF, Hegedus L, Mandel SJ, Paschke R, Rago T, et al. 2013 European Thyroid Association Guidelines for cervical ultrasound scan and ultrasound guided techniques in the postoperative management of patients with thyroid cancer. Eur Thyroid J. 2013;2:147-59.

9. Sutton RT, Reading CC, Charboneau JW, James EM, Grant CS, Hay ID. US-guided biopsy of neck masses in postoperative management of patients with thyroid cancer. Radiology. 1988;168:769-72.

10. Ahuja AT, Chow L, Chick W, King W, Metreweli C. Metastatic cervical nodes in papillary carcinoma of the thyroid: ultrasound and histological correlation. Clin Radiol. 1995;50:229-31.

11. Baloch ZW, Barroeta JE, Walsh J, Gupta PK, Livolsi VA, Langer JE, et al. Utility of thyroglobulin measurement in fine-needle aspiration biopsy specimens of lymph nodes in the diagnosis of recurrent thyroid carcinoma. Cytojournal 2008;5:1-5.

12. Grani G, Fumarola A. Thyroglobulin in lymph node fine-needle aspiration washout: a systematic review and meta-analysis of diagnostic accuracy. J Clin Endocrinol Metab. 2014;99:1970-82.

13. Torres MRS, Nóbrega-Neto SH, Rosas RJ, Martins ALB, Ramos ALC, Cruz TRP. Thyroglobulin in the washout of lymph-node biopsy: what is the role in the follow-up of differentiated thyroid carcinoma? Thyroid. 2014;24:7-18.

14. Baskin HJ. Detection of recurrent papillary thyroid carcinoma by thyroglobulin assessment in the needle washout after fine-needle aspiration of suspicious lymph nodes. Thyroid. 2004;14:959-63.

15. Snozek CL, Chambers EP, Reading CC, Sebo TJ, Sistrunk JW, Singh RJ, et al. Serum thyroglobulin, high-resolution ultrasound, and lymph node thyroglobulin in diagnosis of differentiated thyroid carcinoma nodal metastases. J Clin Endocrinol Metab. 2007;92:4278-81.

16. Cunha N, Rodrigues F, Curado F, Ilheu O, Cruz C, Naidenov P, et al. Thyroglobulin detection in fine-needle aspirates of cervical lymph nodes: a technique for the diagnosis of metastatic differentiated thyroid cancer. Eur J Endocrinol. 2007;157:101-7.

17. Biscolla RP, Ikejiri ES, Mamone MC, Nakabashi CC, Andrade VP, Kasamatsu TS, et al. Diagnosis of metastases in patients with papillary thyroid cancer by the measurement of thyroglobulin in fine needle aspirate. Arq Bras Endocrinol Metabol. 2007;51:419-25.

18. Sigstad E, Heilo A, Paus E, Holgersen K, Groholt KK, Jorgensen LH, et al. The usefulness of detecting thyroglobulin in fine-needle aspirates from patients with neck lesions using a sensitive thyroglobulin assay. Diagn Cytopathol. 2007;35:761-7.

19. Veliz J, Brantes S, Ramos C, Aguayo J, Caceres E, Herrera M, et al. Thyroglobulin levels in needle lymph node cytology for the detection of papillary thyroid cancer recurrence. Rev Med Chil. 2008;136:1107-12.

20. Borel AL, Boizel R, Faure P, Barbe G, Boutonnat J, Sturm N, et al. Significance of low levels of thyroglobulin in fine needle aspirates from cervical lymph nodes of patients with a history of differentiated thyroid cancer. Eur J Endocrinol. 2008;158:691-8.

21. Kim MJ, Kim EK, Kim BM, Kwak JY, Lee EJ, Park CS, et al. Thyroglobulin measurement in fine-needle aspirate washouts: the criteria for neck node dissection for patients with thyroid cancer. Clin Endocrinol (Oxf). 2009;70:145-51.

22. Zanella AB, Meyer EL, Balzan L, Silva AC, Camargo J, Migliavacca A, et al. Thyroglobulin measurements in washout of fine needle aspirates in cervical lymph nodes for detection of papillary thyroid cancer metastases. Arq Bras Endocrinol Metabol. 2010;54:550-4.

23. Jung JY, Shin JH, Han BK, Ko EY. Optimized cutoff value and indication for washout thyroglobulin detection in fine-needle aspirates of metastatic neck nodes in papillary thyroid carcinoma. AJNR Am J Neuroradiol. 2013;34:2349-53.

24. Spencer C, Petrovic I, Fatemi S, LoPresti J. Serum thyroglobulin monitoring of patients with differentiated thyroid cancer using sensitive (Second-generation) immunometric assays can be disrupted by false-negative and false-positive serum thyroglobulin autoantibody misclassifications. J Clin Endocrinol Metab. 2014;99:4589-99.

25. Boi F, Baghino G, Atzeni F, Lai ML, Faa G, Mariotti S. The diagnostic value for differentiated thyroid carcinoma metastases of thyroglobulin measurement in washout fluid from fine-needle aspiration biopsy of neck lymph nodes is maintained in the presence of circulating anti-Tg antibodies. J Clin Endocrinol Metab. 2006;91:1364-9.

26. Hernandez TM, Cuadro AT, Fernandez PY, Baldrich AG, Galvez MD, Elorza FL, et al. Usefulness of the determination of thyroglobulin in lymph node aspirates of patients with papillary thyroid carcinoma and positive antithyroglobulin antibodies. Endocrinol Nutr. 2009;56:447-51.

27. Jeon MJ, Park JW, Han JM, Yim JH, Song DE, Gong G, et al. Serum antithyroglobulin antibodies interfere with thyroglobulin detection in fine-needle aspirates of metastatic neck nodes in papillary thyroid carcinoma. J Clin Endocrinol Metab. 2013;98:153-60.

28. Nakabashi CC, Biscolla RP, Kasamatsu TS, Tachibana TT, Barcelos RN, Malouf EZ, et al. Development, characterization and clinical validation of new sensitive immunofluorometric assay for the measurement of serum thyroglobulin. Arq Bras Endocrinol Metabol. 2012;56:658-65.

29. Vieira JGH, Tachibana TT, Fonseca RMG, Nishida SK, Maciel RMB. Development of an immunofluorometric method for the measurement of anti-thyroglobulin antibodies. Arq Bras Endocrinol Metabol. 1996:232-7.

30. Weetman AP, McGregor AM, Wheeler MH, Hall R. Extrathyroidal sites of autoantibody synthesis in Graves' disease. Clin Exp Immunol. 1984;56:330-6.

31. Jo K, Kim MH, Lim Y, Jung SL, Bae JS, Jung CH, et al. Lowered cutoff of lymph node fine-needle aspiration thyroglobulin in thyroid cancer patients with serum anti-thyroglobulin antibody. Eur J Endocrinol. 2015;173:489-97.

Permissions

All chapters in this book were first published in AEM, by The Brazilian Society of Endocrinology and Metabolism; hereby published with permission under the Creative Commons Attribution License or equivalent. Every chapter published in this book has been scrutinized by our experts. Their significance has been extensively debated. The topics covered herein carry significant findings which will fuel the growth of the discipline. They may even be implemented as practical applications or may be referred to as a beginning point for another development.

The contributors of this book come from diverse backgrounds, making this book a truly international effort. This book will bring forth new frontiers with its revolutionizing research information and detailed analysis of the nascent developments around the world.

We would like to thank all the contributing authors for lending their expertise to make the book truly unique. They have played a crucial role in the development of this book. Without their invaluable contributions this book wouldn't have been possible. They have made vital efforts to compile up to date information on the varied aspects of this subject to make this book a valuable addition to the collection of many professionals and students.

This book was conceptualized with the vision of imparting up-to-date information and advanced data in this field. To ensure the same, a matchless editorial board was set up. Every individual on the board went through rigorous rounds of assessment to prove their worth. After which they invested a large part of their time researching and compiling the most relevant data for our readers.

The editorial board has been involved in producing this book since its inception. They have spent rigorous hours researching and exploring the diverse topics which have resulted in the successful publishing of this book. They have passed on their knowledge of decades through this book. To expedite this challenging task, the publisher supported the team at every step. A small team of assistant editors was also appointed to further simplify the editing procedure and attain best results for the readers.

Apart from the editorial board, the designing team has also invested a significant amount of their time in understanding the subject and creating the most relevant covers. They scrutinized every image to scout for the most suitable representation of the subject and create an appropriate cover for the book.

The publishing team has been an ardent support to the editorial, designing and production team. Their endless efforts to recruit the best for this project, has resulted in the accomplishment of this book. They are a veteran in the field of academics and their pool of knowledge is as vast as their experience in printing. Their expertise and guidance has proved useful at every step. Their uncompromising quality standards have made this book an exceptional effort. Their encouragement from time to time has been an inspiration for everyone.

The publisher and the editorial board hope that this book will prove to be a valuable piece of knowledge for researchers, students, practitioners and scholars across the globe.

List of Contributors

Diego F. García-Díaz, Carolina Pizarro, Patricia Camacho-Guillén and Francisco Pérez-Bravo
Laboratorio de Nutrigenómica, Departamento de Nutrición, Facultad de Medicina, Universidad de Chile
Ethel Codner and Néstor Soto
Instituto de Investigaciones Materno Infantil (IDIMI), Hospital San Borja Arriarán, Facultad de Medicina, Universidad de Chile

Raquel Munhoz da Silveira Campos
Departamento de Fisioterapia, Laboratório de Recursos Terapêuticos, Universidade Federal de São Carlos (UFSCar), São Carlos, SP, Brasil

Deborah Cristina Landi Masquio
Centro Universitário São Camilo, São Paulo, SP, Brasil

Flávia Campos Corgosinho
Universidade Federal de Goiás (UFG), Goiânia, GO, Brasil

Joana Pereira de Carvalho-Ferreira
Programa de Pós-Graduação Interdisciplinar em Ciências da Saúde, Universidade Federal de São Paulo (Unifesp), Santos, SP, Brasil

Bárbara Dal Molin Netto and Ana Raimunda Dâmaso
Programa de Pós-Graduação em Nutrição, Universidade Federal de São Paulo (Unifesp), São Paulo, SP, Brasil

Marco Túlio de Mello
Programa de Pós-Graduação em Nutrição, Universidade Federal de São Paulo (Unifesp), São Paulo, SP, Brasil
Departamento de Psicobiologia, Universidade Federal de São Paulo (Unifesp), São Paulo, SP, Brasil
Escola de Educação Física, Fisioterapia e Terapia Ocupacional, Universidade Federal de Minas Gerais (UFMG), Belo Horizonte, MG, Brasil

Ana Paula Grotti Clemente
Universidade Federal de Alagoas (Ufal), Maceió, AL, Brasil

Lian Tock
Weight Science, São Paulo, SP, Brasil

Sergio Tufik
Departamento de Psicobiologia, Universidade Federal de São Paulo (Unifesp), São Paulo, SP, Brasil

Fausto Fama, Marco Cicciu and Maria Gioffre'-Florio
Department of Human Pathology in Adulthood and Childhood "G. Barresi", University Hospital of Messina, Messina, Italy

Alessandro Sindoni
Department of Biomedical and Dental Sciences and of Morphological and FunctionalImages, University Hospital of Messina, Messina, Italy

Francesca Polito
Department of Clinical & Experimental Medicine, University Hospital of Messina, Messina, Italy

Salvatore Benvenga
Department of Clinical & Experimental Medicine, University Hospital of Messina, Messina, Italy
Master Program on Childhood, Adolescent and Women's Endocrine Health, University Hospital of Messina, Messina, Italy
Interdepartmental Program on Molecular & Clinical Endocrinology, and Women's Endocrine Health, University Hospital of Messina, Messina, Italy

Arnaud Piquard and Olivier Saint-Marc
Department of General, Endocrine and Thoracic Surgery, Regional Hospital of Orleans, Orléans, France

Alireza Milajerdi
Endocrinology and Metabolism Clinical Sciences Institute, Tehran University of Medical Sciences, Tehran, Iran
Department of Community Nutrition, School of Nutritional Sciences and Dietetics, Tehran University of Medical Sciences (TUMS), Tehran, Iran

Zhila Maghbooli
Endocrinology and Metabolism Clinical Sciences Institute, Tehran University of Medical Sciences, Tehran, Iran

Farzad Mohammadi, Banafsheh Hosseini and Khadijeh Mirzaei
Department of Community Nutrition, School of Nutritional Sciences and Dietetics, Tehran University of Medical Sciences (TUMS), Tehran, Iran

Rossana Corbo, Daniel A. Bulzico, Denise Momesso and Fernanda Vaisman
Serviço de Endocrinologia,Instituto Nacional do Câncer (Inca), Rio de Janeiro, RJ, Brasil

Cleo Otaviano Mesa Jr., Hans Graf, Gisah Amaral de Carvalho and Fabíola Yukiko Miasaki
Serviço de Endocrinologia, Hospital das Clínicas, Universidade Federal do Paraná (UFPR), Curitiba, PR, Brasil

Carolina Perez Chaves and Dominique Cochat Fuser
Serviço de Medicina Nuclear, Instituto Nacional do Câncer (Inca), Rio de Janeiro, RJ, Brasil
Joana Carolina Bernhard, Kely Lisandra Dummel, Éboni Reuter, Miriam Beatris Reckziegel and Hildegard Hedwig Pohl
Departamento de Educação Física e Saúde, Universidadede Santa Cruz do Sul (Unisc), Santa Cruz do Sul, RS, Brasil

Lygia N. Barroso, Dayana R. Farias and Gilberto Kac
Observatório de Epidemiologia Nutricional, Departamento de Nutrição Social e Aplicada, Instituto de Nutrição Josué de Castro, Universidade Federal do Rio de Janeiro (UFRJ), Cidade Universitária, Ilha do Fundão, Rio de Janeiro, RJ, Brasil

Marcia Soares-Mota
Instituto de Nutrição Josué de Castro, Universidade Federal do Rio de Janeiro (UFRJ), Cidade Universitária, Ilha do Fundão, Rio de Janeiro, RJ, Brasil

Heloisa Bettiol,Marco Antônio Barbieri and Milton Cesar Foss
Departamento de Puericultura e Pediatria, Faculdade de Medicinam de Ribeirão Preto, Universidade de São Paulo, Ribeirão Preto, SP, Brasil

Antônio Augusto M. da Silva
Departamento de Saúde Pública, Centro de Ciências da Saúde, Universidade Federal do Maranhão (UFMA), São Luís, MA, Brasil

Preneet Cheema Brar
Department of Pediatrics, Division of Pediatric Endocrinology, New York University School of Medicine, New York, USA

Maria Contreras
Texas Tech University Health Science Center, Department of Pediatrics, Amarillo, Texas, USA

Xiaozhou Fan
Department of Population Health, New York University School of Medicine, New York, USA

Nipapat Visavachaipan
Bumrungrad International Hospital, Bangkok, Thailand

Eliege Carolina Vaz and Vania dos Santos Nunes-Nogueira
Departamento de Clínica Médica, Faculdade de Medicina de Botucatu, Universidade Estadual de São Paulo (Unesp), Botucatu, SP, Brasil

Gustavo José Martiniano Porfírio
Centro Cochrane do Brasil, Disciplina de Medicina de Urgência e Medicina Baseada em Evidências, Universidade Federal de São Paulo (Unifesp), São Paulo, SP, Brasil

Hélio Rubens de Carvalho Nunes
Departamento de Saúde Pública, Faculdade de Medicina de Botucatu, Universidade Estadual de São Paulo (Unesp), Botucatu, SP, Brasil

Bruno Mussoi de Macedo, Rogério F. Izquierdo, Lenara Golbert and Erika L. Souza Meyer
Thyroid Section, Endocrine Division, Irmandade da Santa Casa de Misericórdia de Porto Alegre, Universidade Federal de Ciências da Saúde de Porto Alegre (UFCSPA), Porto Alegre, RS, Brazil

Liliana Rateni
Facultad de Ciencias Médicas, Universidad Nacional de Rosario, Santa Fe, Rosario, Argentina

Sergio Lupo
Facultad de Ciencias Médicas, Universidad Nacional de Rosario, Santa Fe, Rosario, Argentina
Center for Assistance and Comprehensive Clinical Research (CAICI), IICTlab, Mendoza, Rosario, Argentina

Jorge Palazzi
Center for Assistance and Comprehensive Clinical Research (CAICI), IICTlab, Mendoza, Rosario, Argentina

Liliana Racca and Sergio Ghersevich
Facultad de Ciencias Bioquímicas y Farmacéuticas, Universidad Nacional de Rosario, Rosario, Argentina

Camila de Moraes, Camila Andrea de Oliveira, Maria Esméria Corezola do Amaral, Gabriela Arcurio Landini and Rosana Catisti
Programa de Pós-Graduação de Ciências Biomédicas, Centro Universitário Hermínio Ometto, Uniararas, Araras, SP, Brazil

Sema Ciftci Dogansen, Gulsah Yenidunya Yalin, Bulent Canbaz, Seher Tanrikulu and Sema Yarman
Istanbul University, Istanbul Faculty of Medicine, Department of Internal Medicine, Division of Endocrinology and Metabolism, Istanbul, Turkey

Nayara Rampazzo Morelli and Bruna Miglioranza Scavuzzi
Departamento de Pós-Graduação em Ciências da Saúde, Universidade Estadual de Londrina (UEL), Londrina, PR, Brasil

Lucia Helena da Silva Miglioranza
Departamento de Ciência e Tecnologia de Alimentos, Universidade Estadual de Londrina (UEL), Londrina, PR, Brasil
Marcell Alysson Batisti Lozovoy and Andréa Name Colado Simão
Departamento de Patologia, Análises Clínicas e Toxicológicas, Universidade Estadual de Londrina (UEL), Londrina, PR, Brasil

Isaias Dichi
Departamento de Medicina Interna, Universidade Estadual de Londrina (UEL), Londrina, PR, Brasil

Andresa de Santi Rodrigues, Mirian Y. Nishi and Berenice Bilharinho de Mendonca
Unidade de Endocrinologia do Desenvolvimento, Laboratório de Hormônios e Genética Molecular/LIM42, Hospital das Clínicas, Disciplina de Endocrinologia, Faculdade de Medicina da Universidade de São Paulo (FMUSP), São Paulo, SP, Brasil
Laboratório de Sequenciamento em Larga Escala (SELA), Faculdade de Medicina da Universidade de São Paulo (FMUSP), São Paulo, SP, Brasil
Uğur Canpolat, Osman Turak, Fırat Özcan, Fatih Öksüz, Mehmet Ali Mendi, Çağrı Yayla and Sinan Aydoğdu
Türkiye Yüksek Ihtisas Training and Research Hospital, Cardiology Clinic, Ankara, Turkey

Maria Laura Iglesias, Abir Al Ghuzlan, Ludovic Lacroix and Martin Schlumberger
Institut Gustave Roussy, Université Paris-Sud, Villejuif, France

Florent de Vathaire
Institut Gustave Roussy, Université Paris-Sud, Villejuif, France
Cancer and Radiation Team, INSERM Unit 1018, Villejuif, France

Angelica Schmidt
Division of Endocrinology, Hospital de Clínicas, University of Buenos Aires Buenos Aires, Argentina

Sylvie Chevillard
CEA, Institute of Cellular and Molecular Radiobiology, Laboratory of Experimental Cancerology, CEA, Fontenay-aux-Roses, France

Eduardo Ottobelli Chielle and Jeferson Noslen Casarin
Departamento de Ciências da Saúde, Laboratório de Bioquímica Clínica, Universidade do Oeste de Santa Catarina (Unoesc), São Miguel do Oeste, SC, Brasil

Fabián Pitoia
Division of Endocrinology, Hospital de Clínicas, University of Buenos Aires Buenos Aires, Argentina

Angelica Schmidt
Division of Endocrinology, Hospital de Clínicas, University of Buenos Aires Buenos Aires, Argentina
Institut Gustave Roussy, Université Paris-Saclay, Villejuif, France

Laura Iglesias and Martin J. Schlumberger
Institut Gustave Roussy, Université Paris-Saclay, Villejuif, France

Michele Klain
Università Federico II di Napoli, Napoli, Italia

Ricardo de Marchi, Tiara Cristina Romeiro Lopes, Angela Andréia França Gravena, Deise Helena Pelloso Borghesan and Maria Dalva de Barros Carvalho
Departamento de Ciências da Saúde, Pós-Graduação em Ciências da Saúde, Universidade Estadual de Maringá (UEM), PR, Brasil

Sandra Marisa Pelloso
Departamento de Ciências da Saúde, Pós-Graduação em Ciências da Saúde, Universidade Estadual de Maringá (UEM), PR, Brasil
Departamento de Enfermagem, Pós-Graduação em Enfermagem, Universidade Estadual de Maringá (UEM), PR, Brasil

Marcela de Oliveira Demitto, Sheila Cristina Rocha Brischiliari and Cátia Millene Dell'Agnolo
Departamento de Enfermagem, Pós-Graduação em Enfermagem, Universidade Estadual de Maringá (UEM), PR, Brasil

Júnia Maria Geraldo Gomes
Instituto Federal de Educação, Ciência e Tecnologia do Sudeste de Minas Gerais, Campus Barbacena, Barbacena, MG, Brasil

Sabrina Pinheiro Fabrini
Centro Universitário de Belo Horizonte, Campus Estoril, Belo Horizonte, MG, Brasil

Rita de Cássia Gonçalves Alfenas
Departamento de Nutrição e Saúde, Universidade Federal de Viçosa, Viçosa, MG, Brasil

Cláudia Porto Sabino Pinho, Alcides da Silva Diniz and Ilma Kruze Grande de Arruda
Universidade Federal de Pernambuco (UFPE), Recife, PE, Brasil

Ana Paula Dornelas Leão Leite, Marina de Moraes Vasconcelos Petribu and Isa Galvão Rodrigues
Pronto-Socorro Cardiológico Universitário de Pernambuco, Recife, PE, Brasil

Roberto Cesareo, Alessandro Casini and Giuseppe Campagna
Department of Internal Medicine "S. M. Goretti" Hospital, Latina, Italy

Andrea Palermo and Silvia Manfrini
Department of Endocrinology, University Campus Bio- Medico, Rome, Italy

Roberto Cianni, Giuseppe Pelle and Valerio Pasqualini
Department of Radiology, "S. M. Goretti" Hospital, Latina, Italy

Carla Simeoni
Compensatory authority (INAIL), Monte Porzio Catone, Rome, Italy

Rosangela Villa Marin-Mio, Linda Denise Fernandes Moreira, Marília Camargo and Marise Lazaretti-Castro
Disciplina de Endocrinologia da Universidade Federal de São Paulo (Unifesp), São Paulo, SP, Brasil

Neide Alessandra Sansão Périgo and Maysa Seabra Cerondoglo
Disciplina de Geriatria e Gerontologia da Universidade Federal de São Paulo (Unifesp), São Paulo, SP, Brasil

Walter Masson, Salvador De Francesca, Micaela Molinero, Daniel Siniawski1, Andrés Mulassi1, Frank Espinoza Morales, Melina Huerin, Martín Lobo and Graciela Molinero
Council of Epidemiology and Cardiovascular Prevention "Dr. Mario Ciruzzi" of the Argentine Society of Cardiology, Buenos Aires, Argentina

Rui M. B. Maciel and Rosa Paula M. Biscolla
Centro de Doenças da Tireoide e Laboratório de Endocrinologia Molecular e Translacional, Divisão de Endocrinologia, Departamento de Medicina, Escola Paulista de Medicina, Universidade Federal de São Paulo (EPM-Unifesp), São Paulo, SP, Brasil

Carolina Castro Porto Silva Janovsky
Centro de Doenças da Tireoide e Laboratório de Endocrinologia Molecular e Translacional, Divisão de

Endocrinologia, Departamento de Medicina, Escola Paulista de Medicina, Universidade Federal de São Paulo (EPM-Unifesp), São Paulo, SP, Brasil
Centro de Medicina Preventiva, Hospital Israelita Albert Einstein, São Paulo, SP, Brasil

Marcio Sommer Bittencourt
Centro de Medicina Preventiva, Hospital Israelita Albert Einstein, São Paulo, SP, Brasil
Núcleo de Pesquisa Clínica e Epidemiológica, Hospital das Clínicas da Faculdade de Medicina da Universidade de São Paulo (HCFMUSP), São Paulo, SP, Brasil

Maykon Anderson Pires de Novais and Paola Zucchi
Divisão de Economia da Saúde, Departamento de Medicina, Escola Paulista de Medicina, Universidade Federal de São Paulo, São Paulo, SP, Brasil

Teresa S. Kasamatsu and Felipe Crispim
Centro de Doenças da Tireoide e Laboratório de Endocrinologia Molecular e Translacional, Divisão de Endocrinologia, Departamento de Medicina, Escola Paulista de Medicina da Universidade Federal de São Paulo (EPM- -Unifesp), São Paulo, SP, Brasil

M. Cecilia Martins-Costa
Centro de Doenças da Tireoide e Laboratório de Endocrinologia Molecular e Translacional, Divisão de Endocrinologia, Departamento de Medicina, Escola Paulista de Medicina da Universidade Federal de São Paulo (EPM- -Unifesp), São Paulo, SP, Brasil
Departamento de Medicina, Universidade de Fortaleza (Unifor), Fortaleza, CE, Brasil

Rui M. B. Maciel, Rosa Paula M. Biscolla and Claudia C. D. Nakabashi
Centro de Doenças da Tireoide e Laboratório de Endocrinologia Molecular e Translacional, Divisão de Endocrinologia, Departamento de Medicina, Escola Paulista de Medicina da Universidade Federal de São Paulo (EPM- -Unifesp), São Paulo, SP, Brasil
Centro de Doenças da Tireoide, Instituto Israelita de Ensino e Pesquisa Albert Einstein (IIEPAE), São Paulo, SP, Brasil
Fleury Medicina e Saúde, São Paulo, SP, Brasil

Elza S. Ikejiri, M. Conceição O. Mamone, Danielle M. Andreoni and Cleber P. Camacho
Centro de Doenças da Tireoide e Laboratório de Endocrinologia Molecular e Translacional, Divisão de Endocrinologia, Departamento de Medicina, Escola Paulista de Medicina da Universidade Federal de São Paulo (EPM- -Unifesp), São Paulo, SP, Brasil
Centro de Doenças da Tireoide, Instituto Israelita de Ensino e Pesquisa Albert Einstein (IIEPAE), São Paulo, SP, Brasil

Index

www.ingramcontent.com/pod-product-compliance
Lightning Source LLC
Chambersburg PA
CBHW080516200326
41458CB00012B/4223